Centering the Margins in Bioethics

Centering the Margins in Bioethics

A Social Justice Approach to the Ethics of Healthcare and Medicine

First Edition

Santiago Sanchez Borboa

University of Arizona

cognella

SAN DIEGO

Bassim Hamadeh, CEO and Publisher
Peaches diPierro, Acquisitions Editor
Danielle Gradisher, Project Editor
Rachel Kahn, Production Editor
Jess Estrella, Senior Graphic Designer
Kylie Bartolome, Licensing Associate
Natalie Piccotti, Director of Marketing
Kassie Graves, Senior Vice President, Editorial

Printed in the United States of America.

Contents

Preface ix

Introduction xi

Unit I The Shadow of Race/ism and The Ocean of White Supremacy Culture in Healthcare and Medicine 1

Reading 1.1 Race, Religion, and Informed Consent: Lessons from Social Science 11

Dayna Bowen Matthew

Reading 1.2 A Model for Culturally Responsive Health Care 49

Dorothy E. Vawter, Kathleen A. Culhane-Pera, Barbara Babbitt, Phua Xiong, and Mary M. Solberg

Reading 1.3 The Handsome Lake Method: An Introduction 59

Alf H. Walle

End-of-Unit Questions 79

Unit II The Specter of Ableism in Healthcare and Medicine 81

Reading 2.1 "Is She Experiencing Any Pain?": Disability and the Physician-Patient Relationship 89

S. K. Toombs

Reading 2.2 "Not Dead Yet": Changing Disability Imaginaries in the Twenty-First Century 95

Faye Ginsburg and Rayna Rapp

Reading 2.3 Unspeakable Offenses: Untangling Race and Disability in Discourses of Intersectionality 111

Nirmala Erevelles and Andrea Minear

End-of-Unit Questions 127

Unit III The Miasma of Cisheteropatriarchy in Healthcare and Medicine 129

Reading 3.1 Analyzing the Problem: Gender Disparities in Behavioral and Mental Health Care 139

Whitney C. Sewell, Whitney Key, and Sarah Gehlert

Reading 3.2 Somewhere Under the Rainbow: Exploring the Identities and Experiences of Trans Persons 153

Emma Dargie, Karen Blair, Caroline Pukall, Shannon Coyle

Reading 3.3 Thinking Transnationally: Reproductive Justice in a Globalized Era 179

Tanya Saroj Bakhru

Reading 3.4 Whose Bodies? Black Lives Matter and the Reproductive Justice Imperative 187

Sikivu Hutchinson

End-of-Unit Questions 191

Unit IV Morality and Mortality 193

Reading 4.1 "Not Dead Yet" and Physician-Assisted Suicide 201

Doris Fleischer and Frieda Zames

Reading 4.2 Why Suicide Is Like Contraception: A Woman-Centered View 227

Dena S. Davis

End-of-Unit Questions 239

Conclusion 241

ACTIVE LEARNING

This book has interactive activities available to complement your reading.

Your instructor may have customized the selection of activities available for your unique course. Please check with your professor to verify whether your class will access this content through the Cognella Active Learning portal (http://active.cognella.com) or through your home learning management system.

cognella® | ACTIVE LEARNING content

Preface

I decided to write this book in Fall 2021, shortly after finishing my PhD in philosophy while working as an adjunct professor. We were (and still are) facing a global pandemic that has exposed just how broken many social systems and institutions are, especially those of healthcare and medicine. During this crisis, marginalized persons have been and continue to be disproportionately harmed by the failures of those in power. To this, we can add that many assaults continue on the rights/liberties of women and trans persons, and the overpolicing of, police violence against, and mass incarceration of Black and Brown persons, whose labor is superexploited so that the rich continue to get richer, remains a problem (to name just a few of many pressing social problems). In these times of continuing and recurring crises, we need to bring about systemic changes to an unacceptable status quo, and I believe that philosophy can help us do so.

This book covers some key fundamentals of ethics from a social justice perspective in a way that is geared to applying them to bioethical issues. It connects these fundamentals to crucial insights from antiracist, disability, and feminist and queer scholarship. In doing so, it takes an intersectional approach and argues for the need to take a historical, embedded, dynamical approach to understanding social, biomedical, and ethical issues. It thus advocates an approach to bioethics that centers the needs and concerns of marginalized persons (focusing on persons who are marginalized because of their race, ethnicity, or Indigeneity, disability, and/or sex, gender, or sexuality). It differs from other bioethics textbooks in that it does not merely include these voices/perspectives in the bioethical conversation but rather centers their contributions and puts them in systematic conversation with traditional Western (i.e., Eurocentric) philosophical resources. By doing so, it provides readers with

- a critical lens that gives greater understanding of the problems faced by marginalized persons, and
- actionable tools that they can use to build more compassionate, inclusive, and humane social institutions in general and institutions of healthcare and medicine in particular.

Historically, traditional Eurocentric philosophy has excluded or paid mere lip service to these marginalized perspectives, centering white, abled, male, economically privileged, cisgender, and heterosexual bodies/perspectives, but this serves to reinforce an unacceptable status quo. This book intervenes in this historical trajectory and centers these marginalized perspectives in order to help solve some of the pressing problems faced by oppressed persons.

My own positionality is that of a well-educated white-presenting Latinx Mexican immigrant cisgender man in the US who grew up upper-middle class. I have enjoyed different degrees of social privilege, especially male and economic privilege in certain contexts, and have faced different degrees of oppression, especially racism in others (which my privilege has, at times, helped shield me from). I recognize just how many there are who are far more oppressed/disadvantaged than me, and I want to use my privilege to center these perspectives, amplifying their voices, and helping articulate how they can help shape our approaches to ethical and social problems for the better.

There are many people more knowledgeable than me regarding systems of oppression. Indeed, it is only relatively recently in my journey to unlearn key oppressive lessons (and replace them with liberatory ones) that the scales have fallen from my eyes with respect to just how pernicious certain aspects of systems of oppression (e.g., ableism and classism) are. I am humbled and inspired by the scholars whose work I engage with and by the myriad activists working on different fronts against injustice. If I can help others see farther into moral vistas, it is only because we can stand on the shoulders of many insightful thinkers/doers of all colors, shapes, and sizes, each of whom provides us with part of the picture of where we are and where we can go. I see my contribution as centering their crucial insights in the philosophical conversation and showing the powerful synergies that emerge from uniting them with traditional Eurocentric philosophical concepts/theories. I thereby hope to help do my part as a philosopher to give readers some tools they can use to help us dismantle the unacceptable status quo we live under and replace it with more humane, inclusive, and compassionate systems/institutions.

This book was made possible by the support of many individuals, not all of whom I can properly acknowledge here. I do, however, owe special thanks to Peaches diPierro, acquisitions editor at Cognella Publishing, who encouraged me to seriously consider writing this book; to Dani Gradisher, my project editor, who adeptly guided me through the sometimes-winding process of writing an edited anthology; and to my dear wife Taylor Boulware, PhD, one of the many thinkers/doers on whose shoulders I stand in order to see just how much is wrong with the world and just how much better a world is possible. Without their help (and the help of many others), this project would not have been possible.

Introduction

Fundamentals of Moral Philosophy and Bioethics

This textbook is for philosophy nonspecialists who either are working in fields related to medicine and healthcare or are interested in working in fields related to medicine and healthcare, and who want to learn about how systems of oppression negatively shape these institutions. It aims to prepare readers with a greater understanding of the lived experiences of persons facing different forms of oppression and marginalization and to provide these readers with the tools to build more socially just institutions in general—and more socially just institutions of healthcare and medicine in particular.

By amplifying the perspectives of those who have been historically marginalized by the medical and philosophical establishment, this book puts the issues and resources from these perspectives in conversation with traditional philosophical theories and tools.

I first came to philosophy because I saw it as offering the promise that, by using our reason, we could find a way to make our lives and the world better. This is not a promise that everyone believes in. Marx famously wrote, "Philosophers have hitherto only interpreted the world in various ways. The point, however, is to change it." In the Philosophy Department of the Humboldt University of Berlin, I read an insightful reply to Marx's statement. It read something like this: "Politicians have hitherto only changed the world in various ways. The point, however, is to improve it. For that, we need philosophy." I wholeheartedly agree with this sentiment. I still believe in the promise of philosophy, but I now vividly see that we need to understand the world we live in in order to realize this promise. We must recognize that the world we have inherited is one with a long history of deep and systemic injustice and inequality—injustice and inequality that have been exacerbated with the COVID-19 pandemic and ensuing crises. Thus, to the above rejoinder to Marx I would add that to improve the world, we need not only philosophy but also the full spectrum of disciplines, including the sciences, humanities, and others, all working together.[1] Only by uniting all of these disciplines can we get an adequate understanding of the many factors that shape our lives and world and how we can intervene in them to bring about real improvements to people's lives.

We can only make our world better and more just by confronting the history and reality of injustice, inequality, and oppression. To do so, we need to "center the margins." That is, as some Black scholars have pointed out, we need to shift our perspective away from the majority's dominant narratives and toward that of historically underrepresented and marginalized groups and the narratives that have been silenced (Hardeman et al., 2016; Hardeman & Karbeah, 2020). This textbook thus aims to provide readers with a better understanding of the complexities of our social world, as well as the tools that they can use to build a more socially just world in the 21st century.

Bioethics textbooks in the past largely ignored bioethical issues arising from the perspective of marginalized persons. Now, major bioethics textbooks discuss such issues. For example, Seay and Nuccetelli's *Engaging Bioethics* (2017) pays attention to gender, race, and cultural diversity, and the newest edition of Vaughn's *Bioethics* (2022) includes a chapter on race and racial bias in medicine. Including the perspective of marginalized and underrepresented persons is certainly an improvement. However, we do even better when we do not simply include these perspectives but further *center* them. By doing so, we better amplify voices that have long been silenced and/or neglected and that provide a key part of the solution to the problems we all face.

The content of the textbook is organized by units. Unit I treats the issues of race/ism, Indigeneity, and ethnicity in bioethics, centering the perspectives of marginalized racial, Indigenous, and ethnic groups. Unit II turns to the issue of disability in bioethics, centering the perspective of disabled persons. Unit III deals with sex, gender, and sexuality in bioethics, centering the perspectives of women, intersex, and LGBTQ+ persons. Unit IV discusses the topic of morality and mortality, while centering feminist and disability studies perspectives. This last unit focuses on physician-assisted suicide, as Unit III on sex, gender, and sexuality emphasizes reproductive justice and therefore deals with the ethics of abortion from the perspective of the margins.

Each of the core units centers the perspective of persons who have been marginalized due to their race, Indigeneity, and/or ethnicity, their disability, or their sex, gender, and/or sexuality. Each unit begins with a short introduction that frames the oppression that different marginalized groups face using analogies that are meant to give readers a sense of just how pervasive and pernicious the forms of oppression faced by these groups are:[2]

1. Here I mean these labels to be as expansive as possible: to include, for example, natural, social, cognitive, and applied sciences; antiracist scholarship; legal and disability studies; the arts; and even management, design, and cuisine.
2. These metaphors can be found, respectively, in the work of Black scholars (e.g., Gamble, 2016; McLoyd, 2022), disability scholars (Campbell, 2009; Wiener, 2018), and feminist and queer scholars (e.g., Carney, 2021; Glitzen & Chun, 2021).

- the shadow of race/ism and the ocean of white supremacy culture
- the specter of ableism
- the miasma of cis/heteropatriarchy (sexism and homo/transphobia)

These introductions also provide helpful further background and theoretical resources to help engage with the readings. There is an additional introduction to each reading that summarizes, motivates, and contextualizes it. Each unit ends with discussion questions that prompt further reflection from the reader and that connect the readings with traditional Eurocentric philosophical concepts. The book ends with a conclusion that highlights the importance of the content and offers some suggestions for how to translate this content into action.

In order to keep the textbook accessible and manageable, I have included at most four readings under each topic. But it is important to recognize that whole textbooks like this one can be written simply on centering the perspective of, for example, Black, Latinx, or transgender persons. There are many additional readings I would have liked to include, but to do so affected the cost of the textbook. The ones I have included serve as especially accessible and/or helpful jumping-off points for these important conversations.

Highlighted throughout is the importance of taking an intersectional approach to the problems of healthcare and medicine. **Intersectionality** is a theoretical framework originating from Black feminism that emphasizes the complexity of identity and oppression when we consider the intersections of race, Indigeneity, ethnicity, gender, class, dis/ability, socioeconomic status, and other social categories as well as how these intersections shape our lived experiences of systems of privilege and oppression (e.g., Collins, 2015; Crenshaw, 1991). Intersectionality helps us see that social identity is *not* a neat hierarchy of social properties that simply get added onto one another. Rather, it is an intersectional set of properties whereby different aspects of our identities "interlock around systems of power, privilege, and disadvantage" (Linker, 2015, p. 59) to shape our experience in complex ways. Only by adopting such a framework can we adequately contend with the complex realities of social identity, privilege, and oppression.

A key lesson from these discussions is that the many systems of oppression that cause health inequities are complex and multifaceted. Thus, we need to tackle these problems by engaging in research at the intersections of different fields (including policy, social psychology, economics, sociology, medicine, and public health) and by implementing intersectoral interventions that target different aspects of systemic oppression (e.g., across housing, education, labor, media, healthcare, criminal justice, and legal sectors) guided by transdisciplinary frameworks (e.g., Assari, 2018; Bailey et al., 2017). Here, I have developed one transdisciplinary framework to help this cause by putting traditional Eurocentric philosophical resources in conversation with insights from the work of scholarship from historically underrepresented and marginalized groups. I hope that readers are inspired to engage in more transdisciplinary research, to find other such frameworks, and to develop nuanced and intersectoral interventions that can effectively dismantle forms of systemic oppression. The ideas in this book are tools that readers can arm themselves with to build more humane and inclusive institutions of medicine and healthcare. They are tools that reckon with the evils, traumas, and injustices of our history and society and provide more ethical and humane care to all humans (especially to those who have been historically marginalized and oppressed), tools to create a more just world.

Fundamentals of Ethics

Ethics/moral philosophy is the critical and systematic study of the moral life.[3] The moral life is the shared practice of evaluating things, actions, and persons according to ethical standards and prescribing how to act, how to live, and what should be. Ethics thus fundamentally investigates how to live, what matters, and what should be. It delves into the meaning, source, and significance of moral/ethical concepts and evaluates the merits of ethical judgments/standards.

There are three main branches of ethics:

- **Normative ethics**—the search for and justification of ethical/moral standards, such as principles and values

This branch asks questions like "Is this action right?" "Is that person good?" "Is this a bad thing?"

- **Metaethics—**the study of the nature of ethical phenomena, our access to them, and the meaning and source of our ethical concepts

This branch asks questions like "What *is it* for a person to be good?" "What does it *mean* for an action to be right?" "How can we *know* that something is bad?"

- **Applied ethics—**the use of ethical theories and concepts to resolve practical ethical problems

This branch asks questions like "How should one distribute the profits in a company?" "How should one deal with one's sources?" "How should one conduct oneself in a trial when there is a conflict of interest?" Applied ethics employs moral concepts to try to

3. I use the adjectives "ethical" and "moral" interchangeably. Some philosophers think of morality as a subset of ethics concerned with interpersonal relations, duties, and expectations, but this is unnecessary given the social justice focus of this textbook.

answer concrete questions that confront people every day, and many such questions relate to particular professions such as business, law, and journalism.

How Does Bioethics Fit In?

- **Bioethics—**applied ethics focused on the practical ethical problems of healthcare and medicine

This subfield of applied ethics asks questions like "Should physicians help terminally ill patients commit suicide?" "How should we decide who gets life-saving organ transplants?" "How can medical research and practice be improved to combat the harmful effects of systems of oppression?

Bioethical questions are faced by (and therefore relevant to) all kinds of persons, not just philosophers; this includes healthcare professionals, lawyers, and policy specialists, but also patients, families, friends, and clergy. Bioethics inevitably employs ethics, but fully informed bioethics requires a good understanding of the relevant nonmoral facts, especially medical, scientific, technological, and legal ones.[4] Moreover, an approach to bioethics that is adequate to the problems we face in the 21st century has to contend with how the moral and nonmoral facts are further complicated when we center the perspectives of those who have been underrepresented, underserved, and marginalized by the medical establishment. Our approach accordingly centers the perspectives, experiences, and concerns of persons who are marginalized because of their race, Indigeneity, and/or ethnicity; their disability; or their sex, gender, and/or sexuality. In order to inform this approach, I first articulate some of the fundamentals of ethics.

Basic Ethical Dimensions/Categories

Ethical concepts can be classified under three basic categories covering different dimensions of the moral life: the right, the good, and moral worth.[5]

The Right (Deontic Concepts)

This first dimension of moral experience consists of evaluations of actions that employ deontic

4. Indeed, many problems in bioethics have both a legal side and a moral side. Note that we must distinguish between what is legal/illegal and what is morally right/wrong. Although morality and the law overlap significantly, they are distinct and come apart, for example, in cases of immoral laws.
5. This section is partially inspired by Timmons (2012, Chapter 1), who himself follows Rawls (2013).

concepts (from *deon*, the Greek word for "duty"). These determine whether actions are right, wrong, or optional.[6]

- **Obligatory/required/right actions**—actions that one morally ought to do or that one has a moral duty to do

Candidates for required actions include maximizing the good of all concerned and respecting the autonomy of each person.

- **Forbidden/wrong actions**—actions that one morally ought not to do or that one has a moral duty not to do

Candidates for forbidden actions include making false promises and torturing someone for fun.

- **Optional/permissible actions**—actions that are neither obligatory nor forbidden or that one has neither a duty to do nor a duty not to do

Candidates for optional actions include what particular career to choose and one's preferred leisure activities.

The Good (Value Concepts)

This second dimension of moral experience consists of evaluations of things. These determine whether things are good/beneficial/valuable/worth choosing, are bad/harmful/disvaluable/worth avoiding, or are neutral/have no value. Here it is useful to make two distinctions: (1) between final value and instrumental value, and (2) between intrinsic value and extrinsic value.[7] The final versus instrumental distinction concerns whether something is worth choosing (or avoiding) as an end or merely as a means to some other end. The intrinsic versus extrinsic distinction concerns whether something has value (or disvalue) because of its own properties or because of its relation to something else. Thus, we get the following:

- **Final good (evil)**—something that is worth choosing (worth avoiding) for its own sake as an end
- **Instrumental good (evil)**—something worth choosing (avoiding) as a means to something else that is of final value (disvalue)
- **Intrinsic good (evil)**—something worth choosing (avoiding) because of its own

6. Note that "right" is used in both a narrow (what is obligatory) sense and a broad (what is not wrong) sense.
7. This section follows Korsgaard's (1983) discussion of these two distinctions.

(intrinsic) properties, "in itself."

- **Extrinsic good (evil)**—something worth choosing (avoiding) because of its relation to something else that is of final value (disvalue).

Note then that all instrumental values are extrinsic (as an instrumental relation is inherently an extrinsic relation), but not all extrinsic values are instrumental. There can be final extrinsic values: things that are worth choosing (avoiding) as ends because of their relationship to something else (e.g., because one has taken an interest in it or because it is part of a project or a greater good). Given this, we have the following possibilities:

- **Final intrinsic goods**—Plausible examples include pleasure, knowledge, achievement, virtue, health, and fulfilling personal relationships.
- **Final intrinsic evils**—Plausible examples include pain, ignorance, failure, vice, illness, and social isolation.
- **Final extrinsic goods**—Plausible examples include personal projects we take a deep interest in and "growing pains" that are inevitable parts of improving one's life or a community as a whole.
- **Final extrinsic evils**—Plausible examples include beliefs, attitudes, and actions that may seem harmless in isolation but that in their social context help to reinforce systems of oppression.
- **Instrumental goods**—Plausible examples include money (its goodness comes from its being a means to things of final value).
- **Instrumental evils**—Plausible examples include inefficiency (its badness comes from its being an impediment to things of final value).

Note that things can be both final and instrumental goods (evils). For example, health, virtue, and fulfilling personal relationships are all worth choosing for themselves but are also good as means to other final goods; and illness, vice, and toxic personal relationships are all worth avoiding for themselves but also because they impede our pursuit of final goods and are means to other final evils.

Moral Worth (Aretaic Concepts)

The third dimension of moral experience consists of evaluations of responsible agents who can legitimately be held accountable for how they live (for what they do and the kind of person they are) and who can therefore be praised and blamed. These evaluations employ aretaic concepts (from *arete*, the Greek word for "virtue"), and they determine whether persons are morally good or bad.

- **Morally good/virtuous person/character**—a person/character who possesses and lives by positive character traits that we call virtues

Plausible candidates for virtues include honesty, beneficence, courage, generosity, and justice. These are all positive character traits that are arguably final intrinsic goods.

- **Morally bad/vicious person/character—**a person/character who possesses and lives by negative character traits that we call vices

Plausible candidates for vices include dishonesty, malice, cowardice, selfishness, and injustice. These are all negative character traits that are arguably final intrinsic evils.

These characterizations of the above basic moral categories are not offered as explanatory or illuminating definitions. Instead, they are meant to equip readers with a working understanding of these basic ethical concepts so that they can apply them in their own moral and bioethical reasoning.

With these basic dimensions of moral experience in hand, I articulate some helpful points about values and moral principles that will give us a better sense of the rich texture of lived moral experience.

The Non-Additivity of Value

When we're discussing different values, it is natural to wonder how to compare them (i.e., when they conflict with each other, which one should take precedence). However, there is also the issue of how the values of goods and evils (considered as negative goods) combine when they are part of a common whole. Here we find at least two possibilities:

- **Additive combination—**The values of parts of a whole are simply added together (with the value of evil things counting as negative value), so the value of the whole equals the sum of the value of the parts.
- **Dynamic/Non-Additive combination—**The values of parts of a whole combine in non-additive ways, so the value of the whole does not equal the sum of the value of the parts.

Although it is perhaps plausible to claim that certain values combine in additive ways (plausibly, some pains and pleasures "cancel out"), it is implausible to hold that all value-combinations are additive. Consider the value of a well-executed curry. It is implausible to hold that the value of this dish, with its complex combination of flavors and textures, is equal to the value of the ingredients simply added together. Rather, what makes such a curry so good is precisely the way the ingredients are skillfully combined to create dynamical interrelations between them that make the dish greater than the sum of its parts. The value of a dish is determined not merely by the value of its parts but also by the dynamical relations between the parts. Aristotle argues that the same point holds for the different parts of a life as a whole (2019, pp. 8–11).

G. E. Moore called these wholes whose value-combinations are non-additive "organic unities" (1993, p. 82). Discussions of organic unities in the literature often get highly technical, but we need not delve into those technicalities. For our purposes, what matters is that organic unities are a key part of lived moral experience: a good community makes the lives of those who are a part of it even better than they would be by themselves, and a toxic romantic relationship makes the lives of the lovers worse than they would be by themselves.

The take-home lesson from this discussion is the idea that goods/evils can form organic unities and thus can enter into **non-additive relations**. That is, things can come together as parts of a whole such that the resulting value of the whole does *not* equal a mere addition of their values.

This is because the whole manifests either

- **Synergistic relations**, which make the whole more valuable than the (mere) sum of its parts, or
- **Antagonistic relations**, which make the whole less valuable than the (mere) sum of its parts.[8]

Organic unities that manifest synergistic relations between their parts are **synergistic organic unities**. Organic unities that manifest antagonistic relations between their parts are **antagonistic organic unities**. Note that in practice, many if not most organic unities are mixed, that is, they manifest both synergistic and antagonistic relations. For example, part of what can make a toxic romantic relationship alluring and hard to escape is that there are often synergistic aspects to it (e.g., the deep passion that the lovers feel when they are together).

What is important for our purposes is that we look out for synergistic and antagonistic relations that complicate the values inherent in our lives and systems/institutions. I argue that to the extent that our healthcare institutions are subject to and perpetuate forms of structural oppression such as racism, ableism, and sexism, they manifest antagonistic relations that diminish the final value of these institutions.

Generally, the concept of organic unities provides us with a lens to look more critically at the value inherent in relevant ethical wholes like our social, political, and medical institutions, including the healthcare system. The concept allows us to see that the way in which value is combined and distributed in our social world is far from being a simple, additive affair. Rather, it consists of complex interactions between multiple factors.

8. As Thomas Hurka (1998) has argued, it is possible to give either holistic or conditional interpretations of organic unities, where in some cases one interpretation may be more appropriate than another. A holistic interpretation of an organic unity holds that the synergistic (antagonistic) relations themselves are the bearers of the non-additive final value in the organic unity, while a conditional interpretation holds that these relations increase (decrease) the final value of the parts in the context of the whole.

Thinking in terms of organic unities requires taking the non-additivity of value seriously, which in turn helps us resist zero-sum thinking. This kind of thinking relies on an additive view of the combination of values and uses it to pit the goods of different parts of a community against each other. It argues that anyone's benefit is equivalent to another's harm, so that the total benefits and harms "cancel out," or sum to zero, and it has been used to justify oppressive classist and racist policies that pit the benefit of different oppressed goods against one another (e.g., economically disadvantaged persons of color and economically disadvantaged white persons).[9]

With these considerations in hand concerning the way values can combine in complex and dynamic ways, I review some moral principles that have been highly influential in ethics and bioethics.

Influential Moral/Bioethical Principles

Moral principles are general moral statements that claim that a thing is morally relevant (by relating it to the above basic ethical categories).[10] There are different kind of moral principles:

- **Absolute principles—**apply without exception, invariantly relating to things or actions.
- **Prima facie principles—**apply when only they are at issue, but they warrant exceptions when other prima facie principles are relevant.

Examples of absolute principles include the claim that lying is always wrong or that maximizing utility is always right.

Examples of prima facie principles include some of a physician's duties:

- **Truthfulness—**to tell their patients the truth
- **Beneficence—**to promote their welfare

In some cases where prima facie principles conflict (e.g., when telling a patient about their condition would worsen this condition), a physician may decide that truthfulness should yield to beneficence. This is compatible with the physician deciding that in other cases (e.g., where patients value honesty above all else) truthfulness is more important.

There are many moral principles, but the following seem to capture key aspects of moral experience, and they can be interpreted as either absolute principles or prima facie principles:

9. Heather McGhee provides an illuminating and well-researched extended argument for this claim in *The Sum of Us* (2022).
10. This section is partially inspired by Vaughn (2022, Chapter 1).

- **Nonmaleficence—**The fact that an action/rule/policy/institution (intentionally or unintentionally) harms someone makes it (to some extent) wrong.[11]

This principle holds that the fact that an action/rule/policy/institution does evil to someone counts morally against it; that is, it is a moral reason against doing the action. This is perhaps the most plausible and widely recognized bioethical principle.

- **Beneficence—**The fact that an action/rule/policy/institution benefits someone makes it (to some extent) right.

This principle holds that the fact that an action/rule/policy/institution does good to someone counts morally in favor of it; that is, it is a moral reason for doing the action. Some have thought this principle to be the core of morality. Ethical human research requires balancing this principle with the value of knowledge gained by experimenting on humans.

- **Utility—**The fact that an action/rule/policy/institution maximizes the benefits minus harms of all concerned makes it (to some extent) right.

This principle claims that the fact that an action/rule/policy/institution maximizes goodness on the whole counts morally in favor of it. This principle recognizes that in practice, we often cannot do good without doing some harm, and it prescribes us to strike the right (good- or utility-maximizing) balance. This principle is especially relevant when deciding how to pursue human research and how to allocate scarce healthcare resources that can often decide matters of life and death (e.g., organ transplants).

- **Autonomy—**The fact that an action/rule/policy/institution violates someone's autonomy makes it (to some extent) wrong, and the fact that an action respects everyone's autonomy makes it (to some extent) right.

This principle highlights the moral integrity of each individual as a self-determining person and claims that the fact that an action/rule/policy/institution respects (violates) this integrity counts morally in favor of (against) it. This principle is key to the bioethical issues of:

    - **Paternalism (and patient autonomy)—**the overriding of a person's autonomy for

11. In general, if we interpret these principles as prima facie, then we should include the "to some extent" parenthetical, but we should leave this parenthetical out if we interpret them as absolute principles.

their own good

- **Informed consent—**the act of agreeing to submit to medical treatment/experimentation by an informed, autonomous person. This is an ethical ideal and requirement for medical treatment and research.

- **Justice—**The fact that an action/rule/policy/institution is just/gives people their fair due makes it (to some extent) right; the fact that an action/rule/policy/institution is unjust/fails to give people their fair due makes it (to some extent) wrong.

This principle claims that the fact that action/rule/policy/institution treats people fairly (unfairly) counts morally in favor of (against) it. It is often relevant when distributing benefits/burdens—for example, when deciding which hospitals get funded and who gets scarce life-saving resources. Different theories of justice offer different explanations of what constitutes fairness. Egalitarian theories of justice perhaps fit best with the social justice focus of this textbook. They argue that equality is a key part of what makes fairness and a just distribution, and they hold that treating people justly requires ensuring that everyone has equal access to certain minimal goods and services.

These principles are regularly used in bioethics to design, evaluate, and restructure healthcare programs, policies, and strategies. Moreover, many concrete bioethical problems emerge from conflicts between these principles. With these considerations considering the texture of the moral life and of bioethical reasoning, I review some essentials of moral theory.

Moral Theories

Moral theories aim to systematically explain the moral life with its three basic categories/dimensions. Moral theories can thus be classified according to how they prioritize/relate these basic categories.

- **Deontic theories** focus on the evaluation of actions. They guide us as to what we ought to do, thus centering deontic concepts.
- **Aretaic theories** focus on the evaluation of persons. They guide us as to what kind of persons we ought to be, thus centering aretaic concepts.

Deontic theories themselves are divided by how they relate value and deontic concepts.

- **Value-Based/Consequentialist theories** concern the nature of final value (disvalue). They aim to explain right (wrong) action by how actions affect what is of final value, thus seeing value concepts as basic and explaining other ethical concepts in terms of value concepts.

- **Duty-Based/Deontological theories** concern the nature of right (wrong) action. They hold that duties (thus deontic concepts) are at least as basic as values, not seeking to explain right (wrong) action solely in terms of how actions affect final value.

These different kinds of moral theories all aim to offer systematic guidance for how to live, albeit in different ways. We can further make sense of them by giving examples of influential moral theories falling under them.

Value-Based Deontic Theories

- **Consequentialism—**What makes an action/rule/policy/institution morally right is the fact that it maximizes the good.

Consequentialist theories take different forms. One key distinction (between act-consequentialism and rule-consequentialism) contends how to evaluate the value/rightness of the consequences of things.

- **Act-consequentialism** holds that
  - the value of things depends on the consequences of individual things, and
  - the rightness of actions/rules/policies/institutions depends solely on the good produced in individual instances.
- **Rule-consequentialism** holds that
  - the value of things depends on the consequences of following rules consistently, and
  - the rightness of actions/rules/policies/institutions depends on whether they conform to a (possibly higher-order)[12] rule that, if followed consistently, would maximize the good (create the greatest net balance of good/benefit minus evil/harm).

These two approaches to consequentialism lead to different approaches to bioethics. Consider the case of a child who has a condition that forces them to live in extreme agony without hope for improvement and whose parents beg a physician to end the child's suffering. An act-consequentialist might argue that painlessly ending the child's life would maximize the good, looking only to the consequences of this individual act to argue that the right action is to end the child's life. By contrast, a rule-consequentialist would look to the consequences of consistently following a rule that claims it is morally permissible to kill children if they are in

12. A higher-order rule is a rule about what rules to follow. This parenthetical applies to what the rightness of individual rules depends on, according to consequentialism (cf. Rawls, 1955).

agony with no hope for improvement. This rule-consequentialist might worry that following such a rule would have disastrous consequences (e.g., widespread distrust in pediatricians), and would thus argue that the right action is not to end the child's life.

Particular consequentialist theories (whether they take an act approach or a rule approach) offer different ideas of what the good is that should be maximized. One influential form of consequentialism called utilitarianism holds that the good consists of utility, that is, pleasure and the absence of pain. Readers who are inclined toward consequentialism should feel free to explore/adopt other substantive theories of the good besides utilitarian ones.[13]

Duty-Based Deontic Theories

- **Kantian ethics—**What makes action/rule/policy/institution morally right is the fact that it treats the moral autonomy/integrity of every person as an end in itself; what makes an action/rule/policy/institution morally wrong is the fact that it treats someone as a mere means.

This approach to ethics is based on the moral philosophy of German philosopher Immanuel Kant (1724–1804).[14] The fundamental principle of this philosophy is the categorical imperative. This can be formulated in a variety of ways, but arguably the most fruitful formulation is the one used above (in terms of respecting the humanity or autonomy of persons).[15]

So far, the approaches to ethical theory we have seen are *monistic* (basing their theories on a single moral standard (e.g., utility, autonomy). However, there are also pluralist approaches to moral theory, such as this:

- **Principlism—**There is more than one basic moral principle that determines what makes something morally right/wrong.

This view, based on W. D. Ross's (2002) moral philosophy, accepts a plurality of prima facie moral principles that may be relevant in any given case. It argues that the moral life is too complex to be captured by a single moral standard and instead argues that many (prima facie) principles of duty (e.g., nonmaleficence, beneficence, utility, autonomy, and

13. Included in other such theories are pluralist theories about the good that hold that different kinds of things are all intrinsically good (e.g., pleasure, kindness, knowledge, achievement, virtue).
14. Kant's own philosophy is highly intricate and systematic (combining theoretical and ethical aspects) and lies beyond the scope of this work, but it has inspired contemporary approaches to ethics that are distinct from it.
15. Other formulations are, roughly, in terms of acting for reasons that all others could accept and of acting in such a way that you regard yourself as part of an ideal community of autonomous moral agents. For our purposes, we need not delve into these issues.

justice) are relevant, using judgment to determine how to resolve conflicts between these principles in particular cases.[16]

Aretaic Theories

- **Virtue ethics—**A theory that guides us in the development of our character, inviting us to aspire to moral excellence by cultivating virtues like humility, generosity, kindness, and courage and avoiding vices like pride, avarice, meanness, and cowardice.

This theory approaches bioethical problems by focusing not so much on actions but rather on whether our decisions manifest virtues or vices, asking us to decide and respond to bioethical problems with virtue.

- **Feminist ethics—**An approach to ethics aimed at eliminating aspects of traditional ethics that ignore or devalue women's perspectives, experiences, and contributions, like the following problematic assumptions often inherent in traditional moral theories:
    - Women are less rational and more emotional than men (and so are less adept at moral theory).
    - Domestic or private moral problems (historically relegated to women) are less important than public ones (historically reserved for wealthy men to tackle).
    - Virtues considered feminine in Eurocentric cultures (e.g., feeling, sharing, and interconnectedness) are not central to morality.

This approach to ethics emphasizes that moral reflection must focus on the social realities that shape moral problems and solutions, which include social practices, values, and norms; personal relationships; social, political, and economic institutions; and power asymmetries.

Importantly, feminist ethics is *not* defined by shared doctrine or ideology (like utilitarian or Kantian ethics) but rather by a distinctive focus on feminist issues. This leads to significant variation in feminist views concerning specific moral and bioethical issues.

- **Ethics of care—**A distinct moral perspective that centers interpersonal relationships,

16. An influential version of this view that is widely used in bioethics was developed by Tom Beauchamp and James Childress in *Principles of Biomedical Ethics* (1979).

their demands, and the virtues and feelings that are central to them, such as care, compassion, and empathy.[17]

This approach to understanding the moral life holds that the heart of morality is not impartial reasoning according to general principles but rather feeling and caring for particular people with whom we are connected. This approach thus challenges core elements of traditional moral theories by focusing on the demands of specific situations. Its approach to bioethical problems asks us to attend to the specifics of the particular personal relationships of people facing such problems in order to articulate adequate solutions to them.

There are other moral theories that have appealed to philosophers, but these are among the most influential, especially in bioethics. Readers should think for themselves about what approach to ethics they find most attractive as they learn more about particular bioethical problems.

Note that part of whether one finds a particular moral theory attractive depends on what one thinks the aim of moral theory should be. One aim of moral theory can be to provide a method or a decision procedure that can be used by suitably informed agents to reach correct moral verdicts in their reasoning about particular cases. Another aim of moral theory is to explain the features of things that make those things morally relevant (i.e., what makes them good/right or bad/wrong). A particular theory might be well-suited to meet one aim without being able to meet another aim.[18] How plausible a person finds particular theories depends on which of these aims the person thinks is more important.

With these fundamentals of ethics and bioethics on the table, the next chapter centers the bioethical problems faced by persons who are marginalized because of their race, Indigeneity, or ethnicity.

References

Aristotle (2019). *Nicomachean Ethics* (T. Irwin, Trans.; 3rd ed.). Hackett Publishing Company.

Assari, S. (2018). Health disparities due to diminished return among Black Americans: Public policy solutions. *Social Issues and Policy Review*, *12*(1), 112–145.

Bailey, Z. D., Krieger, N., Agénor, M., Graves, J., Linos, N., & Bassett, M. T. (2017). Structural racism and health inequities in the USA: Evidence and interventions. *The Lancet*, *389*(10077), 1453–1463.

Campbell, F. A. K. (2009). *Contours of ableism: The production of disability and abledness*. Springer.

17. Although the ethics of care and feminist ethics are not always explicitly described as such, they are aretaic theories to the extent that they encourage us to be certain kinds of persons, viz., who navigate personal relationships and engage with their sociopolitical context in a certain way.
18. For example, opponents of consequentialism argue that it is a bad decision procedure for actually bringing about the best consequences, but some consequentialists reply that their theory is best interpreted as concerned solely with the aim of explaining the nature of value/rightness.

Carney, T. (2021). *Solving the crimes of patriarchy: Meta-lucidity and middle-aged women in* Happy Valley & Broadchurch. Mai: Feminism & Visual Culture. https://maifeminism.com/solving-the-crimes-of-the-patriarchy-meta-lucidity-and-middle-aged-women-in-happy-valley-broadchurch/

Collins, H. P. (2015). *Black feminist thought.* Routledge.

Crenshaw, K. (1991). Demarginalizing the intersection of race and sex: A black feminist critique of antidiscrimination doctrine, feminist theory, and antiracist politics. In K. T. Bartlett and R. Kennedy (Eds.), *Feminist legal theory* (pp. 57–80). https://doi.org/10.4324/9780429500480-5

Gamble, V. N. (2016). Under the shadow of Tuskegee: African Americans and health care. In E. D. Whitaker (Ed.), *Health psychology* (pp. 434–441). Routledge.

Glitzen, T., & Chun, W. (2021). *Pandemic surveillance and homophobia in South Korea.* The Social Science Research Council. https://items.ssrc.org/covid-19-and-the-social-sciences/covid-19-fieldnotes/pandemic-surveillance-and-homophobia-in-south-korea/

Hardeman, R. R., Medina, E. M., & Kozhimannil, K. B. (2016). Structural racism and supporting black lives—the role of health professionals. *New England Journal of Medicine, 375*(22), 2113–2115. https://doi.org/10.1056/NEJMp1609535

Hardeman, R. R., & Karbeah, J. (2020). Examining racism in health services research: A disciplinary self-critique. *Health services research*, *55*(Suppl 2), 777–780. https://doi.org/10.1111/1475-6773.13558

Hurka, T. (1998). Two kinds of organic unity. *The Journal of Ethics, 2*(4), 299–320.

Korsgaard, C. M. Two distinctions in goodness. *The Philosophical Review*, *92*(2), 169–195.

Linker, M. (2015). *Intellectual empathy: Critical thinking for social justice.* University of Michigan Press.

Moore, G. E. (1993). *Principia ethica.* (T. Baldwin, Ed.). Cambridge University Press.

McGhee, H. (2022). *The sum of us: What racism costs everyone and how we can prosper together.* One World.

McLoyd, V. C. (2022). Spotlighting black adolescent development in the shadow of racism: A commentary. *Journal of Research on Adolescence, 32*(1), 295–301.

Rawls, J. (1955). Two concepts of rules. *The philosophical review*, *64*(1), 3–32.

Rawls, J. (2013). The independence of moral theory. *American Philosophical Association Centennial Series*, 283–298. https://doi.org/10.5840/apapa2013245

Ross, W. D. (2002). *The right and the good* (Philip Stratton-Lake, Ed.). Oxford University Press.

Seay, G., & Nuccetelli, S. (2017). *Engaging bioethics: An introduction with case studies.* Routledge.

Timmons, M. (2012). *Moral theory: An introduction* (2nd ed.). Rowman & Littlefield Publishers.

Vaughn, L. (2022). *Bioethics: Principles, issues, and cases* (5th ed.). Oxford University Press.

Wiener, D. (2018). Review of the book *Resistance and hope: Essays by disabled people: Crip wisdom for the people*, edited by A. Wong. *Wordgathering: A journal of disability poetry and literature.* https://wordgathering.syr.edu/past_issues/issue48/reviews/wong.html

Unit I

The Shadow of Race/ism and The Ocean of White Supremacy Culture in Healthcare and Medicine

Introduction to the Unit

In this unit, we discuss how bioethical issues are complicated when we center the perspectives/experiences of persons marginalized because of their race, Indigeneity, or ethnicity. It aims to

- educate readers as to the meaning, history, and significance of the concepts of race, Indigeneity, and ethnicity;
- give readers a sense of the systemic oppression that people marginalized because of their race, Indigeneity, or ethnicity face; and
- acquaint readers with some insightful solutions to the problems of healthcare and medicine that emerge from centering the perspectives/experiences of marginalized racialized, Indigenous, and ethnic groups.

What Race *Is* Versus What Race *Does*

Many have asked "What is race?" In the past, people were attracted to **biological** views/models of race, which hold that race is a biological category concerning people's genetics and phenotype/physical traits/ancestry. These views have proved implausible.[1] Nowadays, it is standard for people instead to adopt **social constructionist** models of race, which hold that race is a social rather than biological property. As biological anthropologist, sociologist, evolutionary geneticist, and critical race scholar Dr. Shay-Akil McLean argues, many of the social constructionist models from mainstream academics mainly tell us that sex is *not* biological, and then they say it is constructed on the basis of phenotype/physical traits/ancestry (McLean, 2021).

Mainstream social constructionist models are problematic, not just because they are uninformative but also because they do not help improve the experience of people of color. As McLean poignantly puts it, "The social construction of race has done more for advancing white supremacy under covert means than ever killing it off" (2020, pp. 40–41). These models most often serve merely as something that liberal anthropologists use to claim antiracist leanings. But what we actually need is a social constructionist understanding of race that becomes "a larger call for anti-racist practices" (McLean, 2020, p. 40).

In order to provide this antiracist social constructionist understanding, McLean argues that we should adopt a *Du Boisian* theorization of race (named after American sociologist, historian, civil rights activist, and author W. E. B. Du Bois). This theoretical approach explores the concept of race as motivated by race/ism and understands that racialization consists of the social reproduction of racialized distinctions motivated by enactments of political control (McLean, 2020, p. 40).

As McLean insightfully points out, the right question to ask is not "What *is* race?" but rather "How do humans *do* race?" We can answer this question by looking at the historical record and at how race frames and shapes the ways humans interact. Historian, author, and educator Blair Imani provides a good outline of the historical invention and reproduction of race from 1452 to 1950 (2021, pp. 100–106). As McLean points out, different concepts of race were constructed by Eurocolonial imperialists in response to capitalist crises, market disasters, and rebellions they encountered. For example,

- **1492—**People from the Caribbean became "**Native American**" when Columbus arrived (mistaking the land for India).
- **1676—**Bacon's Rebellion (in which African and European indentured servants rebelled against European landowners) prompted worries about worker solidarity that, by 1700, led to the racialization of the chattel slavery principle and the treatment of Africans as "**Black**," a distinct enslaved status that extends from mother to child.
- **1691—**The legal category of "**white**" is first used in the Virginia colony to pass a law prohibiting marriage between "whites" and "Blacks."
- **1803—**Colonial officer John Sullivan of the East India Company suggested the Trinidad Experiment: the creation of the concept of a "**Far East Asian**" "free race" to be used as a "racial barrier" between British and "Blacks."

Asking "How do humans *do* race?" leads to asking different questions concerning race and how it

1. As McLean notes, many biological anthropologists have studied human osteology and genetics and concluded that what we call race does not fit models of human genetic variation nor human evolutionary history (2020, p. 41).

affects people's lives. It reveals that people of color (and other oppressed) persons exhibit systematically different environmental stressors because of oppressive social institutions (that are responsible for things like the race/ist and gender wage gaps as well as many well-documented health inequities) (McLean, 2021).[2]

Through this Du Boisian approach, McLean argues for a **historically grounded social constructionist** definition/model/understanding of race, one that is grounded in actual (historical) practice. This approach reveals that our modern concept of race is a relatively recent Eurocolonial invention in our long evolutionary history, one that "arose as a justification for Euro-Western colonialism and enslavement" (McLean, 2020, p. 41). As McLean eloquently puts it: "Race/ism was created by European colonizers in order to seize land, labor, and gain control of the means of production" (cited in Imani, 2021, p. 98).[3]

A historically grounded social constructionist model of race helps us grasp that race/ism is not fundamentally about looking different or about people's attitudes. It's fundamentally about having the power and resources to build and manage social institutions and systems in a way that embodies prejudice and injustice against people of color in our material and social practices (McLean, 2021).

If we want to combat the race/ism inherent in our institutions and societies (including the institutions of healthcare and medicine), we need to educate ourselves about the real meaning and history of this concept. And a key part of this is, as McLean puts it, to understand race/ism as a dynamic system of practices that are taught, invested in, and incentivized, and which produce the very conditions in which we live and die (2020, p. 44).[4]

The Shifting Shadow of Race/ism and the Ocean of White Supremacy Culture

By taking this dynamic, historical approach to understanding race/ism, we learn that race/ism is like a shadow cast over every aspect of our social world: our policies, institutions, practices, language, and even our thinking.[5] This shadow is an antagonistic organic unity over our social world, including the institutions of healthcare and medicine, making them less valuable as wholes than the sum of their parts. This shadow is long and wide and has created race/ist institutions, structures, and ideologies all around us that unfairly privilege (and thus create synergies in the lives of) white persons and unfairly disadvantage (and thus create antagonisms in the lives of) people of color. This unjust distribution of synergies and antagonisms

2. As McLean points out, taking this kind of approach reveals the connection between environmental stressors, biology, and lived experience and shows that there is no sharp distinction to be drawn between mental and physical health: both are aspects of our health as living human beings (McLean, 2021). This textbook follows this insight and deliberately includes readings concerned with mental health and substance abuse.
3. I follow McLean in using the term *race/ism* to highlight that race is a racist social construction.
4. Modeling race/ism as a dynamical system can help provide a more precise, formal articulation of the analogy of the shadow of race/ism, and how it impacts our social world and lives.
5. This metaphor can be found in the work of certain Black scholars (e.g., Gamble, 2016; McLoyd, 2022).

across racial lines itself yields overall antagonisms in society as a whole because of the injustice and inefficiency of this unequal distribution of synergies and antagonisms. This shadow manifests itself in different forms, including these:[6]

- **Individual race/ism**—interpersonal interactions designed to denigrate people of color who are viewed as inferior in society; these interactions can be either
    - **Overt**—for example, a race/ist insult in public, or
    - **Covert**—for example, not giving as much consideration to a Black candidate in a hiring decision
- **Institutional race/ism**—practices, norms, and policies that perpetuate inequality by restricting opportunities for people of color
    - Examples: redlining housing practices, race/ist credit institutions, predatory loaning practices directed at people of color
- **Cultural race/ism**—symbols, ideologies, and practices used to reinforce the notion that people of color are inferior to white people
    - Examples: race/ist stereotypes, Blaxploitation, underrepresentation of people of color in media

It is important to highlight that these different kinds of race/ism are distinct, but not isolated. In fact, they are interrelated and mutually reinforcing. For example, institutional overpolicing of Black bodies is partially enacted/justified through race/ist stereotypes in culture and media that inculcate race/ist beliefs in individuals that make them more likely to call the police on Black persons. One additional noteworthy manifestation of race/ism takes the form of **racial microaggressions**: subtle, everyday (intentional or unintentional) verbal/behavioral/environmental expressions of oppression (e.g., dismissive, insulting, disrespectful treatment) based on one's race (Sue et al., 2007). Note that the term *micro* does not indicate that microaggressions are minor. Rather, they add up in a manner like "death by a thousand cuts" that is detrimental to people's health and welfare (Imani, 2021, p. 117).

The way this shadow manifests itself in harmful ways is complicated by the fact that it is a *shifting* shadow, one that transforms itself as we shine the light of understanding and justice on it. As El-Hajj Malik El-Shabazz once put it,[7] race/ism "is like a Cadillac, they bring out a new model every year" (cited in McLean, 2020, p. 43). This shifting elusiveness is worth reflecting on. As McLean points out, although it is well-known that race lacks explanatory utility as a scientific category, the world still grapples with racial difference. The concept of race, then, is slippery, elusive, and capable of conforming itself to different sets of conditions to reproduce white supremacist conditions. And McLean argues that this is because, ultimately, "the utility of race is its stabilization of colonial and imperial power amassed through historical and ongoing displacement and dispossession in an expanding processual global fashion" (McLean, 2020,

6. Following J. M. Jones's tripartite model of race/ism (Jones, 1997).

7. This is the name that Malcolm X became known by after he completed the traditional Muslim Hajj pilgrimage to Mecca.

p. 43). That is, racial differences persist because they are a historically useful tool for the (generally white, abled, male, rich, straight, cisgender) few to accumulate and maintain power as they have displaced and dispossessed more and more people throughout a history of imperialism and colonialism.

Note that "white supremacist" does not refer simply to, for example, Nazi ideology. Rather, as antiracist scholars and activists like Kenneth Jones and Tema Okun have pointed out, white supremacy is a certain kind of culture that permeates our social world in pernicious ways. This culture socially constructs whiteness and white culture as the "default" way of being human (and thus as a position of power) in a way that is made possible by the creation of other racialized groups (Imani, 2021, pp. 106–108). It partially consists of the following interconnected mutually reinforcing characteristics:[8]

- fear
- perfectionism
- urgency
- defensiveness
- quantity over quality
- worship of the written word
- paternalism
- either/or thinking
- individualism
- avoidance of discomfort
- objectivity (there is one right way that is perfect, attainable, and desirable for everyone)

In their *Dismantling Racism* workbook, Jones and Okun identify these characteristics, noting that they "are used as norms and standards without being pro-actively named or chosen" in a way that "makes it difficult, if not impossible, to open the door to other cultural norms and standards" (cited in Villanueva, 2018, p. 45). These characteristics shape every aspect of our social world. As Cristina River Chapman notes, white supremacy is "the invisible ocean we all must tread" in a way that "deeply informs what we think and feel and even how we think and feel" (cited in Okun, 2021). The message this culture seeks to reinforce in all of us is a version of **zero-sum thinking**: "The only way for me to swim is someone else has to sink" (cited in Okun, 2021). This false narrative implies that for someone to do well, others must be diminished, and it leads us to see the value of humans not as something inherent but as something relative that must be proved.

Given the pervasive way that white supremacy and the shadow of race/ism permeate and shape our social world, "It is crucial to understand that whiteness is a position of power within the system of race" (Imani, 2021, p. 108). It is that which is considered default and normal, and part of that which tends to

8. Much helpful information about white supremacy culture and its characteristics can be found on the White Supremacy Culture website (Okun, 2021).

be centered (together with wealth, maleness, ableness, heterosexuality, and cisgender) in the dominant culture.[9]

Race/ism and white supremacy ultimately harm all of us—but in importantly unequal ways. For example, McGhee (2021) points out that although race/ism has harmed all people in the US (including white people) by draining the social pool of public goods that can serve as a springboard for a thriving middle class, "our people are not all standing at the same [social, economic, or political] depths today" (p. 271). And because of this, as McGhee argues, we cannot look for one-size-fits-all solutions. Rather, we must take seriously the experiences of marginalized racial groups (and other marginalized persons) as giving us knowledge of different, complex problems requiring nuanced, tailored solutions, solutions informed by the perspectives of people of color (and other marginalized people).

The Shadow of Race/ism in Medicine and Healthcare

Given our bioethical focus, we must underscore that the shadow of race/ism is deeply entangled with medical history, especially in the US. For example, as journalist Nikole Hannah-Jones points out, after the Civil War, Black people in the US have continuously faced white ambivalence toward their plight as well as race/ist beliefs and attitudes that have severely limited their access to healthcare (Hannah-Jones, 2019). This included the American Medical Association's refusal to protest the separate but equal clause that legalized hospital segregation and their waging a race/ist propaganda war against proposals for universal insurance. Additionally, medical research has often been conducted on Black bodies without the informed consent of Black persons who were experimented upon. The notorious 40-year Tuskegee syphilis experiment by the US government, in which 399 Black men were deliberately denied effective treatment for syphilis in order to document the disease, serves as just one particularly stark reminder of the race/ist violence that medical research has visited upon Black and Indigenous bodies for the sake of furthering medical knowledge.[10]

More generally, medical research and practice has a deeply race/ist history of creating pseudoscientific classifications and hierarchies based on race that were used to justify race/ist imperialist practices and even to argue that humans of different races belonged to different species altogether (Nieblas-Bedolla et al., 2020). And this race/ist history is part of the long shadow of race/ism cast over the institution of medicine, with effects that continue to this day (e.g., medical education continues to pathologize race, decades into the 21st century).[11]

9. An intersectional framework helps us see that women and economically disadvantaged white persons experience white privilege, but the form this privilege takes differs depending on the person's gender, class, etc.
10. As Davis (2018) points out, other examples include the experiments that J. Marion Sims conducted on enslaved women without anesthesia to correct vesico-vaginal fistulas (Cooper Owens, 2017) (experiments that have had a pernicious lasting impact on physicians' perceptions of Black women's pain) as well as US doctors' finding it appropriate to administer an experimental contraceptive to healthy Native American and Black patients even after finding it caused breast cancer in beagles (and refusing to fund the testing of its use as a contraceptive) (Washington, 2006).
11. Nieblas-Bedolla et al. (2020) point out that race is treated in deeply problematic ways in medical education, including the fact that

Much more can be, should be, and has been said (by antiracist scholars and activists) to articulate the aspects of this shifting shadow and omnipresent ocean and how they create antagonisms in our social world that disproportionately harm people of color in myriad ways.[12] But our discussion so far provides us with an initial critical lens we can use in more informed and nuanced ways to tackle the bioethical problems faced by people of color, a lens that can be further articulated.

Race, Indigeneity, and Ethnicity

At this point, it is important to distinguish between the related concepts of race, Indigeneity, and ethnicity. As we have seen, race is a relatively recent Eurocolonial invention. As Imani points out, Indigeneity, like race, is a relative position within a colonial system (2021, p. 99). People become "Indigenous" when settling colonizers arrive on the already-occupied land. Note that this term is often exclusively applied to people within the Americas, Australia, and New Zealand. Importantly, Indigenous persons are often racialized in certain marginalizing ways, but the identity of Indigenous persons is not reducible to their racial identity, and thinking this way problematically erases aspects of the oppression they face. As Roxanne Dunbar-Ortiz points out, the identity of Indigenous persons in the US is territorial and treaty-based, which brings important complications to our thinking about their intersectional identities (2021, p. 271).[13]

Ethnicity is yet another distinct intersection of identity that concerns the common cultural background or descent that may be shared by a population. Thus, there can be different combinations of ethnicities and races, say, white Irish and white French or Black Italian and Black Haitian. Like Indigeneity, ethnicity can be racialized in marginalizing ways, and it has been used to discriminate. For example, Irish Catholics were racialized as non-white under English colonial rule in a way that followed many Irish famine refugees to the US (Dunbar-Ortiz, 2021, p. 128).[14] These different axes of identities all intersect in complex, contextual ways to which we must be sensitive.

medical students are encouraged and rewarded as part of their education for using race as a diagnostic tool without consulting other relevant factors, which can perpetuate the very social inequities that need to be addressed in medicine.

12. For example, critical race scholars have pointed out that (in an unsettling echo of the Trinidad Experiment's suggestion of creating an Asian buffer "free race") Asian Americans can be seen as occupying a "racial bourgeoisie" or middle status between whites and other people of color (Matsuda, 1993; Chou and Choi, 2013). Furthermore, Black women face particular forms of oppression, including (interpersonal, institutional, and cultural) *gendered race/ism* and a racial form of misogyny, or **misogynoir** (Lewis, 2022). More information can also be found at McLean's Decolonize ALL the Things website (McLean, 2014).
13. Dunbar-Ortiz rightly observes that multiculturalism in the US has historically distorted Indigenous nations and communities, as their territorial and treaty-based identities do not fit neatly into the "grid of multiculturalism" (2021, p. 271). They were distorted by being "included by transforming them into an inchoate, oppressed, racial group," while oppressed Mexican Americans and colonized Puerto Ricans were dissolved into another such group, variously called "Hispanic," or "Latino," and more recently "Latinx" (2021, p. 271).
14. Scholars such as Noel Ignatiev (1995) theorize how the Irish became white, but as Dunbar-Ortiz (2021, p. 131) points out, this development is complex and must be seen in the context of how the Irish became settlers in the US in part by receiving not just what W. E. B. Du Bois calls the "psychological wage" of white privilege but also the material rewards of maintaining the wedge between white and Black workers.

Antisemitism

In discussing the relationship between race and ethnicity, it is worth mentioning antisemitism, which is older than race and race/ism. Jewish identity is nuanced, relating to religion, ethnicity, shared ancestry, history, secular traditions, and culture, and we cannot do justice to the ancient and complex history of the Jewish people here. Nonetheless, our margin-centering approach requires us to make some basic points about antisemitism. As Imani points out, discussing antisemitism as merely religious persecution can be harmful because it erases the ethnic discrimination and racialized discrimination that are dimensions of antisemitism, so we should understand it as inherently racialized in the context of white supremacy (2021, pp. 108–109).[15] Moreover, antisemitism includes not just violence but also a dehumanized perception of Jewish people stemming from white supremacy, as well as the denial of the reality and pervasiveness of antisemitism either throughout history or in the present (including denying the reality and consequences of the Holocaust). Just as pseudoscience has been used to justify and implement race/ism, it has also been used to justify and implement antisemitism, with German racist Wilhelm Marr popularizing the term antisemitism in order to make anti-Jewish hate appear scientific and legitimate, falsely claiming that Jewish people were a racial group called "Semites" (Imani, 2021, p. 111). Exploring the history of antisemitism thus reveals that it is another current of the oppressive ocean of white supremacy we must be aware of and work to resist and dismantle.

Obstetric Race/ism and Black Women's Reproductive Health

In the wake of the recent Supreme Court decision to dismantle federal protections of abortion rights (and the attack this constitutes against the bodily autonomy of women in general, but especially economically disadvantaged women, Indigenous women, and women of color), our intersectional approach to bioethics requires us to articulate our critical lens by emphasizing the phenomenon of obstetric race/ism. As Dána-Ain Davis has pointed out, this is something Black women in particular face when dealing with the way their reproductive lives intersect with the healthcare system and mainstream medical practice.

Obstetric race/ism is the mechanisms of subordination to which reproducing Black women are subjected that track along histories of anti-Black race/ism, consisting of beliefs and practices that sit at the intersection of obstetric violence and medical race/ism (Davis, 2018). Obstetric race/ism is both a phenomenon and a theoretical framework that can help us gain a deeper understanding of how this phenomenon negatively impacts Black women in complex ways at different points in their reproductive lives, including pregnancy, childbirth, and postpartum. According to Davis (2018, 2020), its effects include (but are not limited to)

15. This highlights that although our modern concepts or race and race/ism are a recent invention, racialization is older. What our current race concepts do is provide an especially regimented and systematic way of racializing persons that enacts domination and exploitation based on these racialized distinctions (which were constructed through the rise of Eurocolonialism).

- critical lapses in diagnosis;
- neglect, dismissiveness, or disrespect;
- causing pain (intentionally);
- coercion to perform procedures;
- degradation of the patient through embarrassment, humiliation, or shame; and
- medical abuse (e.g., being experimented upon).

The concept of obstetric race/ism provides an articulation of our critical lens that can help us understand the complex ways Black women's reproductive lives are negatively affected by systems of oppression. To quote and paraphrase Davis, "Racism and its entanglement with medical history cannot be removed from" Black women's experience of how their reproductive lives intersect with the institutions of medicine and healthcare (Davis, 2018, p. 62).

With this background in hand concerning race/ism and white supremacy and their relevance to bioethics, I give an overview of the readings from this unit.

Unit Readings

The first reading reviews some problems with the legal doctrine of informed consent, including the ways the doctrine harms patients who belong to underrepresented and marginalized racial, religious, and ethnic groups. Additionally, the reading spells out how the ethical phenomenon of informed consent becomes complicated when we consider that people from different races, ethnicities, and religions value autonomy differently and for different reasons. As Matthew insightfully argues, "Ironically, the solution to the discrimination felt by the excluded members of society may turn out to provide the remedy for the informed consent doctrine as a whole" (2008, p. 150). This reading thus represents a powerful instance of how, by centering the margins, we can find solutions that help improve the lived experiences not just of marginalized persons but of everyone.

The second reading (Culhane-Pera & Xiong, 2003) is from *Healing by Heart*, a book of stories of people's search for culturally responsive healthcare from US providers. It focuses on successful relationships with traditional Hmong patients and families (an ethnic group living mainly in China and Southeast Asia), offering resources to empower providers and institutions to deliver culturally responsive healthcare. The excerpt contains the basics of a general model for delivering culturally responsive healthcare. This model enriches our approach to bioethics by guiding the development of a more humane approach to providing healthcare to cultural groups whose values may be different from our own. Although the model is directed primarily at clinical practitioners, many of the key learning areas apply to healthcare administrators, educators, and health policymakers in different sectors.

The third reading is a chapter from *Recovery the Native Way* on Indigenous/Native persons' experiences of substance abuse and recovery. It spells out a method of recovery from substance abuse inspired by the life and work of nineteenth-century Iroquois leader Handsome Lake, who developed a method to help Indigenous people embrace their heritage as they recovered from substance abuse. The discussion emphasizes the growing recognition that cultural issues impact both dysfunction and recovery and the need to provide recovery programs tailored toward the needs of specific groups. Alf Walle (2008) argues that not only Native Americans but also Native Hawaiians and the Māori of New Zealand face stress and pressure exerted on their cultures that create conditions of cultural disintegration affecting their lives, welfare, and health. Thus, the ideas from this model can potentially be adapted to other Indigenous groups.

All these readings consider how our approach to the ethics of healthcare and medicine needs to become more nuanced when we consider a multiracial and multicultural context of people with different values experiencing different conditions of the social world. These readings therefore provide insightful proposals for solutions to problems faced by marginalized persons—proposals that can inform a more inclusive and humane approach to the problems of healthcare and medicine in general and thus help build a more socially just multiracial/multicultural world.

References

Chou, R. S., & Choi, S. (2013). And neither are we saved: Asian Americans' elusive quest for racial justice. *Sociology Compass*, *7*(10), 841–853.

Cooper Owens, D. (2017). *Medical bondage: Race, gender, and the origins of American gynecology*. University of Georgia Press.

Culhane-Pera, K. A., & Xiong, P. (2003). A model for culturally responsive health care. In K. A. Culhane-Pera, D. E. Vawter, P. Xiong, B. Babbitt, & M. M. Solberg (Eds.), Healing by heart: Clinical and ethical case stories of Hmong families and Western providers. Vanderbilt University Press.

Davis, D. A. (2018). Obstetric racism: The racial politics of pregnancy, labor, and birthing. *Medical Anthropology*, *38*(7), 560–573.

Davis, D. A. (2020). Reproducing while Black: The crisis of Black maternal health, obstetric racism and assisted reproductive technology. *Reproductive Biomedicine & Society Online*, *11*, 56–64.

Dunbar-Ortiz, R. (2021). Not "a nation of immigrants": Settler colonialism, white supremacy, and a history of erasure and exclusion. Beacon Press.

Gamble, V. N. (2016). Under the shadow of Tuskegee: African Americans and health care. In E. D. Whitaker (Ed.), *Health psychology* (pp. 434–441). Routledge.

Hannah-Jones, N. (Host). (2019, September 13). How the bad blood began [Audio podcast episode no. 4]. The 1619 Project. *New York Times*. https://www.nytimes.com/2019/09/13/podcasts/1619-slavery-healthcare.html

Imani, B. (2021). *Read this to get smarter:* About race, class, gender, disability & more. Ten Speed Press.

Ignatiev, N. (1995). *How the Irish became white*. Routledge.

Jones, J. M. (1997). *Prejudice and racism* (2nd ed.). McGraw Hill.

Lewis, J. A. (2022). #SayHerName: The impact of gendered racism and misogynoir on the lives of Black women. In K. Cokley (Ed.), *Making Black lives matter: Confronting anti-Black racism* (pp. 71–86). Cognella.

Matsuda, M. (1993). We will not be used. *UCLA Asian American Pacific Islands Law Journal*, *1*, 79.

Matthew, D. B. (2008). Race, religion, and informed consent—Lessons from social science. *Journal of Law, Medicine & Ethics*, *36*(1), 150–173.

McGhee, H. (2021). *The sum of us*. One World.

McLean, S. A. (2014). *Decolonize ALL the things*. Accessed August 12, 2022. https://decolonizeallthethings.com

McLean, S. A. (2020). Social constructions, historical grounds. *Practicing Anthropology*, *42*(3), 40–44.

McLean, S. A. (2021). *Race/ism: A human ecological system* [Video]. Vimeo. https://vimeo.com/513572771

McLoyd, V. C. (2022). Spotlighting black adolescent development in the shadow of racism: A commentary. *Journal of Research on Adolescence*, *32*(1), 295–301.

Nieblas-Bedolla, E., Christophers, B., Nkinsi, N. T., Schumann, P. D., & Stein, E. (2020). Changing how race is portrayed in medical education: Recommendations from medical students. *Academic Medicine*, *95*(12), 1802–1806.

Okun, T. (May, 2021). *White supremacy culture*. https://www.whitesupremacyculture.info/

Sue, D. W., Capodilupo, C. M., Torino, G. C., Bucceri, J. M., Holder, A., Nadal, K. L., & Esquilin, M. (2007). Racial microaggressions in everyday life: Implications for clinical practice. *American Psychologist*, *62*(4), 271.

Villanueva, E. (2021). *Decolonizing wealth: Indigenous wisdom to heal divides and restore balance* (2nd ed.). Berrett-Koehler Publishers.

Walle, A. H. (2008). *Recovery the Native way: A therapist's manual*. Information Age Publishing.

Washington, H. A. (2006). *Medical apartheid: The dark history of medical experimentation on Black Americans from colonial times to the present*. Doubleday Books.

Race, Religion, and Informed Consent

Lessons from Social Science

Dayna Bowen Matthew

Editor's Introduction

In this reading, Dayna Matthew explores how the ethical phenomenon of informed consent is complicated once we consider the perspectives of people of different races, ethnicities, and religious orientations and the different ways in which they conceive of medical decision-making and value/prioritize autonomy. She draws on this discussion to propose a solution to the problems that the legal doctrine of informed consent tends to visit upon marginalized groups, which can help to remedy well-known problems with this doctrine. Dayna Matthew, JD, PhD is the dean and Harold H. Greene professor of law at the Washington University Law School. She is a leader in public health and civil rights law, and her work focuses on inequities in health and healthcare and the social determinants of health.

So the last will be first, and first will be last.

—Matthew 20:16

The evidence about informed consent is now several decades old. It is mountainous. It is damning. When failure is the norm, it is time to ask whether there are ineradicable reasons for the failure and time to go back to basics.

—Carl E. Schneider[1]

Introduction

Patients belonging to ethnic, racial, and religious minorities have been all but excluded[2] from the legal academy's ongoing conversation about informed consent. Perhaps this is just as well, since the conversation appears to have concluded that the doctrine has failed to serve as a meaningful regulation of clinical relationships.[3] Informed consent does not operate in practice the way it was intended in theory. More than a decade ago, Peter Schuck noted the "informed consent gap" that distinguishes the "proper" law of informed consent "on the books" from the actual consent law in action, and called for a more contextualized approach to informed consent.[4] Susan Wolf later called for a systemic approach to informed consent in order to accommodate multiple decision points in the managed care setting.[5] Some reformers have sought enhancements to expand the doctrine.[6] Mark Hall, on the other hand, proposed limiting the doctrine's intrusiveness by requiring advanced global disclosures that would make disclosures between the physician and patient unnecessary.[7] Some legal analysts have discussed the strengths of the informed

1. C. E. Schneider, "After Autonomy," *Wake Forest Law Review* 41 (2006): 411–444.
2. See L. J. Pittman, "A Thirteenth Amendment Challenge to Both Racial Disparities in Medical Treatments and Improper Physicians' Informed Consent," *St. Louis University Law Journal* 48 (2003): 131–189 (proposing informed consent include physician duty to disclose to African Americans historic disparity between the types of treatments recommended for blacks versus whites).
3. See, e.g., Schneider, *supra* note 1, at 417. (Reviewing empirical evidence that within the informed consent setting, physicians do not convey information effectively, patients do not understand information conveyed, and patients are unable to accurately analyze the information they receive to conclude, "There is already evidence that a perilously large part of the bioethical agenda has fallen intolerably and irremediably short of the expectations that inspired and would justify it....Consider first informed consent, perhaps the oldest and most basic legal implementation of bio-ethical principles.") See also J. Katz, *The Silent World of Doctors and Patients* (Baltimore: Johns Hopkins University Press, 2002): at 3 (commenting that the development of informed consent law ended as soon as it began).
4. P. H. Schuck, "Rethinking Informed Consent," *Yale Law Journal* 103 (1994): 899–959.
5. S. M. Wolf, "Toward a Systemic Theory of Informed Consent in Managed Care," *Houston Law Review* 35 (1999): 1631–1681.
6. See, e.g., F. H. Miller, "Health Care Information Technology and Informed Consent: Computers and the Doctor-Patient Relationship," *Indiana Law Review* 31 (1998): 1019–1042 (urging to enlarge the required scope of physicians' disclosure to include internet information); see also J. H. Krause, "Reconceptualizing Informed Consent in an Era of Health Care Cost Containment," *Iowa Law Review* 85 (1999): 261–386 (proposed statutory changes to compel physicians to disclose non-covered alternatives to patients).
7. M. A. Hall, "A Theory of Economic Informed Consent," *Georgia Law Review* 31 (1997): 511–536 (global disclosures by managed

consent doctrine.[8] Others have focused on its defects and failings.[9] Most recently, several commentators have realized the shortcomings of the model that relies exclusively on patient autonomy and instead have called for reforms to bolster the ideal of patient involvement and collaboration with physicians in medical choices.[10] In the final analysis, however, the ideal of shared decision making remains a rare and illusive bird.[11]

That minority patients have not figured at all in the literature about informed consent is an egregious omission which this [reading] begins to repair. Moreover, the [reading] demonstrates that by addressing identifiable harms which informed consent law now causes to racial, religious, and ethnic minority patients, the law may also better address many of the concerns legal commentators have been discussing for years with only majority patients in mind. Ironically, the solution to the discrimination felt by the excluded members of society may turn out to provide the remedy for the informed consent doctrine as a whole.

The key is found in the medical, ethics, and social science literature that has attentively considered the impact of informed consent on minority patients. A host of medical and social science disciplines boast a large literature containing strong empirical evidence that the current doctrinal structure of informed consent law actually harms minority patients. The evidence shows that in practice, our current law violates minorities' legally protected dignity interests, reduces the quality of the health care minority patients receive, and widens the disparity between the health treatment and outcomes experienced by minority and majority patients in this country. This literature is a sub-set of the social science data that reveals problems with the operation of informed consent generally.

Clarence Braddock, for example, has shown that consent discussions between doctors and their patients yield incomplete information, and that patients often did not understand their role in medical decision making.[12] Moreover, researchers have seen that even after discussion and full disclosure, the majority of patients—even well-educated ones—routinely misunderstand the goals, benefits, and risks of their proposed treatment.[13] It is not altogether clear that patients on the whole yearn for the participatory

care organizations would inform patients of cost containment measures and reduce physician obligation to disclose expensive alternatives at treatment).

8. E.g., M. A. Bobinski, "Autonomy and Privacy: Protecting Patients from Their Physicians," *University of Pittsburg Law Review* 55 (1994): 291–387.
9. E.g., G. P. Smith, II, "The Vagaries of Informed Consent," *Indiana Health Law Review* 1, no. 1 (2004): 109–129.
10. See, e.g. J. S. King and B. W. Moulton, "Rethinking Informed Consent: The Case for Shared Medical Decision making," *American Journal of Law & Medicine,* 32, no. 4 (2006): 429–502; see also, Katz, *supra* note 3, at 102; J. Wennberg and P. Peters, "Unwarranted Variations in the Quality of Health Care: Can the Law Help Medicine Provide a Remedy?" *Wake Forest Law Review* 37 (2002): 925–931.
11. A. Meisel, "From Tragedy to Catastrophe: Lawyers and the Bureaucratization of Informed Consent," *Yale Journal of Health, Policy, Law & Ethics* 6 (2006): 479–483, at 480.
12. See C. H. Braddock et al, "Informed Decision Making in Outpatient Practice: Time to Get Back to Basics," *JAMA* 282, no. 24 (1999): 2313–2320, at 2313.
13. See, e.g., G. S. Fischer et al., "Patient Knowledge and Physician Predictions of Treatment Preferences after Discussion of Advance Directives," *Journal of General Internal Medicine* 13, no. 7 (1998): 447–454, at 447; see also D. A. Herz et al., "Informed Consent: Is It A Myth?" *Neurosurgery* 30, no. 2 (1992): 453–458, at 453.

model of medical decision making that informed consent doctrine advances.[14] On the other hand, it is clear that the medical profession is perplexed by the vast disconnectivity between the ideal of informed consent doctrine, and what is plausible and possible to execute in "the real world."[15]

This [reading] brings together the research data that describes the experience minority patients have had with informed consent. That literature confirms the deficiencies common to most patients, and goes further to chronicle special harms the doctrine currently visits upon underrepresented patient groups. Together, this evidence provides the basis for the three conclusions reached in this [reading]. First, the core problem with informed consent is that the doctrine fails to embody the broad spectrum of ethical values that it was originally intended to serve. The law began as a pragmatic expression of a balance of ethical values including honoring patient autonomy, encouraging physician beneficence, discouraging malfeasance, and ensuring just, even-handed treatment of all patients. Yet over time, it appears that jurists began to distrust the broader ethical foundations of consent law, and departed to pursue a fascination with one single value—autonomy—which began to overwhelm all other values originally served by the law.

Second, the doctrine's departure from service to a balanced spectrum of ethical values has resulted in law that visits injustice upon racial, ethnic, and religious minority patients. A brief sample of the social science literature confirms the unique harm currently caused by this law's singular focus on autonomy goals to the exclusion of all other values. The legal rules that implement the autonomy focus are contradictory and inconsistent. My third conclusion is that a unifying legal approach that addresses the injustice done by the current law will serve all physicians and all patients while addressing the special harms that minorities now suffer under the present rule. This [reading] seeks to reverse what one commentator has called "the suffocating hegemony of the autonomy principle"[16] in order to improve health care for minority and majority patients alike.

Part I explores the ethical norms that originally gave rise to the informed consent doctrine. This section provides an historical overview of the ethics literature, to demonstrate that ethical values of beneficence, non-malfeasance, autonomy, and even justice once provided the original foundation for the legal doctrine, but have been abandoned in favor of a doctrine narrowly focused only on the protection of individual autonomy. The next section demonstrates the harm of this shift. While all patients suffer the impact of an ethically skewed informed consent doctrine, Part II examines social science literature to illustrate the special impact this change has had on patients belonging to racial, ethnic, and religious minority groups. These patients are harmed most frequently by malfeasance and injustice that exists in American health care. They depend more directly than other patients on physician beneficence, and also experience a greater affront to their autonomy and human dignity when informed consent fails to protect them.

Physicians, anthropologists, and other social scientists have developed substantial data that

14. See, e.g., W. Strull et al., "Do Patients Want to Participate in Medical Decision Making?" *JAMA* 253, no. 21 (1984): 2990–2994, at 2990; see generally, C. E. Schneider, *The Practice of Autonomy: Patients, Doctors and Medical Decisions* (Oxford: Oxford University Press, 1998).

15. See, e.g. C. E. Schneider, "After Autonomy," *Wake Forest Law Review* 41 (2006): 411–444.

16. *Id.*, at 413.

demonstrates that racial, ethnic, and religious minorities often do not subscribe to the autonomy model. These patients wish to include family, community, and religious members in their medical decisions. In some cases, they prefer to defer to physicians or others to make medical decisions on their behalf. When minority patients rely on physician disclosures, they seek different information content in those disclosures than white patients want, and their reasons for obtaining information is different than reasons given by most other patients. Even the methods of communication preferred during disclosure by minority patients differ from methods preferred by others. Therefore, the "one size fits all" autonomy model of informed consent not only fails to protect the justice, beneficence, and non-malfeasance interests of minority patients, but also disrespects the autonomy interests of these vulnerable patient populations.

Part III of this [reading] explains why the current legal doctrine is powerless to correct the ills of a stunted informed consent policy. In this section I review an exemplary selection of informed consent cases to identify the source and nature of the miscommunication between the law and ethics communities. Analysis of a sample group of informed consent cases reveals inconsistencies in the legal doctrine, erroneous outcomes, and the impact the current doctrine has on vulnerable patient populations. Part IV argues that recognizing the core agency nature of the physician-patient relationship in the consent transaction compels the conclusion that fiduciary protections would best correct the defects in this law. A fiduciary model would unify informed consent doctrine, return balance to the range of ethical values it serves, and restore credibility to the doctrine's ability to operate in the real world occupied by providers and patients.

I. The Departure

The Western origins of the informed consent doctrine are summarized in the oft-quoted pronouncement from *Scholendorff v. Society of New York Hospitals.*[17] "Every human being of adult years and sound mind has a right to determine what shall be done with his own body; and a surgeon who performs an operation without his patient's consent commits an assault." Today we understand this statement to evince a fierce protection of patients' interest in self-determination. Consent law awards patients the right to protect their physical bodies from unpermitted medical intrusion.

Our current doctrine compels physicians to disclose information sufficient to allow patients to make voluntary, knowledgeable choices about their care. The contemporary, stated objective, in both legal and ethical literature, is to protect patient dignity and autonomy. In order to give legal protection to the ethical interests of bodily integrity, human dignity, and self-determination, our informed consent doctrine focuses physicians' attention on the quantity and quality of information required to escape liability. The law directs that some exchange of information occur, but focuses only minimal attention on the actual level of communication or understanding between the parties. This is with good reason. The law is ill-suited to police conversations for their genuineness, or thoroughness, or even their effectiveness. Therefore, our legal rules settle for penalizing providers who dole out insufficient quantities of information or fail to cover

17. *Scholendorff v. Society of New York Hospitals*, 105 N.E. 92, 93 (N.Y. 1914)

topics that are germane to patient decision making by an objective, professional standard,[18] or a patient-centered, autonomy standard.[19] Yet, in the clinical setting, between patient and physician, the doctrine of informed consent seems powerless to encourage the conversation and collaboration between equals. It is ineffective as a tool to accomplish a level of understanding that would necessarily precede any rational decision to accept or forego medical treatment. The uncertainty of future events associated with medical treatment about to be undertaken makes the notion of "sufficient and accurate disclosure" an abstraction. Moreover, the limits of time and the realities of patients' posture and relationship to providers in the clinical practice setting make truly knowledgeable choice a fiction.

While the law remains focused on ensuring patients' choice and autonomy, the consent doctrine does little to protect against physicians who affirmatively misrepresent or conceal information from patients. It is ineffective at policing physician self interest. While our laws of informed consent have elevated patients' status and authority by protecting their decisional capacity, we have done so at the expense of monitoring the physician overreaching that informed consent was originally intended to address. The next section traces the history of this transition.

1. Ethical Origins

Ethicists began to offer guidance for physicians in their interactions with patients and with one another long before the common law tradition began. The Greek ethicist, Hippocrates, advised physicians that "[a]s to diseases, make a habit of two things—to help, or at least to do no harm."[20] Later, Hippocrates penned his famous Oath, in which physicians are repeatedly encouraged to work "for the benefit of the sick" while "remaining free of all intentional injustice, of all mischief and in particular of sexual relations with both female and male persons, be they free or slaves." Even today, graduating medical professionals swear to uphold the principles of beneficence—"I will use treatment to help the sick…" non-malfeasance—"but I will never use it to injure or wrong them"—repeating the ancient Greek pronouncement of a physician's ethical duty. Thus, from antiquity, the ethical principles for physician-patient relations were laid. First, beneficence—for physicians, the moral obligation to contribute to the welfare of their patients,[21] and second malfeasance[22]—the obligation to refrain from and even prevent harm to patients—fundamentally motivated the earliest health care providers.

18. See *Canterbury v. Spence*, 464 F.2d 772 (D.C. Cir. 1972) *cert. denied*, 490 U.S. 1064 (1972) (enacted by a slight majority of states).
19. See *Nathanson v. Kline*, 350 P.2d 1093 (Kan. 1960).
20. Hippocrates, *Of the Epidemics*, Book I, Section II, Paragraph 5 (400 B.C.), a treatise on the cause, effect and treatment of epidemic diseases. This phrase is often misquoted "*First* do no harm" and incorrectly attributed to Hippocrates' Hippocratic Oath. The Oath mentions neither any obligation to refrain from harm, nor any duty for a physician to obtain permission or consent before doing a procedure.
21. See T. L. Beauchamp and J. F. Childress, eds., *Principles of Biomedical Ethics,* 5th ed. (Oxford: Oxford University Press, 2001): at 173. ("The implicit assumption of beneficence that exists in medical and health care professions and their institutional contexts: Promoting the welfare of patients—not merely avoiding harm—expresses medicine's goal, rationale, and justification.")
22. Philosopher William Frankena adds the obligations to 1) prevent evil; 2) remove evil; and 3) do good as elements of malfeasance. See W. Frankena, *Ethics* (New Jersey: Prentice Hall, 1973): at 47.

According to James F. Childress and Tom L. Beau-champ, "[T]he idea that beneficence expresses the primary obligation in health care is ancient." The principle requiring respect for patient autonomy is at least as old as those of beneficence and non-malfeasance. In fact, in 360 BCE, another Greek philosopher wrote an application of patient autonomy that spoke directly to the question of what might be a patient's role in medical decision making.

But the doctor, who is a freeman, attends and practices upon freemen—he enters into a discourse with the patient and with his friends—and he will not prescribe for him until he has first convinced him; at last, when he has brought the patient more and more under his persuasive influences and set him on the road to health, he attempts to effect a cure.[23]

Despite the similar origins of all three ethical principles—beneficence, non-malfeasance, and respect for patient autonomy—these values have operated in tension and competition with one another in Western medical ethics. The evolution of our informed consent doctrine is exemplary. The first English language text of bioethics was published in 1772 by Scottish physician John Gregory. In *Lectures on the Duties and Qualifications of a Physician*, Gregory writes to offer an ethical code that will guide a profession he wishes to redeem. According to Professor L. B. McCullough, Gregory wrote in response to a "crisis in intellectual and moral trust" which was due to the poor conduct and practices of self-interested physicians of the 18th century.[24] Gregory therefore wrote to correct the behavior of physicians toward their patients and to establish norms to guide relationships with the sick.

> I come now to mention the moral qualities peculiarly required in the character of a physician. The chief of these is humanity; that sensibility of heart which makes us feel for the distresses of our fellow-creatures, and which, of consequence, incites us in the most powerful manner to relieve them. Sympathy produces an anxious attention to a thousand little circumstances that may tend to relieve the patient; an attention which money can never purchase: hence the inexpressible comfort of having a friend for a physician. Sympathy naturally engages the affection and confidence of a patient, which, in many cases, is of the utmost consequence to his recovery. If the physician possesses gentleness of manners, and a compassionate heart, and what Shakespeare so emphatically calls "the milk of human kindness," the patient feels his approach like that of a guardian angel ministering to his relief.[25]

Gregory's objective was to return the professional to compassion, sympathy, and humility. These had been lost to the profession, as evidenced, in Gregory's day, by the pervasive practices of physicians providing better care to the wealthy, who were able to pay handsomely for medical services, while neglecting poor patients because their poverty offered no possibility for the physician's personal gain. In the end,

23. Plato, *The Laws* (Kalispell, Montana: Kessinger Publishing, 1997).
24. L. B. McCullough, "John Gregory's Medical Ethics and the Reform of Medical Practice in Eighteenth Century Edinburgh," *Journal of the Royal College of Physicians Edinburgh* 36, no. 1 (2006): 86–92.
25. L. B. McCullough, ed., *John Gregory's Writings on Medical Ethics and Philosphy of Medicine* (Dordrecht: Kluwer Academic Publishers, 1998): at 38.

McCullough concludes that while Gregory wrote to urge his colleagues to a higher standard, he did not seek reform out of any notions of respect for patient autonomy. In fact, McCullough sees Gregory's motives as quite the opposite:

> However, if I am right about the conservative nature of Gregory's accomplishment, his concept of medicine as a profession is not a modern, egalitarian idea but a pre-modern idea of a disciplined life of service to those subordinate to one's influence and power.... The physician—patient relationship is not egalitarian or contractual, but a fiduciary obligation of service and protection in which physicians know more about what is in our health-related interests, as a rule, than we their patients do. This is not an egalitarian concept; indeed, it is anti-egalitarian. From its vantage point...with its strong emphasis on individual autonomy and, in its postmodern incarnation, deep distrust of claims to intellectual and moral authority by physicians (or anyone else, for that matter), bioethics has de-professionalized medical ethics.[26]

Gregory sought to constrain physicians' exercise of power over their patients. In this original Gregorian articulation of western medical ethics, the concept of patient autonomy appears to have had no place. Instead, Gregory's *Lectures* reveal the view that physicians stood in a fiduciary relationship to their patients, and in this role, owed them duties of loyalty, compassion, sympathy, and to always act for their benefit.

It was an English physician, however, not Gregory, who wrote the ethical code that ultimately the entire profession adopted. In 1803, Thomas Pervical published *Medical Ethics,* which he subtitled "A Code of Institutes and Precepts Adapted to the Professional Conduct of Physicians and Surgeons." This book formed the basis of the American Medical Association's Code of Ethics, first published in 1847.[27] Section 4 of that original AMA Code of Ethics provides one of the earliest articulations of the doctrine of a physician's disclosure obligations in Western medical ethics. There, a physician is encouraged to disclose only "if absolutely necessary." Moreover, owing to the obligation to be the minister of "hope and comfort to the sick," the doctor's ethical obligation is to find another to make "gloomy prognostications" to the ill.

> A physician should not be forward to make gloomy prognostications because they savour of empiricism, by magnifying the importance of his services in the treatment or cure of the disease. But he should not fail, on proper occasions, to give to the friends of the patient timely notice of danger, when it really occurs; and even to the patient himself, if absolutely necessary. This office, however, is so peculiarly alarming when executed by him, that it ought to be declined whenever it can be assigned to any other person of sufficient judgment and delicacy. For, the physician should be the minister of hope and comfort to the sick; that, by such cordials to the drooping spirit, he may smooth

26. L. B. McCullough, "John Gregory's Medical Ethics and the Reform of Medical Practice in Eighteenth Century Edinburgh," *Journal of the Royal College of Physicians Edinburgh* 36, no. 1 (2006): at 92.
27. A full text PDF version of *The Code of Medical Ethics of the American Medical Association*, adopted in May 1847, is *available at* <http://www.ama-assn.org/ama/upload/mm/369/1847code.pdf> (last visited January 8, 2008).

> the bed of death, revive expiring life, and counteract the depressing influence of those maladies which often disturb the tranquility of the most resigned, in their last moments. The life of a sick person can be shortened not only by the acts, but also by the words or the manner of a physician. It is, therefore, a sacred duty to guard him carefully in this respect, and to avoid all things which have a tendency to discourage the patient and to depress his spirits.[28]

Pervical's writings do guide physician disclosures to patients, but there is not, in his advice, any hint that the purpose of disclosure is to allow patients to engage in discussion and decision making about the direction of their treatment. Pervical does not speak to the idea of equipping patients to make decisions about their care. Certainly there was not any duty expressed or implied that the physician was obligated to respect a patient's autonomy in this professional code. Instead, Pervical places the physician in almost a diestic posture relative to "his" (most certainly not "her") patients, making reference to the "*sacred* duty to avoid all things" that might harm the patient's emotional and mental health. The positive obligation of the physician was no less than to "revive life." It is no wonder that the translation of Pervical's moral code, motivated largely by a lofty beneficence, took on a distinctly paternalistic hue when they appeared in the original AMA Code of Ethics. Referring to the patient's role in medical decision making, the AMA Code's section 6 advises patients to obey their physicians' prescriptions. Moreover, as to the quality of any contribution a patient might make to influence what might be done in the course of treatment, the AMA provided as follows:

> The obedience of a patient to the prescriptions of his physician should be prompt and implicit. He should never permit his own crude opinions as to their fitness, to influence his attention to them. A failure in one particular may render an otherwise judicious treatment dangerous, and even fatal.[29]

Here, paternalism awards to the physician the exclusive right to decide what methods of cure are appropriate, while relegating the patient's views to the level of "crude opinions." Moreover, this ethical provision admits of no temporary or exceptional circumstances that specially justify overriding a patient's own will. At the same time, perhaps this formulation does make room for Joel Feinberg's distinction between weak and strong paternalism.[30] If, for example, "crude" opinions are only those which are uninformed, skewed by addiction, depression, or otherwise compromised, then the advice to ignore such impulses may not be paternalism at all. At least it is paternalism, it may be a form that is justifiable either because it appeals to the *patient* to subordinate his own opinions,[31] or because it beneficently seeks

28. A. Flint, *Medical Ethics and Etiquette* (New York: D. Appleton and Company: 1893): at 21.
29. J. Jih Chin, "Doctor-Patient Relationship: From Medical Paternalism to Enhanced Autonomy," *Singapore Medical Journal* 43, no. 3 (2002): 152–155, at 152.
30. J. Feinberg, "Legal Paternalism," *Canadian Journal of Philosophy* 1, no 1 (1971): 105–124, at 113 (cited in Beauchamp and Childress, *supra* note 21).
31. Beauchamp and Childress define "paternalism" as "the intentional overriding of one person's known preferences or actions by

to avoid the possibility of dangerous and fatal outcomes that may result from corrupting a considered course of treatment. On the other hand, if all opinions held by patients are "crude" by definition, then the groundwork for a patient autonomy "backlash" was firmly laid in 1847. Indeed, by 1957, language about "gloomy prognostications" and "crude opinions" had given way to the language of patient rights and dignity and self-determination. The 1957 preamble read, "The principal objective of the medical profession is to render service to humanity with full respect for the dignity of man."[32]

2. The Turning Point

It is important to note that in 1957, the California Court of Appeals also decided *Salgo v. Leland Stanford Jr. University Board of Trustees,* in which the term "informed consent" was first used. In *Salgo*, the consent claim was actually discussed only in dicta, as an erroneous *res ipsa* instruction had already provided the basis for the court's reversal of the plaintiff's verdict below. Nevertheless, the *Salgo* court went on to discuss the parameters of a legally sufficient disclosure. The court called upon physicians to disclose

> all facts which are necessary to form the basis of an *intelligent consent* by the patient to the proposed treatment.... At the same time, the physician must place the welfare of his patient above all else and this very fact places him in a position in which he sometimes must choose between two alternative courses of action. One is to explain to the patient every risk attendant upon any surgical procedure or operation no matter how remote; this may result in alarming a patient who is already unduly apprehensive.... The other is to recognize that each patient presents a separate problem, that the patient's mental and emotional condition is important and in certain cases may be crucial, and that in discussing the element of risk a certain amount of discretion must be employed consistent with the full disclosure of facts necessary to an *informed consent.*[33]

That case proved to be a watershed. *Salgo* turned the focus in consent cases toward the content and quality of information given to patients. The court called on physicians to provide "full disclosure of facts necessary to an informed consent." Such disclosure gave substance to the process of autonomous decision making; as a practical matter, the court required that patients had "all" the information necessary to decide whether to consent. At the same time, the *Salgo* decision emphasized the primacy of the physicians' beneficence obligation. Under *Salgo,* the physician must "place the welfare of his patient above all else." Also, *Salgo* reminded physicians to avoid causing patients "alarm" or apprehension, thus fulfilling the duty of non-

another person, where the person who overrides justifies the action by the goal of benefiting or avoiding harm to the person whose preferences or actions are overridden." See Beauchamp and Childress, *supra* note 21, at 178. Accepting this definition, admonishing a patient to sacrifice their own opinions in order to accept those of their physician, may be seen as a non-paternalistic suggestion that restricts no autonomous choice whatsoever.

32. V. Herbert, "Informed Consent—A Legal Evaluation," *Cancer* 46, no. 4 (1980): 1042–1044, at 1043.

33. *Salgo v. Leland Stanford Jr. University Board of Trustees*, 54 Cal. App.2d at 576, 317 P.2d at 180 (emphasis added).

malfeasance. In this way, the *Salgo* court managed to balance three ethical values in its version of informed consent.

Yet, although the *Salgo* case itself lays a firm ethical foundation for the informed consent doctrine, neither the legal nor ethical progeny of this case followed suit. Informed consent did not grow thereafter as a reflection of three ethical principles at work together. Rather, the beneficence and non-malfeasance objectives quickly fell away; informed consent became a doctrine justified principally by the obligation to respect patient autonomy.[34] For example, while the 1980 version of the AMA's Code of Ethics added a provision, calling physicians to respect patient "rights,"[35] by 2001 the ethical obligation for physicians to place patient welfare above all and avoid causing patient harm had disappeared entirely from the Medical Code of Ethics. In place of these now out-dated ethical values, the current 2006 version of the AMA Code shrinks the physician's obligation to beneficence and non-malfeasance to merely demonstrating competence and compassion but enlarges the physician's obligation to serve patient autonomy.

The code now declares, "A physician shall be dedicated to providing competent medical care, with com passion and respect for human dignity and rights."[36] As Appelbaum, Lidz, and Meisel write, modern day "[i]nformed consent is justified almost exclusively under the principle of autonomy."[37] Similarly, according to Peter Schuck, "The most fundamental normative argument in favor of requiring health care providers to obtain patients' informed consent to medical treatments proceeds from the principle of autonomy—the notion that each mature individual has a right to make the basic choices that affect her life prospects."[38] Mark Hall and Carl Schneider characterized the transition by saying that ethicists have "crept toward what could be called 'mandatory autonomy'—the view that patients *should* make their own decisions whether they want to or not."[39]

The medical profession alone is not responsible for this shift of values. Ruth Faden and Tom Beauchamp trace the transition to the "politics of regulation" that arose and "consumed" the profession during the early 20th century, in a way that caused medicine to lose its moral direction.[40] Others decry

34. See Beauchamp and Childress for discussion of Allan McCoid's attempt to survey all consent cases to distinguish negligence and battery claims. Beauchamp and Childress, *supra* note 21, at 127.
35. The 1980 Code provides, "A physician shall respect the rights of patients, of colleagues, and of other health professionals, and shall safeguard patient confidences within the constraints of the law." American Medical Association, *Principles of Medical Ethics,* June 1980, *available at* <http://www.ama-assn.org/ama1/pub/upload/mm/369/1980_principles.pdf> (last visited January 8, 2008).
36. American Medical Assciation, Medical Code of Ethics, Preamble, 2006, *available at* <http://www.ama-assn.org/ama/pub/category/2512.html> (last visted January 22, 2008); see also F. W. Hafferty, "Toward the Operationalization of Professionalism: A Commentary," *The American Journal of Bioethics* 4, no. 2 (2004): 28–31 at 29.
37. P. S. Appelbaum, C. W. Lidz, and A. Meisel, *Informed Consent Legal Theory and Clinical Practice* (Oxford: Oxford University Press, 1987): at 22.
38. P. H. Schuck, "Rethinking Informed Consent," *Yale Law Journal* 103 (1994): 899–959, at 924.
39. See M. Garrison and C. E. Schneider, *The Law of Bioethics: Individual Autonomy and Social Regulation* (Eagan: Thompson West, 2005): at 143.
40. R. Faden and T. Beauchamp, *A History and Theory of Informed Consent* (Oxford: Oxford University Press, 1986): at 85 (explaining that the 1903 and 1912 revisions of the AMA Code of Ethics was "almost wholly consumed" with controlling quackery and competition. Having met with limited success, the profession turned to legal regulation.")

consumerism as evinced by direct to consumer marketing.[41] Jay Katz pointedly asserts that the change in traditional norms governing physician-patient communication came not from medicine but from law.[42] David Rothman points more directly towards "social forces" in America particularly, that gave rise to the language of rights, and the pervasive influence of lawyers on the medical profession. Rothman identifies the cause and effect as follows:

> [The Civil Rights movements were] characterized in the first instance by a profound suspicion and distrust of constituted authority.... The movements shared an unwillingness to accede to the discretionary authority of whites, men, husbands, parents, clinical investigators, mental hospital superintendents, elected officials, and of course, doctors, especially when they were males practicing obstetrics, gynecology, or psychiatry. Also movements subscribed to a fierce anti-paternalism, a dogged rejecting of the principles of beneficence, a persistent determination to let constituents speak for themselves and define their own interests. Autonomy and consent became the bywords.[43]

Beauchamp and Faden add further that the spectacular developments in medical technology, as well as publicity about Nazi experiments, Tuskegee, and other medical atrocities, led to a deep distrust of the medical profession, and also gave rise to a legally driven approach to medical ethics. In short, I think it is time to recognize and acknowledge the role the law has played in skewing the development of the informed consent doctrine. Who could deny the powerful tug of the legal pronouncements of autonomy, individual choice, and self-determination that have issued forth from courts of law during the latter half of the 20th century? The abortion decisions, for example, have commanded national attention as the Supreme Court in *Roe v. Wade* declared that the right to individual, personal, and private choice is a "fundamental" and constitutionally protected one.[44] These claims are, in the words of Justices O'Conner, Kennedy, and Souter, "urgent claims of the woman to retain the ultimate control over her destiny and her body, claims implicit in the meaning of liberty...."[45] In another powerful line of cases, the "right to die" decisions also confirmed the centrality of the individual's autonomy rights under the law.

In 1976, the plight of Karen Ann Quinlan brought national and international attention to the right to refuse life-sustaining treatment. Thereafter, the Supreme Court's decision in *Cruzan v. Director, Missouri Dep't of Health*,[46] which sought to balance state interests in preserving life with a common law "right of every

41. See A. Holmer, "Direct-To-Consumer Marketing of Prescription Drugs: Creating Consumer Demand," *JAMA* 281, no. 4 (1999): 382–384.
42. See Katz, *supra* note 3.
43. *Id.*
44. *Roe v Wade*, 410 U.S. 113 (1973).
45. See *Planned Parenthood of Southeastern Pennsylvania v. Casey*, 505 U.S. 833 (1992).
46. (In this case involving a patient in persistent vegetative state following injury from automobile accident, Supreme Court denied parents' petition to withdraw artificial feeding tube and hydration absent clear and convincing evidence of incompetent patient's intent regarding medical treatment.)

individual to the possession and control of his own person, free from all restraint or interference of others, unless by clear and unquestionable authority of law." These words gave vivid centrality to Justice Cardozo's 1914 declaration that "[e]very human being of adult years and sound mind has the right to determine what will be done with his own body...."[47] Surely the pervasive influence of law on the balance of ethical values reflected in medical ethics literature and practice cannot be denied.

II. The Impact

Social scientists have studied and described the impact of informed consent law on a wide range of patient and provider populations. There is a substantial body of empirical evidence that reflects the knowledge gained as physicians,[48] ethicists,[49] and other social scientists have wrestled to determine how the Western, Anglo notions of individual autonomy, self-determination, and rights play out with minority groups

The Western autonomy model of informed consent rests upon the principle that the individual patient is best suited to make medical decisions on his or her own behalf. Thus, the model requires medical providers to give patients the information they need to decide whether or not to accept proposed medical treatment. The legal obligation is designed to compel disclosure of information by physicians to patients so that patients can intelligently and voluntarily direct their medical care. Though the ideal is "shared" medical decision making, legal liability rests on proving that the *patient* would have decided upon an alternative treatment if adequate disclosure about the treatment performed had been provided. Therefore, the law of informed consent directly reflects the notion of patient control and self-determination. The law operates to protect these values, to the effective exclusion of all other values.[50] Where minority patients are concerned, there are at least four problems with this exclusivity.

First, informed consent law errs by assuming that all patients need, want, and should have autonomous control over their medical decision making. This assumption is purely a cultural one, and the fact that it is particularly inapplicable to minority patients means that ironically, rather than respecting these patients' autonomous decision making rights, the informed consent doctrine violates them.

Second, informed consent law governs the conversation between physicians and patients without regard to whether or not these are, in fact, the appropriate parties to discuss and decide courses of

47. *Scholendorff v. Society of New York Hospitals*, 105 N.E. 92, 93 (N.Y. 1914).

48. Robert J. Levine, for example, has observed that the autonomy centered approach to consent reflects an American and thus minority viewpoint. See R. J. Levine, "Informed Consent: Some Challenges to the Universal Validity of the Western Model," *Law, Medicine, and Healthcare* 19 (1991): 207–213, at 207; see also T. P. Duffy, "Agamemnon's Fate and the Medical Profession," *Western New England Law Review* 9 (1987): 21–31.

49. J. Katz, "Informed Consent—Must It Remain a Fairy Tale?" *Journal of Contemporary Health Law & Policy* 10 (1993): 69–89 (Katz advances the ideal of informed consent that actively involves shared discussion and decision making between physician and patient).

50. Others have noted that the narrow focus of the doctrine eliminates consideration of values such as family integrity and physician competence. See, L. J. Blackhall, S. Murphy, G. Frank, V. Michel, and S. Azen, "Ethnicity and Attitudes Toward Patient Autonomy," *JAMA* 274, no. 10 (1995): 820–825.

medical treatment. Again, the social science literature is revealing. Many minority patients want to involve different decision makers than most majority patients wish to include, and more than medical providers typically allow. Third, the law of informed consent prescribes a list of disclosure deemed material to the "reasonable patient" making informed medical choices but ignores the fact that not all patients want the same information content in disclosures, and not all information is sought for the purpose of medical decision making. In the case of majority patients, the social science literature confirms that most minority patients want different types of information than majority patients want and that the majority providers offer.

Finally, although the law of informed consent understandably says little about the method of communicating legally required disclosures, studies show that many minority patients favor different forms and methods of communicating medical information used to make treatment decisions. Each of these issues is addressed in the sections that follow.

1. Ethnicity and Autonomy

The most glaring oversight of the informed consent model is that it assumes that all Americans share the passionate dedication to protecting autonomous patient control over medical decision making that underlies our law.[51] This assumption is empirically false. Different racial and ethnic groups hold different views about the importance of autonomous medical decision making. In a seminal study of 800 patients, Dr. Leslie Blackhall examined and compared the attitudes of European-, African-, Mexican-, and Korean-Americans towards patient autonomy in medical decision making.[52] Her findings were remarkable.

Logistic regression analysis[53] showed that "Korean-American and Mexican-American subjects were less likely than European-Americans and African-American subjects to believe that the patient should be told the truth about the diagnosis and prognosis of a serious illness and were less likely to believe that the patient should make decisions about the use of life-support."[54] Furthermore, when Blackhall examined other demographic factors such as age, gender, and socio-economic status, she found that "[f]or all three measures of attitudes toward patient autonomy, the primary factor related to attitude was ethnicity."[55]

Blackhall next explored the preferences each ethnic group expressed towards the question of who should be involved in a patient's medical decision making. Ethnicity again proved a dispositive variable. "The decision making style exhibited by most of the Mexican-American and Korean-American subjects in our study might best be described as family-centered. Although the patient autonomy model does

51. See e.g., *Canterbury v. Spence*, 464 F.2d 784 (D.C. Circ. 1972) (where it is insisted that informed consent is required to secure "the patient's right of self determination" or the Patient Self-Determination Act passed of 1990 codified as Omnibus Budget Reconciliation Act of 1990, Pub. L. No. 101–508, §§4206, 4751).

52. See Blackhall et al., *supra* note 50, at 823.

53. Logistic regression analysis is an analytical approach used by economists to determine the relationship between several independent variables when the dependent variable or outcome is dichotomous or can limited to two, mutually exclusive choices.

54. *Id.*

55. *Id.*, at 823.

not exclude family involvement, in the strictest version of the family-centered model preferred by some ethnic groups, it is the *sole* responsibility of the family to hear bad news about the patient's diagnosis and prognosis and to make the difficult decisions about life support."[56] After reviewing several other studies where Italian-, Chinese-, and Ethiopian-American patients exhibited similar decision making preferences, Blackhall concluded,

> Autonomy is not viewed as empowering. Rather, it is seen as isolating and burdensome to patients who are too sick and too ignorant about their condition to be able to make meaningful choices.... Thus, belief in the ideal of patient autonomy is far from universal.... Allowing patients to choose from the range of treatment options available ensures that the treatment will conform to their preferences. However, the high value placed on open expression of emotion and on the rights of individuals to control their destiny are not necessarily shared by all segments of American society.[57]

Blackhall readily admits that many unanswered questions remain despite the conclusiveness of her findings. For example, there is considerable variation in views within ethnic groups; they are not homogenous and stereotyping would be inappropriate.[58] Also, the preference she called the "family-centered model" is ill defined and varies from group to group and from family to family. Nevertheless, Blackhall's findings are not only significant in their own right, but they have been further explained in a follow-up study Dr. Blackhall conducted in 2001 to explain the reasons behind the differing perspectives minority patients hold.

In the second study, Dr. Blackhall interviewed 10 percent of the patients who participated in the first phase of her study to identify qualitative reasons for the different views they concerning patient autonomy. Specifically, Blackhall's interviews focused on the participants' views of whether physicians should or should not disclose the truth about terminal diagnoses and poor prognoses to their patients. As in the first study, European- and African-American patients expressed views that differed from those expressed by Korean- and Mexican-American patients. While European- and African-Americans largely favored disclosure,[59] Koreans and Mexicans believed that doctors should not give patients a terminal diagnosis because such a disclosure cruelly eliminates hope for the patient. Rather, Korean-American and

56. *Id.*, at 824.
57. *Id.*, at 285.
58. See Blackhall et al., *supra* note 50, at 825.
59. Interestingly, Blackhall found that although European and African Americans more often believed that patients should know the truth about a terminal diagnosis, they had different reasons for their beliefs. European American participants in the study explained that disclosure was important to allow dying patients' time to get their affairs in order. African American participants often expressed the view that disclosure was important to allow dying patients in time to communicate with God, either to seek forgiveness or to pray for healing and recovery. See, L. J. Blackhall et al., "Bioethics in a Different Tongue: The Case of Truth-Telling" *Journal of Urban Health* 78, no. 1 (2001): 59–71. (This is part two of the study reported in "Ethnicity and Attitudes toward Patient Autonomy").

Mexican-American participants preferred that family members receive news of a terminal diagnosis so that the patient could then rely on family members, not on him- or herself, to make medical decisions.[60]

The Blackhall studies clearly support the conclusion that individual autonomy is not the highest valued ethical principle among non-European ethnic groups making medical decisions. Instead, other cultural and ethical values prevail. For example, Korean-Americans emphasize the principle of filial piety—called "*hyodo*"—rather than autonomy to direct their approach toward medical decision making. Thus, the disclosure of bad medical news should reach a patient through indirect communication with family members, or through experience and intuition—called "*numchi*"—rather than through frank conversations between physician and patient.[61]

In an article examining the views of Chinese-Canadian patients, Kerry Bowman and Edwin Hui considered the Chinese view of autonomy in medical decision making.[62] Bowman and Hui do not advance a separate branch of expressly Chinese bioethics, but they do find a marked distinction between the core ethical values that motivate Chinese patients when compared to their European counterparts.

> The concept of autonomy best highlights the contrast between Western and Chinese cultures. In the West, the principle of autonomy implies that every person has the right to self-determination. In the context of health care this means that the patient is the best person to make health care decisions. Within Chinese culture, however, the person is viewed as a "relational self"—a self for whom social relationships, rather than rationality and individualism, provide the basis for moral judgment. From this perspective, an insistence on self-determination erodes the value placed non personal interconnectedness and the social and moral meaning of such relationships.[63]

60. See generally, *id.*

61. While we might say that a Korean-American's choice to rely on family members is itself an expression of autonomous self-determination, the Blackhall studies reveal that we would have to impose the importance of autonomy on Koreans in order to reach this explanation since this culture places little value on the Western notion of individual self determination.

62. K. W. Bowman and E. C. Hui, "Bioethics for Clinicians: 20. Chinese Bioethics" *Canadian Medical Association Journal* 163, no. 11 (2000): 1481–1485.

63. *Id.,* at 1481–1482. See also C. Y. Tse et al., "Breaking Bad News: A Chinese Perspective," *Palliative Medicine* 17, no. 4 (2003): 339–343. (Reporting similar findings among Chinese patients from Hong Kong to conclude, "The concept of self is a relational one in Chinese culture and family relationship emphasizes harmonious interdependence." But warning that "although autonomy is not a traditional Chinese concept, veracity is.") See also, X. Huang, P. Butow, B. Meiser, and D. Goldstein, "Attitudes and Information Needs of Chinese Migrant Cancer Patients and Their Relatives," *Australian and New Zealand Journal of Medicine* 29 (1999): 207–213 (confirming same findings among 36 Chinese-Australian cancer patients). However, see also S. Tzuh Tang and S.-Y. Lee, "Cancer Diagnosis and Prognosis in Taiwan: Patient Preferences Versus Experiences," *Psycho-Oncology* 13, no. 1 (2003): 1–13, at 8. (Despite authors' assertion that Asian cultures hold different views towards individuality and personal rights than Westerners, the study of 364 Taiwanese cancer patients data did not fully support this conclusion. There, Taiwanese patients "strongly proclaimed their superior rights to be informed about their disease over the family. In general, cancer patients had a higher preference for health-care professionals to inform them than to inform their family members. They also preferred to receive information before their family members did....The argument that cancer patients from an Asian culture [i.e. Chinese/Taiwanese culture] have different preferences regarding being informed of their diagnosis and prognosis and that family members have legitimate superior power in decision making could not be supported by data from this group of cancer patients.")

The Western view of patient autonomy also stands in sharp contrast to the beliefs of traditional Navajo patients. In a study interviewing 34 Navajo informants, Dr. Joseph Carrese reported a contrast between principles of autonomy and Navajo culture. Dr. Carrese described patient self-determination as "centrally important" to the informed consent requirement that physicians disclose bad news and the possibility of serious future illness. In contrast, Carrese found that the Navajo ideals of '*Hozhó*' defined the "traditional Navajo way of thinking, speaking, behaving and relating to other people and the surrounding world."[64]

The *hozhó* principle describes a concept of beauty, blessing, goodness, and order that informs the core Navajo belief that it is important to both think and speak only in a positive way because words have the power to shape reality. "This theme of thinking and speaking in a positive way often emerged when informants reflected on how doctors should communicate with patients; it reflects the Navajo view that health is maintained and restored through positive ritual language."[65] The Navajo culture regards discussion of negative information with a patient as potentially harmful. Thus, Carrese concluded that the Western physician's obligation to comply with principles of patient autonomy and self determination are "ethically troublesome."[66]

> This study further demonstrates that the concepts and principles of Western bioethics are not universally held (*citations omitted*). In our pluralistic society there are communities of patients who do not identify dominate values as their own, a fact that health care providers and institutions need to appreciate.[67]

Dr. Robert Hahn describes cultural versions of informed consent among Italian-, Puerto Rican-, and Vietnamese-Americans and Navajos to compare to the American values for this doctrine.[68] Hahn's findings are insightful. For example,

> The individualism central to the doctrine of informed consent is absent in the traditions of Vietnamese thought. Self is not cultivated, but subjugated to cosmic orders. Information, direct communication, and decision may be regarded as arrogant. Although informed consent may thus be neither understood nor valued, Vietnamese interests and concerns should still be pursued in medical encounters.

64. J. A. Carrese and L. A. Rhodes, "Western Bioethics on the Navajo Reservation—Benefit or Harm?" *JAMA* 274, no. 10 (1995): 826–829.
65. *Id.*
66. *Id.*, at 828.
67. See Carrese, *supra* note 64, at 829. But see also J. S. Taylor, "Autonomy and Informed Consent on the Navajo Reservation," *Journal of Social Philosophy* 35, no. 4 (2004): 506–16. (Taylor examines the same traditional Navajo principle that admonishes physicians not to speak negatively and concludes the underlying ethical principle of autonomy is nevertheless shared by Navajo patients. However, Taylor asserts that protecting the well being of the Navajo patient is the core ethical value served by informed consent models rather than protection of patient autonomy and therefore applying a lower standard of informed consent to Navajo patients than to others does not violate principles of autonomous decision making shared by Navajos and non-Navajos alike).
68. R. A. Hahn, "Culture and Informed Consent: An Anthropological Perspective," Appendix F in *Making Health Care Decisions: The President's Commission for Ethical Problems in Medicine and Biomedical and Behavioral Research* 3, no. 3 (1982): 37–57.

Even in cultures that do adopt autonomy as an important ethical value, the degree of emphasis now placed on this above all other values in the informed consent context conflicts with the place given to other ethical values of equal importance by many minority patients. Dr. Alexia Torke studied African-American patients' perspectives on medical decision making and reported that the dominant place given individual autonomy by our consent law is inconsistent with the African-American patients she interviewed.[69]

Dr. Torke's study identified and asked questions about five issues patients consider in medical decision making. The issues were 1) what information patients consider in decision making; 2) what amount of information do patients desire in decision making; 3) to what extent do patients desire to participate in decision making; 4) what importance do patients place on trusting their provider; and 5) what are patients' perspectives on the degree of control they wish to exercise over their own bodies.[70] Patient responses to questions concerning control over one's body shed considerable light on African-American views of patient autonomy.

First, Dr. Torke found that most patients (80–90 percent) want their physicians to participate in making medical decisions in clinical settings. The range reflects that some patients want physician-led decision making[71] while others preferred the collaborative model.[72] However, the overwhelming majority did not express preference for a patient-only or even a patient-directed model. Second, the reason patients in this study gave for wanting information from their providers was not related to an overwhelming desire to control what was done with their own bodies. Rather, these patients sought information for reassurance, understanding, and to mitigate their fears. They did not seek information to exercise their right of self-determination.[73]

> This finding has implications for the concept of autonomy in the patient-physician relationship. Patient autonomy has been emphasized in recent years, largely as a response to paternalistic models of the patient-physician relationship that guided medical practice in a previous era (*citations omitted*).... The doctrine of informed consent has largely grown from such autonomy-based modes of the patient-physician relationship. These models exclude certain values that are important to the patient-physician relationship, such as the physician's guidance and caring.... In fact, many older African American patients in our study regard the recommendation of the physician as one of the most important factors in their decision making.[74]

69. A. M. Torke, G. M. Corbie-Smith, and W. T. Branch, "African American Patients' Perspectives on Medical Decision Making," *Archives of Internal Medicine* 164, no. 5 (2004): 525–530.
70. *Id.*, at 527.
71. Nearly half the African-American patients in this study—12 of 25 respondents—wanted their provider to make medical decisions; five respondents wanted a joint decision; three patients wanted to make the decision themselves; and five responses could not be classified. *Id.*, at 528.
72. *Id.*, at 529.
73. *Id.*, at 529.
74. See Torke et al., *supra* note 69, at 529.

This section presents samples from a large body of medical and social science literature that appears to have escaped the legal academy's attention. Studies abound that question the myopic focus on individual autonomy that characterizes informed consent law.[75] This literature comfortably concludes that autonomy is a cultural perspective and not a universal right or principle.[76] Studies presented in this section show not only that perspectives of autonomy are strongly correlated with ethnicity, but that several ethnic groups, including Mexican-Americans, Korean-Americans, Chinese-Americans, Navajo Native-Americans, and African-Americans simply do not share the Western, Anglo notion of patient self-determination and autonomy. Of course, the empirically demonstrated correlation between ethnicity and alternative perspectives on autonomy must be handled with sensitivity. Generalizations and stereotypes must not overwhelm the usefulness of these observations.

2. Religion and Autonomy

Without question, ethnicity correlates with perspectives on autonomy more directly than age, socioeconomic status, gender, or other demographic factors.[77] Yet precisely because of the strength of this correlation, Dr. Erika Blacksher, warns of the "risk of serious misuse...that will reinforce a reliance on stereotypes and introduce into clinical practice a very dangerous set of rules."[78] Jurists and medical practitioners alike must be aware that ethnic groups are not homogeneous and therefore must not be treated uniformly when applying the insights contained in the research reviewed here.

Often, the diversity of viewpoints within ethnic or racial groups arises from a variety of religious viewpoints that may be present within the group. For example, different religious sub-groups within the Chinese community will have differing views on the levels of patient and family involvement they wish to have in medical decision making.[79] A Confucian believer may adopt a social hierarchical perspective that holds the family, and not the patient, responsible for medical decisions, even if the patient is competent and capable. On the other hand, this hierarchical view may not be shared by a religious Taoist or Buddhist. Chinese patients do not uniformly hold a single view toward patient autonomy.

Similarly, Dr. Abdallah Daar has found that subtle differences in perspective towards autonomy may

75. See e.g., A. Sehgal, A. Galbraith, M. Chesney, P. Schoenfeld, B. Charles, and B. Lo, "How Strictly Do Dialysis Patients Want Their Advance Directives Followed?" *JAMA* 267, no. 1 (1992): 59–63; J. L. Nelson, "Taking Families Seriously," *Hastings Center Report* 22, no. 4 (1992): 6–12.

76. See I. Hanssen, "From Human Ability to Ethical Principle: An Intercultural Perspective on Autonomy," *Medicine, Health Care and Philosophy* 7, no. 3 (2005): 269–279, observing, It is important to distinguish between respect for a patient's *right* to be autonomous and autonomy as a *cultural phenomenon.* To respect a patient's right to be autonomous is correlated to respecting a patient's right to choose. "As will be discussed later, this *right* to choose does no equal a mandatory *duty* to choose, although it seems to do just that in the minds of many nurses. It seems that the law of consent, like the minds of nurses Hanssen describes above has transformed the merely Western cultural notion of autonomy, into a mandatory, legal obligation.

77. See generally, Blackhall et al., *supra* note 50, at 59–71.

78. See E. Blacksher, "Desperately Seeking Difference," *Cambridge Quarterly of Healthcare Ethics* 7, no. 1 (1998): 11–16, at 11.

79. Bowman and Hui, supra note 53, at 1483–4.

exist among Islamic patients.[80] Thus, consent preferences may differ among those who belong to the Sunni branch of Islam, where public interest and local custom are emphasized, and those belonging to the Shia branch of Islam, where authority and methodology concepts may prevail. A wide diversity of viewpoints may emanate in some religious traditions, from differences in adherents' age, geographic location, divergent levels of conformity with traditional versus contemporary doctrine, and even political differences.[81] Dr. Hazel Markwell noted such a range of bioethical views towards organ donation among Catholic patients.[82] Markwell clearly sets out traditional Catholic doctrine and teaching that may affect patients' views towards autonomy:

> Within Catholicism, the individual has a duty to promote his or her own health, and thus may be seen as having a moral obligation to seek treatment even if he or she does not meet legal criteria for...treatment. Failure to use ordinary measures to preserve life is regarded as morally equivalent to suicide within the Catholic tradition.[83]

Patients who hold these traditional Catholic beliefs may see themselves as having little autonomous choice to withhold consent for medical treatment. On the other hand, Catholic patients with more contemporary views may exercise their autonomous decision making powers more freely. Further, some Catholic patients may discard notions of autonomy completely, in favor of other ethical values.

> Although the principles of beneficence, non-malfeasance, autonomy and justice are compatible with Catholic beliefs, some patients will be guided by the theological requirements of faith, hope, love and fidelity and by more specific religious requirements that are not completely captured in the principles of secular bioethics.[84]

Judaism has extensively developed a long history of bioethical reasoning within the faith. Yet Jewish bioethics admits a range of viewpoints and interpretation of doctrines and teachings. Dr. Gary Goldsand notes that the degree of orthodoxy or observance can influence a Jewish patient's clinical preferences and their views on autonomy.[85]

80. A. S. Daar, et al., "Bioethics for Clinicians: 21. Islamic Bioethics," *Canadian Medical Association Journal* 164, no. 1 (2001): 60–61 (although Dr. Daar ultimately concludes Sunni and Shia bioethics differ little).
81. See e.g., J. Davidson, "Generations Have Different Views of the Church," *National Catholic Reporter* (October 29, 1999) (online journal reporting results of survey of Catholic believers) *available at* <http://www.natcath.com/NCR_Online/archives/102999/102999o.htm#TOP> (last visited January 8, 2008); see also, C. Harper, "Catholic Pluralism Is Subject of One Creighton Study," *Center for the Study of Religion and Society Newsletter* 7 (1994) *available at* <http://puffin.creighton.edu/human/CSRS/news/S96-1.html> (last visited January 8, 2008); see also, W. D'Antonio, "Autonomy and Democracy in an Autocratic Organization: The Case of the Roman Catholic Church," *Sociology of Religion* 55, no. 44 (1994): 379–396.
82. H. J. Markwell and B. F. Brown, "Bioethics for Clinicians: 27. Catholic Bioethics," *Canadian Medical Association Journal* 165, no. 2 (2001): 189–191.
83. *Id.,* at 191.
84. *Id.,* at 190.
85. G. Goldsand et al., "Bioethics for Clinicians: 22. Jewish Bioethics," *Canadian Medical Association Journal* 164, no. 2 (2001): 219–221, at 221.

> In general, the process of consent used in Western countries is also applicable to Jewish patients. Orthodox Judaism requires that a patient follow medical directions, but it is also expected that the best information be disclosed before the patient agrees to a procedure or treatment. Judaism promotes a strong commitment to the sanctity of life; as a result, there may be some difficulties when discussions take place about the withdrawal or withholding of treatments.... Jewish people have a long tradition of asking a rabbi for advice when faced with difficult decisions. Families may present physicians with the result of rabbinical deliberations which must be taken into account when decisions are made.[86]

However, while an orthodox Jewish believer may look to include their religious leader and family in medical decision making, Jewish patients from liberal Reform, Conservative, and even secular Jews are likely to hold widely divergent views on their autonomy and the role of others in medical decision making.[87]

As we examine the ways in which an overly simplistic doctrine of informed consent ignores ethnic, racial, and religious diversity, it is vital to avoid the equal danger of stereotyping ethnic and racial groups.

> There are inherent limitations to considering culture as a predictive variable, simply plugging race or ethnicity into your multiple regression analysis; or in the clinical context, using someone's name, appearance, or national origin as a predictive factor.... In our data, culture is not evident as a set of rigid "beliefs" that can be biopsied or extracted from individuals, but is only meaningful when analyzed and interpreted in particular local sites and within a particular political and historical context.[88]

The key lesson to be gleaned for the data sampled above, however, remains salient: it is that by acknowledging generally held views within minority groups, researchers reveal ways in which law based on an Anglicized, Western tradition may ignore or even mistreat patients from non-western backgrounds. Yet, despite intra-group diversity, it is clear that religious, ethnic, and racial minorities hold dramatically different views of patient autonomy from their white, Western counterparts. It is clear, moreover, that these patients' preferences are largely overlooked by American medical providers. These empirical facts have profound implications for clinical practice generally, and specifically for the application of informed consent law.

A. Clinical Implications

Informed consent law defines a physician's duty to disclose a requisite list of material information in order to allow reasonable patients to determine what shall be done with their own bodies. This law presupposes

86. *Id.*, at 221
87. *Id.*, at 220.
88. H. E. Hern, Jr., et al., "The Difference That Culture Can Make in End-of-Life Decision Making," *Cambridge Quarterly of Healthcare Ethics* 7, no. 1 (1998): 27–40.

a single model: the physician[89] discloses to the competent patient; the information disclosed comports with a legally prescribed list; and the patient assumes the ultimate decision making role to determine the course of treatment. Again the social science and medical literature empirically reveal that these legal assumptions are at odds with both the reality of medical practice and the preferences of some patients. Moreover, once again the social science literature pertaining to the racial and ethnic minority patient population most dramatically illustrates the shortcomings of the current informed consent legal model.

3. Ethnicity and Decision-Making Preferences

The standard articulation of consent law presumes that patients, and patients only, should receive disclosures of medical information. Yet studies have shown that patients vary widely in the level of participation they wish to have in receiving and applying medical information to make treatment decisions. Several studies have shown that while most patients want to receive information about their treatment from their doctors, the majority of patients prefer to delegate ultimate medical decision making to their physicians.[90]

In the largest of these studies, Dr. Wendy Levinson surveyed of over 2,700 patients from Caucasian, His-panic, and African-American backgrounds. Levinson's study showed that although the collaborative model of medical decision making produced better health outcomes for patients, fully half of the patients surveyed (52 percent) preferred to leave final medical decisions to their physicians. Hispanic and African-American respondents were more likely than white patients to rely on their physicians, both for gathering medical knowledge, and for treatment decisions.[91] This ethnic disparity remained even after controlling for socio-economic and health insurance status. Levinson's study could not explain the source of the observed disparity, but suggested some interesting possible explanations, including that physicians may communicate with or engage minority patients differently in decision making.[92] Alternatively, minority patients may have different models for managing their health. In fact, there is considerable evidence that ethnic minority patients not only prefer heightened physician participation in medical decision making, but they also are more likely than white patients to include family and community in their decision making.[93]

89. Beyond the scope of this paper, but also of interest to any considered evaluation of our informed consent law must be the question of whether it is physicians or other actors in the clinical setting that should be charged with disclosure of medical information. Understandably, the law identifies a single medical actor who has control over the relationship and can be held accountable for the behavior of others to charge with the informed consent duty to disclose. However, in another setting it would be fruitful to consider whether the model for a more extended informed consent conversation should admit for discussion (which already occurs) between patients and health professionals besides and in addition medical doctors.
90. See W. Levinson et al., "Not All Patients Want to Participate in Decision Making: A National Study of Public Preferences," *Journal of General Internal Medicine* 20, no. 6 (2005): 531–535, at 533 (citing studies by Deber, Charles, and others, finding the majority of patients prefer to rely on physicians to make treatment decisions.)
91. *Id.*, at 533–534.
92. See e.g., Hern, *supra* note 88, at 33–34 (medical staff hold Western perspective that non-disclosure harms patients rights, deprives patient of opportunity to set affairs in order and compromises patients' self-care.)
93. Hispanic, Native American, Italian, Greek, Russian, and many Asian societies may prefer a decision-making model that reflects

In many cultures, patients may choose to include or even delegate medical decision making to family members.[94] In one study of 36 Chinese cancer patients, researchers found that half of the participants believed their family members should advise physicians concerning how much information patients should receive. Most patients studied preferred to have one or two close family members with them to receive medical information.[95] This researcher explained Chinese patients' familial preferences by distinguishing three patient decision models. The first group included patients who wanted the family to participate in medical decision making. The second group included patients who asked the family to decide on their behalf. The third category belonged to Chinese patients who preferred the Western autonomy model, and chose to discuss and decide their medical treatment with no interference from either physician or family.[96]

Dr. Leslie Blackhall's follow-up study of 800 patients also addressed family roles in medical decision making. Blackall's second study confirmed that Korean-American decision making is influenced by the obligation called "*hyodo,*" or filial piety owed by grown children who take care of their parents. *Hyodo* informs the question of who receives patient information and who controls medical decision making.[97] In another study, Dr. Goldstein reported the same "primacy of the family and the family's role in editing information provided to the patient" among Greek immigrant patients.[98] Another researcher explained the role of family and community in decision making as follows:

> In many non-Western countries, the family stays in the hospital with the patient, bringing food and providing actual bedside care. Although this may be partly because of the hospital system of care, it also is an avenue for the family to show love and protection. This notion of family as guardians of the patient extends to other groups in America as well.... African Americans [are] more likely to perceive the family as protectors against physicians than Hispanic Americans or whites. Chinese society inculcates great respect and reverence for elders.... Even in Japan, which is the most "westernized" Asian country, only 13% of physicians report informing their patients of their diagnosis.[99]

However, the racial and ethnic distinctions do not stop here. Not only do ethnic and racial minority patients

the "collectivist" traditions dominant in their culture. See J. Oliffe, "'Truth Telling' and Cultural Assumptions in an Era of Informed Consent," *Family and Community Health* 30, no. 1 (2007): 5–15.

94. See J. Car and M. R. Partridge, "Cross-cultural Communication in Those with Airway Diseases," *Chronic Respiratory Disease* 1, no. 3 (2004): 153–160 (encouraging physicians to improve cultural competency to reduce health care disparities and inequality).
95. X. Huang et al., "Attitudes and Information Needs of Chinese Migrant Cancer Patients and their Relatives," *Australian and New Zealand Journal of Medicine* 29 (1999): 207–213, at 211.
96. C. Y. Tse, "Breaking Bad News: A Chinese Perspective," *Palliative Medicine* 17, no. 4 (2003): 339–343, at 340.
97. L. J. Blackhall et al., "Bioethics in a Different Tongue: The Case of Truth-Telling," *Journal of Urban Health: Bulletin of the New York Academy of Medicine* 78, no. 1 (2001): 59–71.
98. D. Goldstein, "Communicating in a Multicultural Society II: Greek Community Attitudes Towards Cancer in Australia," *Internal Medicine Journal* 32, no. 7 (2002): 289–296, at 295.
99. A. Lapine et al., "When Cultures Clash: Physician, Patient, and Family Wishes in Truth Disclosure for Dying Patients," *Journal of Palliative Medicine* 4, no. 4 (2001): 475–480, at 477.

differ from white patients in determining *to whom* medical information should be communicated, but also in deciding *what information* should be shared.

While the second element of informed consent law presupposes a standardized disclosure—proposed treatment, its risks, benefits, and alternatives—will serve all patients equally well, the empirical literature reveals varying preference for information content, especially among minority patients. Medical researchers have assembled a large body of literature that confirms this. The strongest evidence of these disparities concerns what social scientists have learned about patient preferences for disclosing truthful diagnosis and prognosis information to terminally ill patients.

The second part of Dr. Leslie Blackhall's study of ethnicity and autonomy remains the seminal empirical evidence that minority ethnic groups prefer not to disclose a terminal diagnosis while white patients, who more readily adopt the autonomy model, favor full disclosure. Again, ethnicity appears to be the most important variable to determine preferences for disclosure. When compared to African- and European-American patients, only 47 percent of Korean-Americans and 65 percent of Mexican-Americans believed that terminally ill patients should be told the truth about their diagnoses.[100] A Stanford University Medical Center interpreter wrote to confirm similar preferences held by the Mexican-American patients she met.[101] Among Greek immigrants in Australia, the reasons participants gave for non-disclosure varied widely. Some explained, "There is a stigma attached to it [cancer] in our culture" so that non-disclosure was seen as a way to avoid shame.[102] Others believed disclosure would hasten a patient's decline. Some believed disclosure caused the patient to lose hope, and a minority of patients believed that disclosure and treatment actually made the cancer itself worse.[103] Finally, depending upon the level of culturization patients had experienced, some preferred non-disclosure to allow patients to choose alternative therapies and traditional medicines.[104]

Dr. Evelyn Chan studied the differences in disclosure preferences among African-American, Hispanic, and Caucasian men being asked to consent to prostate cancer screening.[105] Dr. Chan's research also revealed that content preferences differed by ethnicity.[106] For example, African-Americans in this study were aware that blacks are generally at higher risk for prostate cancer and wanted risk information that expressly compared the mortality rates for black patients compared to whites. Hispanic participants, on the other hands, wanted more detailed information about symptoms, while whites sought more information about the advantages and disadvantages of the proposed screening test.[107] Moreover, Dr. Chan also found

100. See Blackhall, *supra* note 86, at 60.

101. L. Haffner, "Cross-Cultural Medicine A Decade Later," *Western Journal of Medicine* 157, no. 3 (1992): 255–259, at 257 (describing informed consent case where daughters opposed giving mother cancer diagnosis information).

102. See Goldstein, *supra* note 98, at 292.

103. *Id.,* at 294. (Goldstein notes similar fears held by some Italian and Arabic women).

104. *Id.*

105. E. C. Y. Chan, "Cultural Sensitivity and Informed Decision Making About Prostate Cancer Screening," *Journal of Community Health* 28, no. 6 (2004): 393–405, at 393.

106. *Id,* at 397.

107. *Id.*, at 399.

that patients from different ethnic groups understood information differently depending on the way it was communicated. When describing the size of the prostate gland, focus groups reported that white patients understood this information when the size of the prostate was likened to a walnut, while Hispanics understood when the size was likened to a small lime.[108] Insightfully, Dr. Chan related her findings to the current state of informed consent law.

> Differences in the way African Americans, Hispanics, and Caucasians want information about prostate cancer and screening presented suggest that there may be cultural differences in the reasonable person standard of informed consent, a legal standard found in most states. According to the reasonable person standard, physicians ought to disclose information that a hypothetical reasonable person needs to know to make an informed decision. Information ought to be disclosed more from a patient's point of view than a physician's out of a respect for patient autonomy. But our study results suggest that what is reasonable for an African American person to know may differ from what is reasonable for a Hispanic or Caucasian person to know in order to make an informed decision.[109]

Of course, the patient-centered perspective that Dr. Chan advocates is the minority rule articulated in *Canterbury v. Spence*.[110] A slight majority of states adhere to the professional custom or objective standard rule announced in *Natanson v. Kline*.[111] However, in either case, the legal rule is not flexible enough to accommodate the rather dramatic differences based on ethnicity documented here.

The social science literature sampled in this section shows that minority patients care not only *who* receives medical information, but also have strong preferences about *what* and *how* information is communicated. These preferences distinguish minority patients from white patients. The current law does not require providers to take these differences into account when obtaining patient informed consent. Therefore, patients whose preferences depart most dramatically from the common-law disclosure requirements are the patients harmed the most by our current consent laws.

A. Clinical Implications

The narrow focus of current informed consent law harms minority patients, reducing the quality of the medical care they receive and widening the disparity between the quality of health care racial and ethnic minority patients receive, and that afforded to European-Americans belonging to mainstream religious groups. First, there are the obvious harms to these patients' dignity interests. The preferences racial, ethnic,

108. *Id.*, at 397.
109. *Id.*, at 401.
110. Specifically, the *Canterbury* court required disclosure of material risks and defined those thusly: "A risk is material when a reasonable person, in what the physician knows or should know to be the patient's position, would be likely to attach significance to the risk in deciding whether or not to forego the proposed therapy." *Canterbury v. Spence*, 464 F.2d 772 (D.C. Cir. 1972), *cert. denied*, 490 U.S. 1065 (1972).
111. *Nathanson v. Kline*, 350 P.2d 1093 (Kan. 1960).

and religious minority patients express represent deeply held convictions that are relevant to the most intimate and important health decisions people make. However, beyond the dignity harm, minority patients experience a decline in the quality of their health care and outcomes directly related to the operation of informed consent law.

Cultural miscommunication between physician and patient will influence patient compliance with medical treatment, as well as the support patients receive from family and community during recovery.[112] Researchers Bowman and Hui explain that the failure by physicians to acknowledge cultural distinctions among patients results in a complete breakdown in communication between providers, patients, and their families.[113] Two patient case studies reported in the *Journal of Palliative Medicine* vividly illustrate the direct impact that miscommunication may have on patients' health outcomes.[114]

Dr. Anne Lapine reports two case studies that are instructive. The first case involved a Chinese patient diagnosed with primary renal cell carcinoma with brain metastases, and the second, a man from the nation of Georgia suffering from advanced non-small cell lung carcinoma. Both patients presented to medical teams at the Medical College of Wisconsin with terminal illnesses, poor prognoses, and families who requested that the truth of their respective diagnoses not be disclosed to the patients. The Chinese patient's daughter and son-in-law refused to consent to a biopsy intended for the purpose of determining a course of treatment. However, part of the family reticence may have been that the

> resident [physician] truthfully described the patient's poor prognosis and indicated that the biopsy would unlikely affect outcome or treatment.... The neurology resident, who had been raised and educated in Poland, felt it was unethical *or even illegal* to withhold information from the patient and expressed her opinion to the family. Mistrust rapidly developed and tension between the resident and the family escalated to the point where the family would not allow any consultants to see the patient and would only allow primary caregivers into the room under their supervision.[115]

Certainly, while the biopsy itself could not have affected the course of this patient's treatment, longevity, or comfort, it is indisputable that the information gleaned from the biopsy might well have. However, due to the breakdown in trust and communication between patient and family, caused at least in part by the physician's perception of what informed consent law allowed, this patient received an inferior quality of care.

The second patient in Dr. Lapine's study was younger and represented by his wife. As in the first case, the immediate consequence of the cultural biases built into informed consent law in this case was severe:

> She [the patient's wife] explained that in Georgian culture, having a disease such as

112. See J. Mitchell, "Cross-Cultural Issues in the Disclosure of Cancer," *Cancer Practice* 6, no. 3 (1998): 153–160.

113. See Bowman and Hui, *supra* note 62, at 1483. (Emphasis added.)

114. A. Lapine, R. Wang-Cheng, M. Goldstein, A. Nooney, G. Lamb, and A. R. Derse, "When Cultures Clash: Physician, Patient and Family Wishes in Truth Disclosure for Dying Patients," *Journal of Palliative Medicine* 4, no. 4 (2001): 475–480.

115. *Id.*, at 476. (Emphasis added.)

> cancer is seen as a burden on the family. She felt that if he knew the prognosis, he would be at high risk of committing suicide to protect his honor. She pleaded with the team not to disclose the diagnosis. She added that in Georgian culture, the accepted practice is to inform the family, not the patient, of a terminal diagnosis.... [Yet] the oncology consultant expressed significant reservations. He noted that most treatment protocols require informed consent and was concerned that having a surrogate provide consent when the patient was decisional, yet uninformed would be unethical...*and potentially illegal*....[116]

Ultimately, ethics committees met in both these cases and reached cumbersome accords between provider, patient, and families. In both cases reported by Dr. Lapine, physician perception of the informed consent law stood in the way of better care and outcomes in each of these two cases. A better outcome could have been accomplished under current law for the Chinese patient. For example, the patient could have designated a family member or surrogate to make decisions even while competent by signing a medical power of attorney. However, the informed consent law itself—or at least providers' understanding of it—created a barrier to selecting this choice that could have better served the patient in this case study. Therefore, no biopsy was performed and this patient simply returned home without any care—palliative or otherwise—and died.

In the case of the Georgian patient, since informed consent law does not explicitly prohibit physicians from allowing patients to waive their right to decide their medical treatment for themselves, one could argue the current law adequately accommodates ethnic decision-making preferences. However, this argument fails. First, there is ample evidence that in light of the evidence that minority patients' preferences are not being accommodated under the current legal model. Also, some ethnic patients and families mistrust the American medical system and seek care only as a last resort when the quality of their health outcomes have been jeopardized.[117] For these patients, the legal emphasis on autonomy clashes directly with the commitment to provide patients with good medical care. In Dr. Lapine's words, "[A]utonomy conflicts with beneficence, the mandate of physicians to act for the good of the patient."[118]

Defects in current informed consent law has a detrimental impact upon all patients, but disproportionately impacts those patients who are the most likely to hold ethical values and perspectives that diverge from those of Western providers. These patients do not receive the same quality care as majority patients do, and that is unjust. They suffer harm, not good, at the hands of their providers because of the way informed consent law operates. This violates beneficence principles and non-malfeasance. Even autonomy values are not served. The data shows that the prized rights to autonomy, self-determination, and human dignity through control of one's own medical decision making are, in fact, compromised by the current informed consent law, although the law places paramount value on protecting these very interests.

116. *Id.*, at 477. (Emphasis added.)

117. *Id.*, at 478.

118. *Id.*, at 475.

Informed consent law has thus become one further way in which minority patients receive disparate and inferior quality health care in this country, when compared with their white patient counterpart.

Having examined history and the impact of our current law, we are ready to turn our attention to examining the structure of the informed consent law. The next section describes the internal inconsistency of the legal doctrine of informed consent. It demonstrates the need to replace existing, conflicting approaches to this doctrine, with a unified approach to better serve all patients and their providers.

III. Legal Insufficiency of Current Law

We have seen in this [reading] that there is a dramatic incongruity between the autonomy model that underlies informed consent law and the ethical values held by racial, ethnic, and religious minority patients. We have looked at the broad clinical implications of ways the legal doctrine of informed consent misses the mark to narrowly focus on autonomy to the exclusion of other important ethical values.

This section argues courts have struggled with the legal insufficiency of existing theories advanced to support the informed consent doctrine. This section also reviews several representative informed consent cases and concludes that courts have been unsuccessful in finding a cohesive doctrinal explanation for informed consent law primarily because the underlying ethical basis for the law has been over-simplified.

1. The Salgo Case and its Progeny

Prior to the *Salgo* decision in 1957,[119] most bioethicists[120] agree that the ethical values most central to the

119. In *Salgo v. Leland Stanford Jr. University Board of Trustees,* 317 P.2d 170, 181 (Cal. Dist. Ct. App. 1957) (holding a physician violates duty to patient and is subject to liability if physician withholds any facts necessary for patient to form an intelligent basis for consent to proposed treatment and physician may not minimize known dangers in order to induce patient consent).

120. It is outside the scope of this paper to explore the variety of ethical systems that exist to inform the overall field of bioethics, and medical ethics in particular, except to the extent that these ethical systems derive from particular cultural, ethnic and religious minorities used as exemplars herein. Therefore, whether one chooses a utilitarian or consequentialist approach to ethical theory and seeks to maximize good while minimizing harm; or whether one adopts a deontological view of duty and obligation; or whether the more modern approaches such as liberal individualism or case-specific approach of casuistry is most appealing, where the question of informed consent is concerned, the fundamental problem of identifying a common moral system is solved in this paper by relying on the substantial consensus that bioethicists have achieved around three fundamental principles approach to bioethics. The principles of justice, beneficence and autonomy, identified in *The Belmont Report of the National Commission for the Protecting of Human Subjects of Biomedical and Behavioral Research* (1974–1978) represent a consensus foundational to a common theory of medical ethics. In November 1979, *The Belmont Report* was published in the Federal Register, *available at* <http://www.hhs.gov/ohrp/humansubjects/guidance/belmont.htm> and to this day articulates the unifying ethical principles which underlie human subject research and clinical ethics today. See, 45 C.F.R. Pt. 46. While principlism, as this ethical theory has come to be called, is not without its critics (see, e.g., J. D. Arras, "Principles and Particularity: The Roles of Cases in Bioethics," *Indiana Law Journal* 69 (1994): 983–1014, at 991) few would disagree that these three values, applied to clinical and research medicine, constitute the core of Western bioethical theory.

informed consent doctrine were beneficence and non-malfeasance. As the social reform and turbulence that accompanied the 1960s arrived, both the law and the ethics of informed consent took a turn.

The earliest cases to establish America's informed consent jurisprudence were an uneven lot. They combined legal theories of battery, tort, and contract to uniformly hold defendants liable for performing procedures that were not agreed to at the time of consent. Yet these cases each spoke in varying degrees about individual rights and control. In 1904, the Minnesota Supreme Court held a defendant physician liable for battery when he operated on a patient's left ear though the patient's consent permitted a procedure on her right ear.[121] Though the case sounded in battery, the *Mohr v. William* court viewed the physician and patient relationship as a contract.

> Consent, therefore, of an individual, must be either expressly or impliedly given before a surgeon may have the right to operate. There is logic in the principle thus stated, for, in all other trades, professions, or occupations, contracts are entered into by the mutual agreement of the interested parties, and are required to be performed in accordance with their letter and spirit. No reason occurs to us why the same rule should not apply between physician and patient.[122]

Mixing recovery theories still further, the *Mohr* court explained the justification for its holding by saying that surgeons were forbidden to violate patients' "bodily integrity," because "[t]he free citizen's first and greatest right which underlies all others—the right to himself—is the subject of universal acquiescence."[123] In the end, the *Mohr* court could not comfortably explain which legal theory supported its conclusion—contract, tort, or battery. Next, in a 1906 action for trespass on the person,[124] the Illinois Supreme Court refused to imply consent out of a presumed deference to the physician's best judgment. In *Pratt v. Davis*, the plaintiff gave her consent to undergo one operation to remove her ovaries. At the time of consent, the defendant surgeon had described the procedure as "trifling." Nevertheless, the plaintiff awoke after anesthesia to find she had been operated on twice and the defendant had performed a complete hysterectomy. Nothing in the *Pratt* court's language suggests a focus on autonomy, self-determination, or individual rights. Yet, as we know, by 1914, Justice Cardozo has issued the now famous informed consent talisman, declaring everyone to have the right to control one's body.[125]

Three observations about these early cases are in order. First, they suggest little discourse occurred between the legal and ethics communities about the doctrine of informed consent. Recalling the distinctly unegalitarian tilt of the early AMA Codes, while that bias would not necessarily have been preferable, the patients' rights themes raised by *Pratt*, *Mohr*, and *Scholendorff* belie the fact that wholly distinct and unrelated world views operated in law and medicine through the early 20th century. Second, without offering an explanation, it is worth noting that all the early, reported consent cases involve women

121. *Mohr v. Williams*, 95 Minn. 261, 104 N.W. 12 (1905).
122. *Id.*, at 268.
123. *Id.*, at 265.
124. *Pratt v. Davis*, 224 Ill. 300, 79 N.E. 562 (1906).
125. See *Scholoendorff v. Society of New York Hospitals*, 211 N.Y. 125, 105 N.E. 92 (1914).

patients. If this trend ceased after the 19th century, it would be of little moment. However, not only do a large number of informed consent cases appear to involve women plaintiffs, but a survey of cases in which plaintiffs prevail in informed consent litigation suggests that more women win these cases than men.[126] Finally, the early informed consent cases evince a tension between the goals of informed consent law, and selecting the correct legal cause of action. The challenge was and remains to match the informed consent doctrine to a uniform understanding of the ethical principles the cases are meant to apply.

A. Negligence or the Law of Battery?

The choice between treating informed consent cases under negligence or battery law remains unclear. Courts have attempted to outline the terms and conditions under which each respective doctrine is appropriate to the aims of informed consent.

The first attempt was by the Kansas Supreme Court in *Nathanson v. Kline*.[127] The plaintiff in *Nathanson* was diagnosed with breast cancer which the defendants treated with cobalt irradiation but without advising the plaintiff of any of the associated risks or hazards that accompany this treatment. The plaintiff pled her claims based on negligence law, and therefore, the court held the defendant physician had a duty to make reasonable disclosure of known risks and hazards. On a motion for rehearing, the Kansas Supreme Court answered the charge that it had confused the negligence standard for a medical malpractice claim, with the absolute liability standard of an assault and battery case. In order to clarify its analysis, the court reiterated the choice to apply a negligence standard and concluded the defendant physician had breached his duty to make a reasonable disclosure such as a reasonable medical practitioner would make under the same or similar circumstances. Thus, the *Nathanson* court rejected the battery approach.

Later, in *Rubino v. De Fretias,*[128] a Federal District Court construed Arizona law and the state's constitution to determine whether a plaintiff could amend her complaint to add a battery count. The *Rubino* plaintiff sought to recover damages for the defendant physician's unconsented removal of her vaccination mark. The court allowed the amendment, distinguishing a claim for *negligent* failure to obtain informed consent, from an action sounding in *battery to punish an unconsented touching*. The negligence claim, according to the *Rubino* court, alleged the physician failed to disclose a risk of treatment as required by the standard of care. This action, the court said, vindicates the patient's right to receive the standard of care. The battery action, on the other hand, "sustains a patient's right of self determination…." However, the problem with this explanation is that this plaintiff was not alleging the vaccination was negligently removed, but that it should not have been removed at all.

126. There are a host of reasons why this may be true. Perhaps women are represented in the reported cases disproportionately because only the most egregious informed consent fact patterns are tried and women are more often victims of individual rights' violations. Alternatively, perhaps women are the primary consumers of certain types of health care and those providers are more often open to negligence claims due to the nature of their practices. The list of possible explanations is long. And to hazard a guess without further study of these cases, the types of consent cases women bring, the actual incidence of their success and failure, and other empirical data, little more can be said at this juncture.

127. *Nathanson v. Kline*, 187 Kan. 186, 354 P2d 670, 673 (1960 hearing denied).

128. *Rubino v De Fretias*, 648 F.Supp 182, 185 (1986)

Perhaps the most helpful distinctions among the possible cause of actions in informed consent cases were drawn in a Connecticut case, *Logan v. Greenwich Hospital Association*.[129] After giving birth, plaintiff in *Logan* was diagnosed with lupus. Defendant's recommendation for closed needle biopsy did not include disclosure of alternative open kidney biopsy technique that also could have been used to diagnose the extent of her disease. The court held it was error to instruct the jury that the defendant physician had no duty to disclose a more hazardous alternative technique. The court required that all viable alternatives must be disclosed to a patient. The *Logan* holding was based on negligence theory, but the court took the time to distinguish the battery theory of recovery: "The theory of Battery as a basis for recovery against a physician has generally been limited to situations where he fails to obtain any consent to the particular treatment or performs a different procedure from the one for which consent has been given, or where he realizes that the patient does not understand what the operation entails."[130] Negligence claims, on the other hand, address the sufficiency of physicians' disclosures to determine whether the provider has met the standard of care for informing patients prior to treatment. Next, the *Logan* court tackled an issue that continues to be debated in courts today.

Courts have split to take two different approaches to defining what is "material" and therefore subject to disclosure to patients considering whether to consent to a treatment of procedure. The "Lay" or "Patient Centered" standard requires physicians to disclose all information which the reasonable patient would consider material to the patient's decision. This is a stronger autonomy model and emphasizes the patient's need to control not only the treatment decision but also the content of information conveyed to make that decision.[131] On the other hand, the professional model defines the standard of disclosure by what a reasonable physician in like circumstances *would disclose,* based either upon what others in the profession define as the standard for disclosure[132] or based upon what the physician knows or should know that a patient in a similar position would deem material to the consent decision.[133] The *Logan* court chronicles this debate, outlining the choice of several jurisdictions have made in their attempt to emphasize patient autonomy.

The *Logan* court called this dilemma "the essential ambivalence between the right of the patient to make a knowledgeable choice and the duty of the doctor to prescribe the treatment his professional judgment deems best for the patient." Though the court rightly identified the competing values at stake, unfortunately the court was premature in its prediction that courts were close to reaching a resolution to the problem.[134] The law of informed consent is no closer today to choosing a reasoned or uniform

129. *Logan v. Greenwich Hospital Association*, 191 Conn. 282, 465 A.2d 294 (1983).

130. *Id.*, 191 Conn. at 289.

131. See *Wilkinson v. Vesey*, 110 R.I. 606, 627, 295 A.2d 676, 689 ("It is our belief that in due deference to the patient's right to self determination, a physician is bound to disclose all the known material risks peculiar to he proposed procedure.")

132. See *Canterbury v. Spence*, 464 F.2d 772 (D.C.Cir.) *cert. denied* 409 U.S. 1064 (1972).

133. See *Wilkinson v. Vesey*, 110 R.I. at 627, 295 A.2d at 676.

134. *Id.*, 191 Conn. at 289, 264 A.2d at 299.

justification for applying either battery or negligence law to informed consent cases than it was when *Logan* was decided.[135]

B. Negligence, Contract, or Fiduciary Law?

In some cases, courts alternatively chose between contract, fiduciary, and negligence theories to address informed consent claims. A recent and instructive example is found in *Quintanilla v. Dunkelman*.[136] This California court decided the informed consent issue on negligence principles that the evidence was sufficient to support a jury verdict in the plaintiff's favor. The case involved a Spanish-speaking patient who spoke, but could not read Spanish. The patient was a 32-year-old wife and mother who had an 8th grade education. She sought treatment and eventually surgery to address a vaginal lesion. However, according to the plaintiff, the surgery was negligently performed and unconsented. Two physicians and a clinic were named defendants in the lawsuit. The first defendant physician owned the clinic and saw the patient for all of her visits during the year prior to surgery.

The jury concluded, based on the evidence of the physician's disclosure, that the patient reasonably believed this first physician was scheduled to remove the external lesion in an out-patient procedure. Yet, on the date of the surgery, she was given general anesthesia. Moreover, a second physician performed surgery to remove not only an external lesion, but also performed laparoscopic surgery and a D & C to remove another mass. Finally, the jury concluded that the consent forms the patient signed prior to surgery were ineffective because they were written in Spanish and not interpreted for the patient who read neither Spanish nor English. The jury returned a verdict for the plaintiff[137] and awarded damages, later reduced by the court to conform with the state's damages cap. Both parties appealed. Among the questions on appeal, the *Quintanilla* court faced the defendants' allegations that the plaintiff's consent form provided conclusive evidence of informed consent because the doctrine of estoppel by contract applies to written medical consent forms.[138] Also, the plaintiffs challenged the judgment below contending that the trial court erred in failing to instruct on the physician's fiduciary duty to obtain informed consent.[139]

The *Quintanilla* court rejected both allegations of error and affirmed the findings that held both physicians liable for negligence as to the plaintiff and to her husband. Most remarkable, however, is the way in which the *Quintanilla* court grounded its analysis in a series of four ethical principles which the court called "postulates." The four ethical principles were: First, unlearned patients and their physicians are generally not in intellectual parity. Second, an adult of sound mind has the right to exercise control over own body and determine whether to submit to surgery. Third, for a patient's consent to treatment to be effective, the consent must be informed. "And the fourth is that the patient, being unlearned in medical

135. See, e.g., *Rasmussen v. Skagit County*, 448 F. Supp.2d. 1203 (W.D. 2006)

136. *Quintanilla v. Dunkelman*, 34 Cal. Rptr. 3d 557 (2005).

137. Damages for the patient were fixed at $380,000.00 and for her husband, the jury awarded a total of $60,000.00 for present and future loss of consortium.

138. *Quintanilla*, 133 Cal. App. 4th at 116.

139. *Id.*, 133 Cal. App 4th at 100.

sciences, has an abject dependence upon and trust in his physician for the information upon which he relies during the decisional process, thus raising an obligation in the physician that *transcends arms-length transactions. From these ethical imperatives, we derived the obligation of a treating physician of reasonable disclosure of the available choices with respect to proposed therapy and of the dangers inherently and potentially involved in each.*"[140]

Quinttanilla v. Dunkelman teaches two indispensable lessons. First, the case demonstrates a balanced approach to identifying the core goals of the informed consent process. This court chose the negligence model to decide the informed consent question and declined to apply contract or fiduciary theories of law that might control typical "arms-length transactions."[141] It began by first identifying the ethical goals of the law, and then tailoring the doctrine to meet those moral objectives. Thus, out of justice and beneficence concerns, this court found the imbalance of power between patient and physician was significant. The same lack of parity, though, also made the notion of absolute, autonomous decision making inappropriate. Here a patient relied on the authority and beneficence of her physician whom she trusted. By first noting the "abject dependence" of the unlearned patient upon the physician, the *Quintanilla* court also enforced the duties of beneficence and non-malfeasance the physicians in this case owed to their patient. Finally, the court also acknowledged the patient's right to exercise control and the requirement of truly informed consent; both imperatives reflect the ethical value of respect for patient autonomy.

In this case, uniquely, the court's reasoning began from the moral foundations and values important to the relationships and conflicts before it, and then applied those principles using the legal tools that would serve their end. This is the exact reverse of the way in which the *Scholendorff* pronouncement has produced an informed consent jurisprudence based first upon legal rights to control and only second on the ethical principles fundamentally underlie the laws purpose. The *Quintanilla* court turns this thinking on its head to begin by examining the first principles of ethics; in this way, the court lays out a better rule of law.

The second lesson this case teaches is that courts can and should apply informed consent law in a way that reflects the importance of culture and ethnicity. Mrs. Quintanilla was not a patient for whom the Western version of the autonomy ethic has very much meaning at all. That fact was important to this court's disposition of the case. According to the evidence, the plaintiff was a nonassertive person who accepted authority. The fact that she is Hispanic pre-disposed Mrs. Quintanilla, moreover, not to question her physicians. In fact, according to the plaintiff's own words, "[I]f a doctor tells a Hispanic to do something, the Hispanic believes it."[142] The fact that Mrs. Quintanilla was His-panic also had great bearing on the ways in which a meaningful consent might have been obtained. First, the disclosure would have been accessible to her in her own language. Second, Mrs. Quintanilla's husband, Ramon, would likely have been included in the decision to undergo treatment. Mrs. Quintanilla's capacity to understand what was disclosed to her was influenced by her education as well as her culture. The court found the plaintiff had probably not heard

140. *Quintanilla*, 133 Cal. App. 4th at 114. (Emphasis added.)

141. In the section that follows, I argue that the fiduciary model, in fact, is preferable.

142. *Quintanilla*, 133 Cal. App. 4th at 111.

and certainly did not understand the words and phrases continued in the consent form, such as "excision of the vulvar lesion," "laparoscopy, or D & C," "possible biopsy" or "possible aspiration."[143]

The autonomous moral agent that is at the core of Western contemporary informed consent law is an individual who is both capable and desirous of making choices that are untouched and not encroached upon by others. To respect this person, the *Quintanilla* law has sought ways to adhere to the Kantian admonition: "So act as to treat humanity, whether in thine own person or in that of any other, in every case as an end withal, never as a means only." This conceptualization of autonomy clashes irreconcilably with sociological information we have about the Hispanic patient such as Mrs. Quintanilla.

> [Traditionally,] Hispanics are familistic: that is, they value family relationships so highly that family well-being takes priority over individual well-being. But the word "family means not only the nuclear parent-child family, but an extended family of several generations, including cousins.... [The] Hispanic family is patriarchal; that is, authority is vested in the male head of the family. There are several corollaries.

Further, operating only from the perspective of Western ideal of autonomous, informed consent would vastly overlook the extent of the damages Mrs. Quintanilla suffered.

> The complex values known as *machismo* is perhaps the best known. *Machismo* is a particular cultural definition of masculinity, with implications for women as well. *Machismo* has been associated with a strong double standard of sexual morality, with masculinity to be demonstrated through displays of physical and sexual prowess....[144]

Mrs. Quintanilla, her husband, and her family were ultimately deprived of quality health care in four ways. The physicians provided treatment that did not meet the standard of care. They violated their ethical obligation to act beneficently toward their patient. They violated the patient's autonomy right to include her family in medical decision making, and to have their cultural preferences respected during her care. Finally, that these violations could only occur to damage the health care received by Hispanic patients is unjust. While the *Quintanilla* court eventually came to a just result in this case, its analysis is aberrational. The question that remains is whether a unifying legal doctrine can be developed to organize and explain the law of informed consent. The following section answers in the affirmative.

IV. A Better Approach—Recognizing a Fiduciary Relationship

This section introduces a new legal paradigm for informed consent. It is well beyond the scope of this [reading] to fully develop the model introduced here. Nevertheless, the outline introduced in this section sets forth an approach to addressing the shortcomings identified in the body of this [reading]. The key

143. See, *Quintanilla*, 133 Cal. App. 4th at 116–17 (court concludes that in absence of translation of consent document cannot know whether recitels were understood.)

144. See J. J. Lindenthal and M. Schneider, *Health Concerns of Hispanics in New York City* (Mellen Research University Press, 1991): 7–8.

to finding a solution to the problems experienced by ethnic, racial, and religious minorities under the current informed consent regime, and to many of the deficiencies experienced by all patients with informed consent, lies in accepting the simple fact that physicians stand in a fiduciary relationship to their patients when disclosing information intended to serve as a basis for patients' medical decision making. If the law of informed consent were modified to recognize this fiduciary relationship, the interests of minority as well as majority patients would be better served, and the disclosures that physicians offer would also be better guided and protected by informed consent law.

The first key to recognizing the fiduciary relationship as an organizing paradigm for consent law lies in abandoning the notion that the relationship between a physician and a patient is an egalitarian one. Physicians and patients do not stand in *informational* equality with one another. A patient consults a physician because the physician is expected to know and be able to do something more than what the patient could do without the physician's expertise and training. Similarly, the patient knows and is in control of personal health information upon which the physician must depend in order to make informed and effective judgments and disclosures. Therefore, the informed consent conversation is not one among equals. It is a conversation on the one hand involving one who has greater medical knowledge than the other, and is directed by the one who has the ability, and indeed the duty, to influence another's decisions and choices. On the other hand, the patient bears ultimate responsibility for determining who is involved in the medical decision, what quantity of information must be shared to reach the medical decision, and the format of the communication that will surround the medical decision. Despite this level of control over the medical decision, the patient is also wholly dependent upon the physician to obtain the information necessary to make a decision. The error of informed consent law has been in oversimplifying the complexity of the relationship between physician and patient by regulating the disclosure rather than the relationship. Fiduciary law provides legal guidance for the conduct and interaction between parties, in contrast to the simplistic regulation offered by current consent rules.

The second key to understanding why the fiduciary model better fits the problems outlined in this [reading], is the fact that the harms that a properly conceived body of informed consent law seeks to prevent are not solely harms to a patient's dignitary interests. The dignitary harm certainly matters. However, informed consent law also seeks to protect against the harm of a physician using her position of power and authority to hurt, rather than help a patient. The law seeks to protect against the harm of a physician lying to a patient. The law seeks to protect against the harm that occurs when a physician places her own interest above the interest of her patient. Moreover, informed consent law also must protect the physician's earnest effort to guide patients in ways that will benefit and not injure their health and well-being. Physicians must be assured, under a broader view of informed consent law, that acting in a way that may reasonably be viewed as serving the best interest of a patient will absolve them from liability for negative outcomes traced to to the medical decision a patient makes. Law that focuses solely on the reasonableness of disclosures alone cannot address these concerns. Rather, informed consent law must be modified to incorporate the fiduciary duties of care and loyalty, requiring physicians to act in the best interest of their patients', while protecting them from liability where they can show they have used their best medical judgment during the consent process.

The effect of these two seemingly simple assertions would be profound if incorporated into the law of informed consent. First, by recognizing the physician-patient relationship as a fiduciary one for consent purposes, the law would hold physicians to a heightened duty of responsibility in their disclosures. Instead of the current wrestling between patient- or professional-standards of materiality, focus would turn to the physician's duty to protect the patient's interests in light of who the individual patient is as a whole person. The physician's duty of care would involve the obligation to both ask and respect patients' cultural and religious beliefs in medical decision making. The emphasis in consent law would turn toward the physician's obligation to exercise care for patients' best interests. Therefore, the law would encourage physicians to inquire as to patient preferences for the level of information, the identity of decision makers, and the respective involvement of both patient and physician in decision making. To satisfy the duty of loyalty, the law would require physicians to permit patients to exercise the level of control the patient wishes to exercise in medical decision making. Where physicians, not patients, are responsible to make treatment choices, the duty of loyalty will obligate physicians to choose in the best interests of their patients. As one court has said, "The relationship of patients and physicians is a fiduciary one of the highest degree. It involves every element of trust, confidence and good faith."[145]

Applying a fiduciary model to the setting in which informed consent is obtained much more correctly reflects the relative positions of patient and physician and therefore would better serve to protect the ethical obligations of physicians to treat patients with beneficence and justice. The fiduciary model correctly addresses the patient's posture of vulnerability and reliance on providers for fair treatment, in the same way that this model protects other parties whose interests are misaligned. The fiduciary model is appropriate for informed consent because patients have no ex ante way to monitor physicians' choices. At the same time, the fiduciary model is far more likely to encourage providers to take self-initiated steps to earn patients' trust. Physicians may incorporate more information, include assistants and extenders on their staff, or develop culturally competent materials to share during the informed consent process. Relieved of the obligation to disclose information so that patients can autonomously make their own treatment decisions, physicians are likely to engage in bonding activities that not only protect patients' interests, but limit physicians' exposure to liability. In short, the fiduciary model would return informed consent law to a beneficence-based doctrine, which at once would be able to serve non-malfeasance, autonomy, and justice values. To be sure, the fiduciary model will change informed consent law to honor minority patients' ethical values in medical decision making which are now being completely ignored. However, minority patients will not be the only beneficiaries of a changed view of consent law. The fiduciary obligation to act in a patient's best interest will hold providers to the highest standards of beneficience when managing health information for the benefit of all patients. Where current law fails to acknowledge either the extent or limitations of patients' control over their medical treatment, fiduciary rules will hold providers to the highest standard of conduct while recognizing that patients are ill-equipped to monitor that conduct. Instead, fiduciary law will give providers incentive and courts the authority to regulate the power that providers' specialized knowledge affords them, thus minimizing malfeasance. Judicial oversight based on

145. In *Lockett v. Goodill*, for example, 430 P.2d 589, 591 (Wash. 1967) a Washington court found "the relationship of patients and physicians is a fiduciary one of the highest degree.

fiduciary principles will provide a better basis for addressing justice concerns, when neither ethical nor legal incentives have proved sufficient to prevent discriminatory paternalism towards vulnerable patients whether they are members of minority or majority groups. At the same time, providers will be justly protected by fiduciary rules that defer to good faith conduct in much the same way that the business judgment rule protects agents in corporate settings.

By correctly identifying the precise nature of the relationship where consent occurs, and the range of harms informed consent law seeks to prevent, courts may broaden the protective reach of the doctrine so that patients need not fit a monolithic "reasonable person" model in order to be protected. Instead, patients of different nationalities, cultural and religious backgrounds may also have their interests protected as well. If courts apply the fiduciary model to resolve informed consent cases, the *Quintanilla* court will no longer be unique. Instead all courts will expect physicians to honor all ethical values for all patients they treat.

V. Conclusion

My objectives in this [reading] are three-fold. I seek to call attention to the injustice that informed consent law visits upon patients who belong to racial, ethnic, and religious minority groups. Also, I hope to encourage jurists and legal theorists to draw upon the vast body of empirical information available from various social science disciplines in an effort to guide and improve medical decision making for all. Finally, I want to encourage courts to apply the fiduciary model to hold providers and patients accountable for their roles in informed consent. Once this is done, then the real work begins. I regard the law as an instrument, capable of being used to accomplish positive social change. Once we lawyers admit our corrective responsibility for what has long been clear as an empirical, ethical, and cultural matter, then legal scholars can join the discourse already underway between ethicists, medical providers, and social scientists seeking new solutions to reform this ailing doctrine.

The United States Census 2000 reports that 12.5 percent (or 35.3 million) Americans are Hispanic or Latino. African-Americans represent 12.3 percent (or 34.6 million) of the total American population. Chinese-, Japanese-, and Korean-Americans together represent 1.6 percent of the population, or 4.3 million people. Together, adherents to Judaism (1.3 percent), Buddhism (.5 percent) and Islam (.5 percent) represent 5 million Americans. These ethnic, religious, and racial minorities are the people that current informed consent law most directly harms. However, they are not alone.

The data presented in this paper reveals that our current law's focus on autonomy, self-determination, and individual control has impact on all patients. Indeed, the law affirmatively harms the racial, ethnic, and religious minority patients, many of whom already suffer significant health care disparities in our system. However, all patients and providers benefit from a decision to require informed consent to protect beneficence, non-malfeasance, autonomy, and justice concerns. All patients will receive improved health care as physicians exercise the duties of good faith, care, and loyalty toward them. Moreover, physicians and other providers will benefit from being free of an artificially constrained list of "do's and don'ts." A fiduciary model of informed consent law will improve the quality of health care for more than 100 million minority patients, potentially at risk under current law, while also regulating the informed consent procedure and practice in a way that will bring balance and justice to all American patients and providers.

Questions

1. Matthew discusses how people of different races, religions, and ethnicities tend to value autonomy differently and for different reasons. We also learned that some legal theorists think informed consent law as it is actually practiced exhibits a "suffocating hegemony" of autonomy. How do these facts affect the way you think about the moral significance of autonomy?
2. Matthew argues that moving to a fiduciary model (as a legal framework for the physician-patient relationship) would help solve the problems with the doctrine of informed consent by providing healthcare providers incentives and courts authority to minimize malfeasance toward all patients, especially marginalized racial, religious, and ethnic groups. Do you agree or disagree that such a framework would help improve the lives of such marginalized groups? Why? Provide at least two reasons for your viewpoint. Can you give an example from your life or someone else's that supports your answer?

A Model for Culturally Responsive Health Care

Dorothy E. Vawter, Kathleen A. Culhane-Pera, Barbara Babbitt, Phua Xiong, and Mary M. Solberg

Editor's Introduction

This reading gives the fundamentals of the *healing by heart* model for culturally responsive healthcare. This is a model developed by the editors of a book of ethical and clinical stories of Hmong families (an ethnic group living mainly in China and Southeast Asia) and Western providers. This model consists of nine interconnected areas of learning and focuses on knowledge and skills in cross-cultural health ethics. It is the result of clinical experience with the Hmong community and ethnographically informed reflection on their health-related cultural beliefs and values. It identifies key ethical issues arising from cross-cultural healing relationships and offers an approach to working through serious cross-cultural ethical conflicts. The editors are a diverse interdisciplinary group of female healthcare providers and scholars whose knowledge and experiences inform the model. Kathleen Culhane-Pera, MD, MA is a family physician who has worked with multicultural communities as a family physician, researcher, and anthropologist. Dorothy Vawter, PhD is a senior ethics and health policy consultant at the Minnesota Center for Health Care Ethics. Phua Xiong, MD is a family practice physician at the St. Paul Family Medical Center in St. Paul, Minnesota. Barbara Babbitt, BSM, RN, MA has spent many years working to improve how healthcare is delivered to culturally diverse families. Mary M. Solberg, PhD, MSW is professor emeritus in religion at Gustavus Adolphus College in St. Peter, Minnesota.

The goal of culturally responsive health care is for patients and providers to feel respected and satisfied with both the healing methods used and the health outcomes (Jecker, Carrese, & Pearlman, 1995). This [reading] presents a model of the knowledge, skills, and attitudes that support the delivery of culturally responsive health care.

The *Healing by Heart* model for culturally responsive health care, as depicted in Figure 1.2.1, identifies nine areas of learning and the interconnections among them. The arrows reflect the way learning in one area supports and influences learning in other areas. Table 1.2.1 provides a more extensive outline of the model, which is distinctive in its attention to knowledge and skills in cross-cultural health care ethics. (For examples of other models, see Betancourt, Green, & Carillo, 2002; Brach & Fraser, 2000; Campinha-Bacote, 1999, 2003; Campinha-Bacote & Munoz, 2001; Cross, Bazron, Dennis, & Isaacs, 1989; Huff & Kline, 1999a; Leininger, 1988, 1995a; Spector, 2000.)

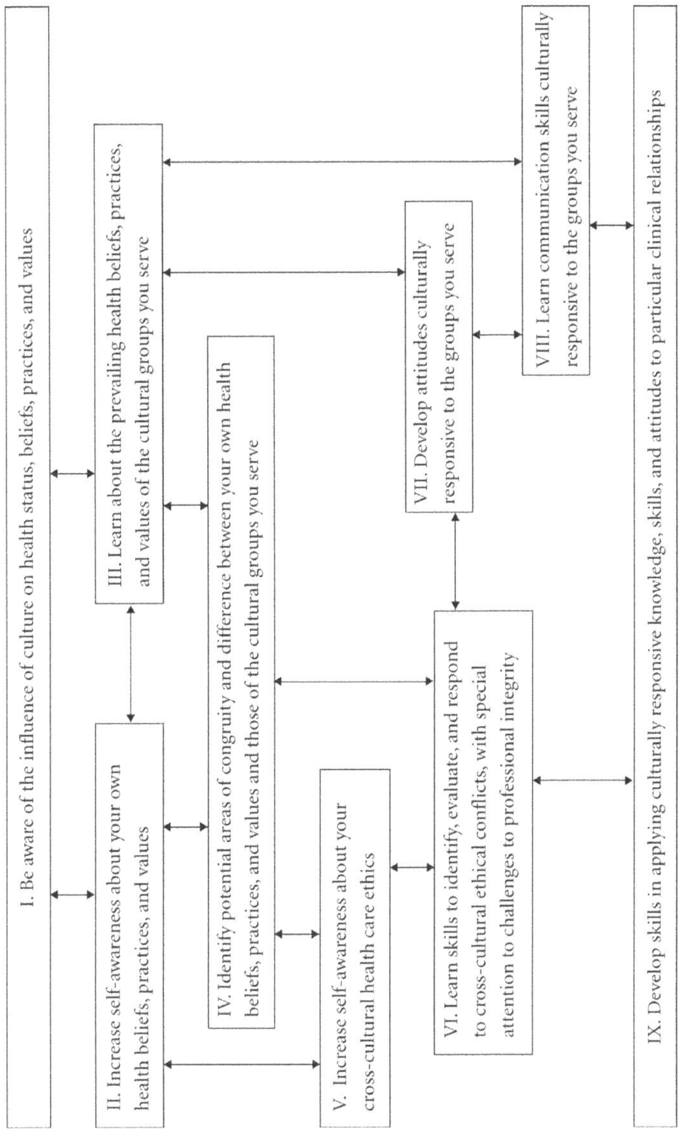

Figure 1.2.1 The Healing by Heart Model for Culturally Responsive Health Care

Table 12.1 Outline of the *Healing by Heart* Model for Culturally Responsive Health Care

I. Be aware of the influence of culture on health status, beliefs, practices, and values

II. Increase self-awareness about your own health beliefs, practices, and values
  - A. *Your health beliefs and practices*
    1. Your concepts of anatomy and bodily functions
    2. Your beliefs about illness causation, illness prevention, and health promotion
    3. Treatment, illness prevention, and health promotion activities you engage in
  - B. *Your health care ethics*
    1. On what basis do you believe health care practitioners are to be trusted?
    2. What behaviors do you believe demonstrate respect for persons, patients, and families?
    3. What do you believe are the ideal roles, responsibilities, and prerogatives of patients, families, practitioners, institutions, and states?
    4. What types of information about a patient do you believe you should disclose, to whom, and how?
    5. What considerations do you believe are relevant when assessing a patient's best interests?
    6. What methods and criteria do you believe support good health care decision making?

III. Learn about the prevailing health beliefs, practices, and values of the cultural groups you serve
  - A. *Past and present contextual influences*
    1. Politics
    2. Economics
    3. Social and family structure (gender, marriage, children, education, class)
    4. Religion
    5. Geographic location
    6. Refugee flight or immigration history
    7. Relationships with other groups (including discrimination)
    8. Culture change, acculturation, variation
    9. Access to health care systems
  - B. *Health-related cultural beliefs and practices*
    1. Traditional and changing concepts of anatomy, bodily functions, and malfunctions
    2. Traditional and changing beliefs about illness causation, illness prevention, and health promotion
    3. Traditional and changing practices for treatment, illness prevention, and health promotion
  - C. *Health-related moral practices and commitments*
    1. On what basis do patients and families from this cultural group tend to trust traditional healers, health care practitioners, and institutions?
       - a. What, if any, are the historical and cultural barriers to trusting practitioners?
       - b. What types of trust and distrust does this group tend to have of U.S. practitioners?
    2. According to this cultural group, what behaviors demonstrate respect for persons, patients, and families?
       - a. What attributes are deserving of respect?
       - b. How important is it to respect persons/patients/families?
       - c. What behaviors demonstrate respect for persons/patients/families, and for patients of different ages and genders?
       - d. What are the privacy needs and expectations of patients?
       - e. What, if any, taboos are there regarding touching, disrobing, examining, or discussing parts of the body?
    3. According to this cultural group, what are the ideal roles, responsibilities, and prerogatives of patients, families, traditional healers, health care practitioners, institutions, and states concerning such matters as:
       - a. identifying the cause of an ailment?
       - b. identifying appropriate remedies and healers?
       - c. engaging in healing activities?
       - d. providing and receiving information from healers and health professionals?
       - e. decision making?
       - f. protecting ill and vulnerable persons?
       - g. conducting follow-up assessments of effectiveness and outcome?

Table 1.2.1 Outline of the *Healing by Heart* Model for Culturally Responsive Health Care

        h. paying for services?
    4. According to this cultural group, what health-related information should be disclosed, to whom, and how?
        a. What importance is ascribed to informing patients of diagnosis and prognosis?
        b. What importance is ascribed to protecting confidentiality?
        c. What, if any, topics or words are taboo?
    5. According to this cultural group, what considerations are relevant to assessing a patient's best interests and the risks and benefits of treatment alternatives?
        a. What types of benefit are important?
        b. What types of risk are acceptable/unacceptable?
        c. What types of evidence are valued and relied on when assessing benefits and harms to a patient?
    6. According to this cultural group, what methods and criteria support good health care decision making?
        a. Which health and non-health-related consequences are important to consider?
        b. Who needs to be involved?
        c. What is the role of the patient?
        d. What is the role of the family, friends, community members, health care practitioners, states, and proxy decision makers?
        e. What standards are proxy decision makers to use?

IV. Identify potential areas of congruity and difference between your own health beliefs, practices, and values and those of the cultural groups you serve (for example, see Table 1.2.2)

V. Increase self-awareness about your own cross-cultural health care ethics
- A. *What is your concept of good cross-cultural health care relationships?*
    1. Provider and patient/family have a trusting and respectful relationship?
    2. Provider and patient/family agree on interventions?
    3. The patient's best interests are secured, as the patient or family understands best interests, except when a patient/family's wish entails a significant and disproportionate ethical challenge to professional integrity? (for further examples, see Figure 1.2.2)
- B. *What are your criteria for assessing decision-making capacity in persons with diverse health beliefs?*
    1. U.S. biomedical criteria?
    2. Criteria of the patient's cultural group?
    3. Both?

VI. Learn skills to identify, evaluate, and respond to cross-cultural ethical conflicts, with special attention to challenges to professional integrity
- A. *Distinguish between types of provider objections to treatment wishes*
    1. Objections based on personal preferences
    2. Objections based on personal moral beliefs, including personal conscience
    3. Objections based on professional integrity
- B. *Learn to evaluate objections based on professional integrity*
    1. Assess the patient's or family's treatment wish
        a. Type of wish?
            - A request or a refusal?
            - A diagnostic, curative, life-sustaining, palliative, or preventative intervention?
            - A standard, prohibited, or experimental intervention?
        b. Decision-making capacity of the patient/family?
            - Child/adult with/without decision-making capacity?
            - Capacity assessment based on: biomedical criteria, criteria of patient's cultural group, or both?
        c. Source and strength of the treatment wish?
            - Deep cultural or religious beliefs or commitments?
            - Deep personal beliefs or commitments?
            - Powerful emotions?

- Socioeconomic conditions?
- Impaired decision-making capacity?
- Misunderstanding or lack of knowledge?

2. Assess the ethical challenge to professional integrity
   a. Strength of empirical support for the health claims and predictions?
   b. Type(s) of challenge to professional integrity? (see Table 1.2.3)
      - Violates human rights?
      - Is cruel?
      - Poses significant harm to identifiable third parties?
      - Poses harm that outweighs benefit?
      - Poses significant risk to public health?
      - Offers no health benefit?
      - Offers low probability of benefit?
      - Serves non-health-related objectives?
   c. Degree of professional agreement about the challenge to professional integrity?
3. Compare the strength and source of the patient's or family's wish with the strength of the challenge to professional integrity

C. *Be aware of the range of possible responses to cross-cultural ethical conflicts*
   1. Accede
   2. Compromise
   3. Educate
   4. Build trust
   5. Persuade
   6. Transfer
   7. Refuse
   8. Override
   9. Impose

VII. Develop attitudes culturally responsive to the groups you serve
   A. *Be open and nonjudgmental*
   B. *Adopt cultural humility, including openness to sharing power*
   C. *Demonstrate patience and empathy*

VIII. Learn communication skills culturally responsive to the groups you serve
   A. *Nonverbal communication*
      1. Greetings
      2. Head movements
      3. Smiling and laughing
      4. Hand gestures
      5. Eye contact
      6. Facial expressions
      7. Tone of voice
      8. Touching
   B. *Verbal communication*
      1. Working with interpreters (see Table 1.2.4)
      2. Greetings
      3. Introductions
      4. Styles of address
      5. Reasons for the visit
      6. Sensitive topics
      7. Risks and benefits
      8. Bad news
      9. Compliments

IX. Develop skills in applying culturally responsive knowledge, skills, and attitudes to particular clinical relationships

Table 1.1. Outline of the *Healing by Heart* Model for Culturally Responsive Health Care

A. *Listen to the patient's or the family's responses to questions about their perspectives*
   1. "What do you [or other people] think is wrong?"
   2. "What do you [or other people] think has caused the problem?"
   3. "How has this problem affected your life?"
   4. "What are you [or other people] afraid of?"
   5. "What healing methods have you tried?"
   6. "What do you [or other people] think will help?"
   7. "Who usually makes [or, helps you make] decisions about your health care?"
   8. "What concerns do you have about seeking U.S. health care services for this problem?"

B. *Explain the biomedical conceptualization of the problem*

C. *Acknowledge similarities and differences between the provider's and the patient's perspective*

D. *Recommend a course of action*

E. *Negotiate options*

F. *Evaluate cross-cultural ethical conflicts and appropriate responses (see Table 1.2)*

The first section of this [reading] presents practical recommendations for how health care providers can apply the *Healing by Heart* model to relationships with Hmong patients and families in the United States. Guidance is offered on cross-cultural health care ethics, communication skills, and applying such knowledge and skills to particular clinical encounters. These recommendations are consistent with the National Standards on Culturally and Linguistically Appropriate Services (CLAS) in Health Care (U.S. Department of Health and Human Services [U.S. DHHS], 2000c, 2001d).

While the model is directed primarily to practitioners in clinical settings, many of the key learning areas are also applicable to health care administrators, educators, and health policy makers working in government, insurance companies, and private organizations. The final sections of the [reading] recommend ways health care administrators, educators, and policy makers can support the delivery of culturally responsive health care. [...]

Recommendations for Public Policy Makers

Social, political, and economic issues influence the major determinants of health in this country. People in the upper socioeconomic class have the best health, the lowest rates of disease, and the best health care, while people in the lower socioeconomic class have the worst health, the highest burden of all diseases, and the worst health care. People of non-European-American heritage have higher morbidity and mortality rates and lower usage rates of health care facilities and procedures than European-Americans. These disparities of health and health care services are unjust. Redressing these disparities requires the development and implementation of supportive policies by government and nongovernment agencies. (For example, see Andrulis, 1999; Brach & Fraser, 2000; Huff & Kline, 1999b; Lavizzo-Mourey & Mackenzie, 1996; Lecca, Quervalu, Nunes, & Gonzales, 1998; New Jersey Legislature, 2003; U.S. DHHS, 2002a, 2002b.)

The U.S. Department of Health and Human Services has taken several steps to improve the quality of health care for people from all racial and ethnic backgrounds. Its efforts include the Initiative to Eliminate Racial and Ethnic Health Disparities (U.S. DHHS, 2000b); Healthy People 2010, a program that puts the goal of eliminating health disparities on the national agenda (U.S. DHHS, 2000a); and the National Standards on Culturally and Linguistically Appropriate Services (CLAS) (U.S. DHHS, 2000c, 2001d). More recently, the Centers for Medicare and Medicaid Services began requiring that Medicare+Choice organizations address either clinical health care disparities or culturally and linguistically appropriate services for their Quality Assessment Performance Improvement project (U.S. DHHS, 2002b; Agency for Healthcare Research and Quality, 2003). For examples of partnerships between governmental and nongovernmental organizations to implement policies to reduce health disparities, see U.S. DHHS, 2002a. At the state level, policy efforts are under way to require mandatory cultural competency training for medical licensure (New Jersey Legislature, 2003). For other, more detailed resources on the responsibilities of organizations and policy makers to support culturally responsive health care see, for example, Andrulis, Goodman, & Pryor, 2002; Brach & Fraser, 2000; Huff & Kline, 1999b; Lavizzo-Mourey & Mackenzie, 1996; and Lecca, Quervalu, Nunes, & Gonzales, 1998.

Policy makers can work toward improving culturally responsive health care by advocating for such policies as:

- Third-party payers (insurance companies, managed care organizations, Medicaid/Medicare funds, etc.) that reimburse for health care interpreters
- Third-party payers that reimburse transportation costs
- Support for the training of qualified health care interpreters and the development of national uniform standards of practice
- Medicaid and Medicare contracts that require health care organizations to provide clear guidelines for culturally responsive care
- Policies that require training in patient-centered communication skills for continued state licensure for physicians, nurses, and other clinicians
- Accreditation requirements that hospitals and professional training programs provide training in the delivery of culturally responsive health care
- Programs to recruit and support members of diverse cultural groups in professional schools and positions of leadership
- Enforcement of federal laws that require institutions to be responsive to constituencies' needs for interpreter services

To redress the root causes of health disparities in this country policy makers should embrace a wide understanding of the social and economic factors that influence health. They need to advocate for political and economic policies that help communities be healthier, with decent housing, living-wage jobs, convenient affordable transportation systems, and clean, safe environments. Refugees and immigrants need help to adjust to their new society, with language classes, job skills training, child care, and financial assistance. Policies and programs are needed to help stem addictions to tobacco, alcohol, gambling, and illicit drugs. In short, advocating for culturally responsive health care can have broad implications for the health of all people and may benefit from close coordination between local, state, regional, and national policy makers.

Conclusion

Those interested in promoting health and improving health care for patients from all cultural backgrounds must act to reduce personal, institutional, political, and economic barriers to delivering culturally responsive health care. Work is needed at the individual, institutional, and public policy levels.

The solutions are multiple. Be aware of the cultural basis for differences in health status and health-related beliefs, practices, and values. Understand the cultural perspectives of the cultural groups served. Learn to communicate effectively across cultural and linguistic differences. Learn to negotiate and to work effectively through serious cross-cultural ethical conflicts. Attend to the policies, procedures, and values of health care institutions where practitioners, patients, and families interact. Advocate for organizational and system changes that support culturally responsive care. Engage in partnerships with community organizations. Together these activities empower patients to seek—and health care professionals to deliver—culturally responsive health care.

References

Agency for Healthcare Research and Quality. (2003). *Oral, linguistic, and culturally competent services: Guides for managed care plans.* Retrieved April 4, 2003, from www.ahrq.gov/about/cods/cultcomp.htm

Andrulis, D. P. (1999). Cultural competence assessment of practices, clinics, and health care facilities. In E. J. Kramer, S. L. Ivey, & Y. Ying (Eds.), *Immigrant women's health: Problems and solutions.* San Francisco: Jossey-Bass, 330–335.

Andrulis, D., Goodman, N., & Pryor, C. (2002, May 6). *What a difference an interpreter can make: Health experiences of uninsured with limited English proficiency.* Boston: The Access Project. Available from www.healthlaw.org/immigrant.shtml

Betancourt, J. R., Green, A. R., & Carillo, J. E. (2002). *Cultural competence in health care: Emerging frameworks and practical approaches.* Field report. Retrieved January 31, 2003, from www.cmwf.org/programs/minority/betancourt_culturalcompetence_576.pdf

Brach, C., & Fraser, I. (2000). Can cultural competency reduce racial and ethnic health disparities? A review and conceptual model. *Medical Care Research and Review, 57* (Supplement 1), 181–217.

Campinha-Bacote, J. (1999). A model and instrument for addressing cultural competence in health care. *Journal of Nursing Education, 38*(5), 203–207.

Campinha-Bacote, J. (2003). Many faces: Addressing diversity in health care. *Online Journal of Issues in Nursing, 8*(1) Manuscript 2. Retrieved February 9, 2003, from http://nursingworld.org/ojin/topic20/tpc20_2.htm

Campinha-Bacote, J., & Munoz, C. (2001). A guiding framework for delivering culturally competent services in case management. *The Case Manager, 12*(2), 48–52.

Cross, T. L., Bazron, B. J., Dennis, K. W., & Isaacs, M. R. (1989). *Towards a culturally competent system of care: A monograph on effective services for minority children who are severely emotionally disturbed.* Washington, DC: Child and Adolescent Service System Program (CASSP) Technical Assistance Center, Georgetown University Child Development Center.

Huff, R. M., & Kline, M. V. (1999a). The cultural assessment framework. In R. M. Huff & M. V. Kline (Eds.), *Promoting health in multicultural populations: A handbook for practitioners.* Thousand Oaks, CA: Sage.

Huff, R. M., & Kline, M. V. (1999b). *Promoting health in multicultural populations: A handbook for practitioners.* Thousand Oaks, CA.: Sage.

Jecker, N. S., Carrese, J. A., & Pearlman, R. A. (1995). Caring for patients in cross-cultural settings. *Hastings Center Report, 25,* 6–14.

Lavizzo-Mourey, R., & Mackenzie, E. R. (1996). Cultural competence: Essential measurements of quality for managed care organizations. *Annals of Internal Medicine, 124*(10), 919–920.

Lecca, P., Quervalu, I., Nunes, J. V., & Gonzales, H. F. (1998). *Cultural competency in health, social, and human services: Directions for the twenty-first century.* New York: Garland.

Leininger, M. (1988). Leininger's Theory of Nursing: Cultural care diversity and universality. *Nursing Science Quarterly, 1*(4), 152–160.

Leininger, M. (1995a). Culture care assessment to guide nursing practices. In M. Leininger (Ed.), *Transcultural nursing: Concepts, theories, research & practices* (2nd ed.). New York: McGraw-Hill, 115–148.

New Jersey Legislature. (2003). Proposed bills in Senate (S411) and Assembly (A2297). Retrieved February 7, 2003, from www.njleg.state.nj.us/bills/BillsByNumber.asp

Spector, R. E. (2000). *Cultural care: Guides to heritage assessment and health traditions.* Upper Saddle River, NJ: Prentice Hall Health.

U.S. Department of Health and Human Services. (2000a). *Healthy people 2010: Understanding and improving health.* (2nd ed.). Washington, DC: U.S. Government Printing Office. Available from www.healthypeople.gov/document/tableofcontents.htm

U.S. Department of Health and Human Services. (2000b). *Initiative to eliminate racial and ethnic disparities of health*. Available from www.raceandhealth.hhs.gov/
U.S. Department of Health and Human Services. Office of Minority Health. (2000c). *National standards on culturally and linguistically appropriate services (CLAS) in health care. Federal Register, 65*(247), 80865–79. Available from www.omhrc.gov/clas
U.S. Department of Health and Human Services. Office of Minority Health. (2001d). *National standards on culturally and linguistically appropriate services (CLAS) in health care: Final report*. Retrieved February 2, 2003, from www.omhrc.gov/omh/programs/2pgprograms/finalreport.pdf
U.S. Department of Health and Human Services. (2002a). *Healthy people 2010: Memorandum of understanding (MOU) goals*. Retrieved February 7, 2003, from www.healthypeople.gov/Implementation/mous
U.S. Department of Health and Human Services. Centers for Medicare and Medicaid. (2002b). *Medicare managed care manual*. Chapter 5, *Quality assessment: Appendices*. Retrieved February 2, 2003, from http://cms.hhs.gov/manuals/116_mmc/mc86c05exhibits.asp#s2003

Questions

The *healing by heart* model holds that culturally responsive healthcare requires (among other things) being aware of the influence of culture on health status, beliefs, practices, and values, and that one should increase awareness about (a) one's own health beliefs, practices, and values, and (b) about one's cross-cultural healthcare ethics.

1. What are some of your beliefs about health and health practices?
2. What are some aspects of your healthcare ethics?
3. What are some aspects of your cross-cultural healthcare ethics?

Reading 1.3

The Handsome Lake Method

An Introduction

Alf H. Walle

Editor's Introduction

In this reading, Alf Walle introduces a method for recovery from substance abuse inspired by the life and work of nineteenth-century Iroquois leader Handsome Lake, who developed a method to help Native people embrace their heritage as they recovered from substance abuse. Walle compares the Handsome Lake method with the twelve steps of Alcoholics Anonymous and relates his discussion to the conditions of other Native groups such as Native Hawaiians and the Māori of New Zealand. Alf Walle, PhD is an anthropologist, folklorist, and literary critic with an eclectic background

1. The author's *The Path of Handsome Lake: A Model of Recovery for Native People* (Walle, 2004) provides an expanded view of these ideas and is recommended.

whose experience as a state-certified substance abuse counselor specializing in the treatment of Alaskan Native clients informs this method.

Diversity and Recovery

Increasingly, substance abuse counselors recognize that cultural issues impact both dysfunction and recovery. This realization follows decades in which differences between people were ignored or discounted. The Twleve Steps Program of Alcoholics Anonymous and Narcotics Anonymous, for example, tends to link substance abuse with a spiritual bankruptcy that can affect people from all cultures and ways of life. Such a vision minimizes the differences between people and focus on their similarities (dysfunctional tendencies triggered by substance abuse.)

Currently, in contrast, the differences between people are being recognized. Thus, the Secular Organization for Recovery (SOS) offers a secular alternative to what is perceived as the religious and spiritual ethos of Alcoholics Anonymous/the Twelve Steps method (Christopher, 1992, 1997). Rational Recovery (Trimpey, 1985) and Self Management and Recovery Training (Hovarth, 1997), also offer nonspiritual and rational alternatives of therapy and self-help.

Other organizations, such as Women for Sobriety (Kirkpatrick, 1978, 1990), tailor themselves around the needs of women, arguing that females, as a group, have a series of special needs and vulnerabilities (that revolve around self-esteem, guilt, etc.) In all of these cases, a universal program of recovery (typified by Alcoholics Anonymous/the Twelve Steps method) is rejected and replaced by techniques that are tailored toward the needs of specific groups.

Cultural differences also need to be addressed. I have been told, for example, that many Hispanic men embrace a "macho" posture and, as a result, they may have trouble admitting to any kind of "powerlessness," even though doing so is a keystone of the Alcoholics Anonymous/Twelve Steps program. Some Native Americans, furthermore, are rather private and reserved and may not be comfortable discussing their misdeeds (or even their positive achievements) within the context of an open forum (as encouraged by the Twelve Steps program.) And since the Twelve Steps method is the brainchild of middle class White men, various groups complain that the approach is not well suited to them. Thus, a number of African Americans have confided to me that they can embrace Alcoholics Anonymous only with difficulty and that much of the rhetoric they hear at meetings is not relevant to them, as members of the Black community. I have heard numerous Native people make similar observations.

Today, universal strategies of recovery are being replaced with an emphasis on diversity. Currently, Lance Dodes (2002) and Stanton Peele (1992) have emerged as particularly vocal critics of Alcoholics Anonymous arguing that substance abusers need methods that help reduce the stress that can trigger dysfunction.

Native Americans and Alcohol/Substance Abuse

Today, there is a recognition that Native people experience a distinct series of vulnerabilities and needs that can trigger dysfunction. As mentioned above, many Native Americans are not well served by universal strategies of treatment, such as those associated with the Twelve Steps program.

Cultural differences appear to contribute to the tendency toward ineffectiveness. This situation is multiplied by the fact that Native Americans in general, consist of a heterogeneous group of diverse cultures, societies, and nations that cannot all be conveniently lumped together (any more than various White cultures—such as the German, English, Italian, and Irish—that are distinctive and need to be accepted as such.) In addition, since some Native Americans live in a reservation setting while others reside within the larger community, different individuals face a varied pressures. As a result, no one strategy of recovery is likely to be universally applicable to all Native Americans.

An appropriate method (or metaphor) for promoting recovery among Native Americans is sorely needed. This technique must be able to transcend the differences that exist between a wide range of Native cultures, while mitigating the socioeconomic pressures that Natives collectively face. Among these impacts are (1) profound encroachments by the dominant culture, (2) economic hardship, (3) the generally reduced status of Native Americans within the mainstream world, (4) being subjected to a ubiquitous process of cultural genocide/the conflict of being caught between worlds, and (5) the relentless undercutting of the cultural traditions that usually bind people together and provide meaning and significance to life.

Therapists and clients often attempt to meld a program of recovery with aspects of the traditional culture. Although recognizing that all cultures can and should evolve and that individual people need to respond to circumstance, counselors and clients should not forget the negative power of unmitigated social change. Both therapists and clients, furthermore, need to recognize that cultures, although evolving, can maintain themselves and continue to function. This is true, even though specific individuals simultaneously have a niche in both the mainstream world and in traditional culture. It is equally vital to remember that when individuals have a niche and a stake in two different (and potentially competing) communities, conflict and stress are likely to develop.

Encouragingly, cultures often respond to challenges in a positive and constructive way, and continue to be a powerful force in people's lives. By recognizing that mental health tends to be nurtured by a strong cultural underpinning, both therapists and clients are reminded of the role that a person's heritage and traditions play in promoting good mental health.

This [reading] deals with that reality by using the example and tools of a nineteenth century Iroquois leader, Handsome Lake, a man who overcame alcoholism while simultaneously helping his culture to adjust to changing times—and, thereby, revitalize itself.

The Caldron of Handsome Lake

The Iroquois of New York State and Ontario, Cananda are (and long have been) an impressive people and a powerful and proud nation. Without the aid of White leadership, the Iroquois created a complex government; some observers even suggest that documents like the Declaration of Independence and the

United States' Constitution were influenced by the example of the Iroquois. If makes no difference if these speculations are fact or legend; in any event, the Iroquois are a complicated nation that has achieved greatness and deserves our respect. The fact that the Iroquois have suffered hard times in recent centuries does not cast a shadow on these achievements.

In the colonial era, the British and the French were competing for control of what is now Ontario, Canada and western New York. Up through and including the French and Indian War, the Iroquois were able to manipulate the situation and enjoy the prosperity that resulted. Good things, unfortunately, do not last forever:

> With the victory of the British in the War with France the Iroquois found themselves outflanked, no longer able to play off the British and French against each other and surrounded by a circle of British forts. (Wallace, p. 442)

When White military leaders no longer needed their Native allies, the situation of the Iroquois declined and the generosity of the British dwindled.

When the Revolutionary War began, the Iroquois again became embroiled in a conflict that was larger than their world. Being caught in the middle (since much of the fighting took place on Iroquois territory), they had to decide which side to support. Realizing that the British wanted Iroquois territory merely for trading purposes and fearing that many Whites would migrate into Iroquois land if the revolution were successful, most Iroquois sided with Britain.[2]

Although the decision to ally with the British was a reasonable choice, it was costly:

> [During the war, the Iroquois homeland] was devastated by the John Sullivan [United States military commander] expedition in 1778, which in a three-pronged offensive managed to burn the houses and the crops in almost every major Iroquois town. Many of the women and children, and the surviving warriors, took refuge at Fort Niagara with the British, who housed them in a refugee camp, inadequately clothed, inadequately fed, inadequately sheltered, and swept by disease. By the end of the war, despite their military successes, the Iroquois population had been cut approximately in half. (Wallace, p. 443)

The war took a terrible toll on the Iroquois, both in the cost of human lives and when viewed in political and economic terms.

After the war, the victorious United States, remembering that the Iroquois had been their enemies in the battle for independence, showed them few favors. As the Iroquois leaders had predicted, furthermore, hordes of White settlers were attracted the area. By the turn of the nineteenth century the Iroquois were beaten in war, decimated by diseases brought by the Whites, and besieged by social and economic rivals.

2. As a nation, the Iroquois did not have a pro-British policy; instead individual groups were allowed to make their own decision regarding the war. Most, however, sided with the British.

The results of this unenviable situation include infighting, personal resignation, and retreat. As is often the case under such circumstances, dysfunctional behavior (including alcoholism) became rampant.

Noted anthropologist, Anthony Wallace observes that many examples of what therapists and psychiatrists recognize as pathological behavior existed; they include rampant violence, uncontrolled weeping and pining, fear of peers (as evidenced by accusations of witchcraft), social disunity, and, widespread alcoholism. Clinical depression was commonplace and Wallace observes that when people were sober, they were likely to be suicidal (1970, 196–201).

Anomie: The Pain of Social and Cultural Disruption

Looking at the situation faced by the Iroquois of the late eighteenth/early nineteenth century, the telltale signs of traumatic social change and cultural disintegration are obvious. These processes, in turn, went hand in hand with an epidemic of alcoholism. Handsome Lake, a forceful Iroquois leader, provides a classic example of that syndrome as well as a demonstration of how the cultural heritage of a people can be instrumental in recovery. The case of Handsome Lake and the Iroquois, furthermore, are hardly exceptions to the rule; indeed, the sociological concept of anomie has long dealt with the disruption and pain caused by social change. It is useful, therefore, to discuss the process of anomie, as distilled by social theorists such as Robert Merton, before dealing with Handsome Lake as a specific example of alienation/alcoholism and readjustment/recovery.

Discussed in layman's terms, anomie has sometimes been equated with "normlessness," although a more theoretical definition indicates that it:

> signifies the state of mind of one who ... has no longer any sense of continuity, of folk, of obligation. The anomic man has become spiritually sterile, responsive only to himself, responsible to no one. (MacIver, 1950, p. 84)

As a result, individuals who experience anomie become alienated and cut off from their heritage. As Dressler observes:

> To put it allegorically, the anomic individual has lost his past, foresees no future and lives only in the immediate which is virtually nowhere. (Dressler, 1969, p. 251)

According to Robert Merton, a major twentieth century social theorist, a key cause and source of anomie is a disparity between the goals that society gives to people and the means of achieving them; when this unhealthy situation arises, anomie is the likely result (Merton, 1957, pp. 121–194). Specifically, Merton argues that the mores and norms of a society provide its members with goals to which they should aspire, on the one hand, and socially acceptable methods for achieving these goals, on the other. Over time, however, the culture (or the socioeconomic milieu in which it exists) may change to such a degree that its members are no longer able to achieve sanctioned and honored goals in a socially acceptable manner. It goes without saying that the plight of the Iroquois in the late eighteenth/early nineteenth century placed them in such a situation.

Merton went on to suggest that when people cannot achieve their goals in socially acceptable ways, the propensity for deviant behavior increases. Thus, mainstream upper middle class people (who have a relatively good chance of achieving their goals in socially acceptable ways) tend to act in accordance with cultural norms, even though some may resort to "white collar crime." Those in less fortunate circumstances, in contrast, are more likely to embrace some sort of deviant response. Members of minority groups and those who are members of cultures that are out of step with the dominant hierarchy (such as Native people who largely embrace their traditional heritage and/or have not mastered "mainstream ways") are particularly likely to act in deviant and/or dysfunctional ways. That was the precise response exhibited by many Iroquois in the late eighteenth/early nineteenth centuries. Many Native people from throughout the world are currently responding in a parallel manner.

The concept of anomie continues to be a useful concept. Representative applications of the concept have been used to explain the formation of teenage gangs (Cloward & Ohlin, 1960; Jankowski, 1991), to explore deviance in seventeenth century Puritan society (Erikson, 1966), and to explain "moral panics" in contemporary Great Britian (Jenkins, 1992). The concept of anomie is one of the keystone theories of social change and deviant behavior and it tends to be commonly used in research that deals with these phenomena. In addition, the concept of anomie has been used to describe the plight of people who, like many Native Americans, are members of hinterland or ethnic/cultural enclaves.

Nonetheless, a cultural heritage typically has the ability to serve, protect, and nurture individuals. As Walle has observed when discussing the impact of economic development upon such populations:

> Ultimately, culture helps people cope with the stresses of "future shock" and rapid social and economic transformations.... [By adopting] a social structural approach ... [it is possible to be aware] that changes in one area of a culture typically trigger other transformations which may be both unanticipated and negative. [A strong traditional culture can mitigate these impacts]. (Walle, 1998, pp. 182–183)

Thus, while individuals may suffer from anomie due to circumstances that are beyond their control, a strong and vital cultural tradition can help to mitigate these negative forces. If the culture is weakened and not functioning in a coherent way, however, it will lose its ability to help people cope with the struggles and challenges they face.

In situations where cultural traditions have been significantly undercut and/or where they are unable to help their members to cope with the problems faced, individuals may begin to act in counterproductive ways. Of special interest to us here is Merton's category of "retreatism" that he presents as one response to anomie. Merton observes that retreatism occurs among people who embrace both the goals of society and the proscribed methods of achieving them, but are unable to succeed in socially accepted ways. Merton suggests that retreatists include hermits, the mentally ill, and *alcoholics, and drug abusers.*

Thus, when the culture (or the circumstances within which the culture operates) no longer provides an appropriate avenue for personal achievement and self-respect, the result is likely to be retreatism, a response that often plays itself out in substance abuse.

Many Native Americans appear to be locked into this hurtful situation societies. The inability of these people to succeed in ways that reflect their traditional culture leads some Native Americans to retreat from society. Drug and alcohol abuse are specific types of retreat. As a result, some substance abuse among Native Americans can be viewed as a response to anomie caused by stresses upon or a breakdown of the traditional culture.

As is common knowledge, many Native Americans have experienced a profound breakdown in their traditional cultures and, on many occasions, no alternative has emerged to fill the void. This is exactly the kind of situation where anomie is predicted to develop and where retreatist responses are likely to lead to substance abuse. Such perspectives coincide with current trends in substance abuse therapy that see a connection between feelings of helplessness and a tendency towards dysfunction. Thus, Lance Dodes, best known for his *Heart of Addiction* states:

> Virtually every addictive act is preceded by a feeling of helplessness or powerlessness. Addictive behavior functions to [mitigate the] ... underlying feeling of helplessness.

In presenting this point, Dodes emphasizes that working to eliminate feelings of helplessness is the key to recovery. Stanton Peele (1992), mirroring Dodes, notes that alcoholics often describe their addiction as a form of "self-medication" that helps them to cope with the pressures of life. Peele, as Dodes, believes that substance abuse is a way of dealing with situational stress and tension.

As can be seen, the concept of anomie deals with the impacts of social change and the disruptions that it causes in people's lives. One specific response to the pressures of anomie is retreatism (withdrawing from the world). According to Merton, alcohol abuse is often a form of retreatism that can be explained as a response to anomie. Many Native Americans who suffer from alcoholism appear to have fallen victim to this kind of counterproductive response to social change and alienation.

The Recovery Continuum of Handsome Lake: An Overview

The story of Handsome Lake is a saga of cultural decay that led to dysfunction and alcoholism, on the one hand, and a return to sobriety and cultural rebirth, on the other. By examining these two different aspects of the Handsome Lake story, it is possible to make some useful observations about anomie and alcoholism and relate them to the circumstances faced by contemporary Native people.

The story takes place among the Iroquois of the late eighteenth/early nineteenth century, a society that, as described above, had suffered grievously due to defeat, disease, cultural disruption, and social change. Because of their situation, the Iroquois suffered from the pain of anomie and they responded in typical ways including a high incidence of dysfunctional behavior. In specific, alcoholism ran rampant.

Within this setting of defeat and despair, Handsome Lake, a once respected member of Iroquois society, had fallen into the abyss of ungoverned alcoholism. Out of control and seriously ill, it appeared that his productive life was over. By the spring of 1799, his drinking and its impacts had grown steadily worse:

> Handsome Lake ... was bedridden, reputedly ... as a consequence of prolonged alcoholic access. (Wallace, 1978, p. 445).

In the June of that year:

> Handsome Lake collapsed ... in the presence of his daughter ... he appeared to have died, but actually he was in a trance state and was experiencing the first of a series of visions in which messengers of the Creator instructed him in his own and his people's religious obligations. (Wallace, pp. 445)

After his recuperation from apparent death, Handsome Lake emerged as a new man, and one who dedicated his life to personal sobriety and to the cultural rebirth of Iroquois society.

Eventually these visions (and Handsome Lake's insights regarding them), were synthesized into a new strategy by which the Iroquois (both as a culture and as specific individuals) could stem their decline.

On the one hand, Handsome Lake encouraged his people to embrace their cultural traditions. The late eighteenth and early nineteenth century had devastated the Iroquois and their culture was in a state of complete disarray. In the midst of this chaos, Handsome Lake forcefully championed his culture, its traditions, and the nobility and worth of the Iroquois heritage.

This embrace and championing of Iroquois culture, however, was not merely envisioned as paying homage to the past. Handsome Lake clearly recognized that if Iroquois society was to be revitalized it would have to transform itself in line with the realities of contemporary life. Thus, Iroquois men had long been hunters and warriors and they left farming to women, viewing it as an unmanly and shameful profession. When White people migrated into Iroquois territory, however, new methods of farming (that included men performing their share of the work) began to outstrip Iroquois farming techniques. As a result, these newcomers further undercut the Iroquois economy. Under these circumstances, Handsome Lake encouraged Iroquois men to take up farming and he urged them to perceive agriculture as a legitimate profession that should not be a source of shame or embarrassment.

In his discussions of anomie, Robert Merton has pointed to "innovation" as one possible response to an environment in which people cannot achieve their goals in socially acceptable ways. It must be noted, however, that Merton was referring to a relatively stable culture and, therefore, he depicts innovation as an illegitimate means of success (such as criminal behavior.) Antisocial or not, embracing the innovation may provide better opportunities for success and, therefore, can help to eliminate the ravages of anomie.

In the case of Handsome Lake, he took illegitimate behaviors (men farming, as a prime example) and transformed them into acceptable and honorable pursuits. As a result of the innovations that Handsome Lake advocated, Iroquois society found itself in a better position to respond to the circumstances faced in the early nineteenth century. It is easy to see the value of Handsome Lake's solution; he offered an alternative to cultural decline and poverty. Providing an option to retreatist responses (such as alcoholism), Handsome Lake offered an innovative alternative that led to a positive cultural rebirth and a firmer economic foundation for Iroquois society.

Handsome Lake coupled the embrace of traditional Iroquois culture (albeit adjusted to circumstance) with an insistence that people cease pursuing activities that were disruptive and dysfunctional. Drinking alcoholic beverages was high on the list of banned behaviors.[3] Being an alcoholic himself, Handsome Lake was well aware of the dangers of alcohol and he strongly discouraged the use of alcoholic beverages. Although Handsome Lake's position is more extreme than that of Alcoholics Anonymous (since Alcoholics Anonymous sees no reason for successful social drinkers to abstain), this response seems to be closely akin to the American temperance movement that was taking root during the nineteenth century and which ultimately flowered into the legalized prohibition movement of the early twentieth century. In addition, Mormonism (another highly successful religion that emerged at approximately the same time and the same location as that of Handsome Lake)[4] places a similar ban on alcoholic beverages. Apparently both White and Native American reformers from Western New York in the early nineteenth century were aware of the devastating impact of alcohol on both individuals and society; as a result, they urged tight controls.

Having embraced and updated his cultural traditions and choosing to abstain from dysfunctional activities, including alcoholic drinking, Handsome Lake insisted that people acknowledge their past errors, sins, and wayward ways in order to refrain from similar misdeeds in the future.

Largely through the example and the message of Handsome Lake, the Iroquois people were able to stem their downward spiral of decline and to reemerge as a vital cultural entity. As a result, many Iroquois who had suffered from alcoholic behavior were able to enjoy what we now call "recovery" (reclaiming their lives through spiritual growth coupled with abstinence.)

This, in a nutshell, is the history of the heritage and legacy of Handsome Lake. His story is recorded in various places[5] and the reader is encouraged to consult both primary and secondary sources for more details about his life, his bout with alcoholism, the accomplishments after his recovery, and the revitalization of Iroquois society that resulted from his leadership.

The Path of Handsome Lake

Having provided an historic overview of the life and contribution of Handsome Lake, it becomes necessary to distill his vision and his achievements into a useable set of principles that are appropriate for therapy.

3. Others include promiscuous sexual behavior and the practice of witchcraft that was also disruptive to society and (according to Iroquois beliefs) injurious to specific people.
4. Handsome Lake was born in Avon, New York and promoted his antidrinking position in the early nineteenth century. He died in 1815 and the Long House religion, which is based on his teachings, began to flower in its present form around 1830. The Mormon religion first became an organized force in the 1830s (Joseph Smith, founder of the religion, reports he had a vision from God around 1820 and that in 1827 an angel helped him locate some manuscripts that became sacred Mormon texts. The religion was formally established in April 1830). This preliminary work of Joseph Smith in establishing the Mormon religion took place in and around Palmyra, New York, within easy reach of Handsome Lake's birthplace.
5. Important primary sources include A. F. C. Wallace's (1952) "Halliday Jackson's Journal to the Seneca Indians"; Thomas S. Abler's (1989) *Chainbreaker: The Revolutionary War Memoirs of Govern Blacksnake*, and Arthur C. Parker's (1913) *The Code of Handsome Lake*. The most extensive (and respected) secondary work is A. F. C. Wallace's (1970) *The Death and Rebirth of the Seneca*. William Fenton and Elisabeth Tooker's (1951) "On the Development of the Handsome Lake Religion" is also insightful. It should be noted that there is an extensive research tradition on Handsome Lake and this is only a suggestive sampling. For those in the counseling profession, however, it is probably adequate.

The model I have distilled will be called the "Path of Handsome Lake." Although the words used are not precisely those of Handsome Lake, the basic message and the way in which it is presented clearly reflect his vision. They form a suggested program of therapy that stems from one of the most revered and influential Native American reformers.

This path, as suggested by Handsome Lake, consists of six components that combine cultural health with individual well-being. It stresses that dysfunction and alcoholism can be overcome by simultaneously focusing on both cultural and individual concerns. Not only were Handsome Lake's methods effective among the nineteenth century Iroquois, they provide a means of combating dysfunction in today's world. The suggested "Path of Handsome Lake" includes:

1. ***Embrace tradition***: "I possess a culture and a tradition. Embracing them is sacred, meaningful, and joyful."
2. ***Transform your tradition to keep it strong***: "All cultural traditions change and all cultural traditions are under attack. I will strive to help my culture evolve and flourish."
3. ***Stop alcohol/substance abuse***: "I will break the cycle of personal and cultural decay by ceasing to abuse alcohol."
4. ***Admit to errors made***: "I recognize my past errors and I will remember them when choosing a more noble and fulfilling path."
5. ***Do not repeat errors of the past***: "Having chosen a more noble and fulfilling path, I will strive to keep my errors in the past and correct them as soon as they occur."
6. ***Heritage and recovery***. "My heritage and my traditions give me a spirituality. By ignoring my heritage and my traditions, I am denying my own self and I may become vulnerable to relapse. By embracing, my heritage, I can better succeed in recovery and in life."

As a useful device, I have culled a six-fold path from the teachings of Handsome Lake in order to affirm how he combined a concern for a healthy society with strategies designed to overcome personal dysfunction. This process goes hand in hand with strengthening and nourishing the cultural, its heritage, and traditions.

Comparing the Path of Handsome Lake and Alcoholics Anonymous

In many ways, the Path of Handsome Lake and the Twelve Steps of Alcoholics Anonymous are parallel. Indeed, these two programs of recovery are in general agreement in many ways. Alcoholics Anonymous, however, does not deal with various issues that are of concern to Native people who are faced with profound cultural stress and disruption. This void seems to be the result of the fact that Alcoholics Anonymous was the product of relatively successful (aside from their alcoholism) middle class White men who were firmly a part of the dominant culture of their era. These individuals, as a group, do not appear to have been victimized by the impact of rampant social/cultural change and anomie (even though they lived through the Depression). Thus, Alcoholics Anonymous was not formed by people who were likely to be suffering from anomie and it does not dwell on the specific issues that impact people who are the victims of the kind of circumstances that triggers retreatism.

Alcoholics Anonymous, however, is not inherently at odds with using the Path of Handsome Lake as a tool of recovery. As a result, although Native people who are suffering from alcoholism can clearly benefit from Alcoholics Anonymous, they may need to devote supplemental attention to the fact that their cultures are under profound attack from pressures that are beyond their control.

Table 1.3.1 compares the Path of Handsome Lake method with those of Alcoholics Anonymous and the Twelve Steps program.

The Path of Handsome Lake and Alcoholics Anonymous Compared

Path	Discussion	Compared With AA
1. ***Embrace tradition***: "I possess a culture and a tradition. Embracing them is sacred, meaningful, and joyful."	People often need to be reminded that they are members of social and cultural traditions that profoundly impact them in both overt and covert ways.	The founders of AA did not think in terms of specific cultural traditions and envisioned their program as universal. They however, did not rule out other programs.
2. ***Help keep traditions strong***: "All cultural traditions change and are under attack. I will strive to help my culture evolve and flourish."	Helps people to understand how cultures may be under attack and that both individuals and the collective society should work to strengthen cultural ties.	The founders of AA do not think in terms of cultural stress, the fact that cultures evolve, or the impact of social stress upon alcoholic behavior.
3. ***Stop alcohol/substance abuse***: "I will break the cycle of personal and cultural decay by ceasing substance abuse."	It is vital to deal with both the individual and the cultural impacts of substance abuse. While substance abuse is an individual disease, it also has cultural causes and implications	AA embraces the disease concept of alcoholism and emphasized that to successfully restructure their lives, total abstinence is essential. The impact of substance abuse upon others is recognized
4. ***Admit to errors made***: "I recognize my past errors and I will remember them when choosing a more noble and fulfilling path."	Under the influence of substance abuse, many individuals act in shameful, careless, or hurtful ways. It is necessary to acknowledge this potential and make amends as appropriate.	Steps 4 through 9 of the 12 Steps of AA specifically deal with recognizing the errors of the past and atoning for them.
5. ***Do not repeat errors of the past;*** "Having chosen a more noble and fulfilling path, I will strive to keep my errors in the past and correct them as soon as they occur."	Developing a pattern of appropriate and noble behavior is essential for both the health of the culture, the recovering individual, and the people with whom the recovering individual interacts.	Step 10 of the 12 Steps of AA recommends that people maintain a vigilant guard against error and to immediately atone for errors when they do occur.

The Path of Handsome Lake and Alcoholics Anonymous Compared

6. ***Heritage and recovery.*** "My heritage and my traditions give me a spirituality. By denying them, I deny my own self and I may become vulnerable to relapse. By embracing, them, I can better succeed in recovery and in life."	The concept of anomie suggests that personal alienation and/or cultural decay can lead to substance abuse. As a result, recovering people will be less prone to relapse if their culture is a powerful force that is able to provide them with support.	The founders of AA did not specifically deal with the impact of the larger culture upon the health of the individual recovering person.
Discussion	The Path of Handsome Lake and the methods of Alcoholics Anonymous and its 12 Step Program dovetail and do not conflict with one another. The Path of Handsome Lake, however, is better able to deal with the impact of cultural stress upon substance abuse and the need for people to be attuned to their cultural traditions.	

The Landmarks and Their Purpose

While the Path of Handsome Lake links personal recovery to cultural health, the Landmarks of the Path introduces more concrete goals and specific targets of action. While the Landmarks do not replace the Path, they provide a method of following its guidelines.

As with the Path of Handsome Lake, the Landmarks of the Path can be presented as a six-step process. These steps include:

1. "We recognize who we are."
2. "We acknowledge that our heritage, culture, and traditions are our strength."
3. "We reject the vulnerability that comes from ignoring our roots."
4. "We realize that others may have their own traditions and we respect them."
5. "We understand that strength that comes from embracing ourselves, not retreating from challenges."
6. "Handsome Lake's example and advice may be useful to all who face personal disruptions."

In this manner, the Landmarks provide a systematic way of addressing the needs of Natives whose drift into substance abuse may be the result of an alienation from their heritage. Each will be briefly discussed.

1. We recognize who we are

In general, progress results when people recognize who they are and act accordingly. People, however, are very complex and are made up of many bits of personality, character, and past experience. Some of these categories may include negative traits (such as a personal vulnerability to substance abuse). People are both individuals and part of a heritage or culture. And they may be torn between different goals, motives, and rival cultural traditions. These are issues that need to be confronted in a positive and constructive way. Native people are often strongly influenced by their cultural origins, even if they are not aware of it. As a result, it is important for Native people to consider the importance of their cultural heritage and think in terms of it.

As people seek recovery, they need to understand who they are. By possessing this vision of their identity, the influences impacting them, and their potentials for the future, people are better able to meet the challenges of life. And overcoming substance abuse is one of the greatest battles anybody will ever fight.

2. We acknowledge that our heritage, culture, and traditions are our strength

Not only do people need to understand who they are and the fact that their Native heritage is a big part of their identity, they also need to recognize that their ethnic identity can give them strength, power, and purpose. A strong and positive cultural connection is a powerful asset even if it is often ignored. Forgetting a cultural identity and thinking it has little effect can prove to be very hurtful.

Those who recognize their cultural identity can avoid be blindsided by failing to understand how their culture is part of them and how it impacts the way they think, feel, and behave.

3. We reject the vulnerability that comes from ignoring our roots

As Native cultures have been drawn into the mainstream world, there has been a tendency for people to ignore their roots. When this happens, Native people are likely to deny their cultural heritage and experience alienation, pain, and sorrow. Doing so can trigger dysfunctional behavior, such as substance abuse. Developing an awareness of their cultural traditions and making them a more conscious part of their lives can be important tools of recovery.

Having recognized the power and importance of their heritage, the value of self-reflection becomes all the more obvious. By rejecting the vulnerability that comes from ignoring their heritage, people can make progress.

4. We realize that others may have their own traditions and we respect them

Cultural traditions touch people in very personal ways. As a result, those from different cultures are apt to experience their own feelings, motives, goals, strengths, and weaknesses. Nonetheless, people who band together in search of recovery often come from different backgrounds. This is true in the mainstream world as well in programs of recovery that are geared around the special needs of Native people. Even specific Native traditions (such as the Athabascan, people of Alaska) are made up of many subgroups that are distinct from each other in significant ways. It is important to develop an appreciation of (and if necessary a tolerance for) other peoples and their way of life. Various programs of recovery attempt, in their own way, to deal with the fact that people band together to combat substance abuse.

People are products of their own heritage; it provides them with a distinct way of being human. Other people, in contrast, have their own traditions. Learning about, acknowledging, and celebrating diversity is important and empowering. It is also essential if different people are to work together for their common well being.

5. We understand that strength comes from embracing ourselves, not retreating from challenges

If people are to put their lives in order, they need to accept themselves for who they are. A part of this identity involves the degree to which Native people fit into the mainstream culture. While the larger world (and people's place within it) may need to be acknowledged and embraced, this represents only a part of personal identity. Aspects of the mainstream world, however, are often more obvious to people than their traditional cultural heritage.

Rapid change takes a hurtful toll. I am reminded of the term "future shock" that was coined by Alvin Toffler many years ago. Toffler noted that modern society is in such a rapid state of change that people, raised in one era, must live in world that has quickly become profoundly different. As a result, people become alienated. Toffler, of course, was inspired by the anthropological idea of "culture shock" in which people entering a foreign society often face stress, confusion, and dysfunction. Native people, of course, are often simultaneously impacted by both future shock and culture shock. Their world is changing quickly and their cultures are often being overpowered by alien ways of life. It should come as little surprise that many Native people exposed to these pressures suffer from substance abuse and other dysfunctions.

By re-embracing their traditions, people can gain the strength they need to meet the problems of life. By understanding and accepting who they are, people can better employ the tools that their culture provides and use them to combat their problems.

Those suffering from substance abuse often drink and drug in order to retreat from the challenges they face. On many occasions, Native people are confronted by crises linked to the fact that their cultures are in a state of disarray and/or because they are not adequately attuned with their heritage. An antidote for these problems is to for people to accept their cultural heritage and work to embrace and strengthen it.

6. Handsome lake's example may be useful to others who face personal disruptions

Programs of recovery typically point to the value of helping others. When people are given a second chance in life, they often want to share their good fortune. While they should do so in a nonforceful and nonjudgmental manner, helping others is beneficial both to the giver and the receiver.

This program is built on developing personal and cultural self-awareness. It suggests that if people better understand who they are and why they respond in the way they do they can better cope with their the pressures of life.

Handsome Lake challenges people to live a sober and moral life. He also emphasizes that this goal can best be achieved when people develop an awareness of, culturally, who they are. Native substance abusers seeking recovery can benefit from Handsome Lake's example and the advice he gives. All people, furthermore, can benefit from acknowledging who they are and by using that reality as a stepping stone toward recovery.

By embracing their cultural heritage and by understanding its impact, recovering substance abusers can gain valuable tools of sobriety. By ignoring their traditions, in contrast, profound triggers to dysfunctional behavior can easily remain unaddressed and sources of strength may remain untapped. The Landmarks are presented in Table 1.3.2.

Landmarks of the Path

Landmark	Significance	Discussion
Recognize who we are	People in recovery need to understand their strengths, weaknesses, and identities.	Although AA's Twelve Steps program focuses on strengths and weaknesses, it does not deal with cultural identities.
Acknowledge power of culture	Recovering people often need to acknowledge their cultural identity and what it impacts.	If people are unaware of their cultural identity, they might not totally understand themselves.
Transcend alienation	When cultures are weakened or ignored, people can become vulnerable to substance abuse. By strengthening these traditions, dysfunction can be attacked	The dysfunctional behavior resulting form alienation can be reversed by strengthening and embracing the culture.
Respect other traditions	Other people possess cultures and traditions that are meaningful to them. These heritages deserve the respect of others.	Recovery often takes place alongside those from different cultures. Understanding and honoring different cultures are important.
Embrace ourselves	Since cultural identity is a crucial part of personality and character, people need to become consciously aware of it and its power.	By better understanding their personality, character, and cultural origins, substance abusers can better restructure their lives and recover.
Many can benefit	Because ignoring a cultural identity potentially impacts all people, those from many different cultures can benefit from following the Path of Handsome Lake.	Many people, some more than others, have suffered grievous impacts from rapid cultural change. They can benefit from this program.
Discussion	The Landmarks of the Path provides a means of applying the Path of Handsome Lake. It can also be used to gauge the degree to which progress is being made. It focuses the power and significance of the cultural heritage and it seeks to unite people of different traditions while acknowledging their distinctiveness.	

Viewed in this way, the Landmarks of the Path emerges as a specific set of strategies that people can employ to rebuild their heritage, affirm their connection to it, and live a productive and fruitful life as they recover from substance abuse. While the Landmarks is not the Path suggested by Handsome Lake, it does provide clues, suggestions, and orientations on how to follow it.

Handsome Lake and Recovery

This [reading] views the example of Handsome Lake as a model of recovery for Native people. Handsome Lake personally dealt with issues concerning the decay and rebirth of cultural traditions and their impact on substance abuse (and other dysfunctional behaviors.) He developed a strategy of recovery centered on cultural issues that transcends, while not totally eclipsing, other therapeutic methods. By taking cues directly from the life and teachings of Handsome Lake, a method tailored around the needs of Native substance abusers who have been impacted by social disruption and anomie is proposed.

Predating, but in complete agreement with modern theories of sociology such as anomie, Handsome Lake recognized the impact of cultural stress on dysfunction. Aware of this connection, Handsome Lake understood that the recovery of the individual and the viability of society go hand in hand. Given this reality, he affirmed that cultures should embrace their traditions and heritage while adjusting them to mesh with existing circumstances. By combining sobriety with appropriate cultural and personal strategies, he provided a path to recovery.

Essentially Handsome Lake:

1. Recognized that pain and suffering are caused by profound and unmitigated social change;
2. Advocated preserving traditions, on the one hand, while updating them to they can function effectively, on the other; and
3. Linked recovery to cultural strength coupled with individual effort.

These perspectives dovetail with many of the components of the Twelve Steps program of Alcoholics Anonymous and Narcotics Anonymous that urge personal responsibility, penance, and ongoing vigilance. Embracing these principles expands beyond generic programs of recovery by dealing with cultural issues.

Guidelines for Counselors and Therapists

A basic premise of this [reading] is that generalized programs of recovery (such as Alcoholics Anonymous/Narcotics Anonymous and the Twelve Steps method) are currently being augmented by specialized alternatives that deal with the specific needs of specific people. Among Native people, alternatives are sorely needed because mainstream, generic programs like Alcoholics Anonymous/Narcotics Anonymous were created without any specific reference to the impact of massive cultural stress and its hurtful impact on people.

The Handsome Lake method deals with these cultural issues by expanding beyond generic programs, on the one hand, while simultaneously dealing with profound and often disabling impacts of social change, on the other. The resulting self-help strategy can be fruitfully employed by Native people who seek to recover from substance abuse.

A benefit of this program is that it acknowledges the impact of social stress while helping people to (1) cope with these pressures and (2) restructure themselves and their cultures in order to deal with the challenges that are faced. Because the founders of the Twelve Steps program were members of the dominant culture of their era, they do not deal in a forceful manner with cultural stress and disintegration. As a result, although the Twelve Steps program is useful, it does not provide a full answer to substance abusers whose cultures are experiencing profound stress, decay, and disruption.

Handsome Lake, in contrast, clearly understood how cultural stress can trigger dysfunctional behavior. As a result, his work and example suggest a self-help program that can be linked to cultural renewal. Because many indigenous people face cultural stress, they will benefit from a program that recognizes and responds to these pressures.

Beyond Native Americans

While Native Americans are distinct in many ways from other Native and traditional people, the stress and pressures exerted on their cultures are mirrored by the experiences of many other ethnic enclaves that are confronted by the outside world. Thus, Harold Napoleon (1996), a Yup'ik (Native Alaskan ethnic group) has noted the hurtful impacts of cultural decline and he has independently suggested strategies of recovery that parallel the suggestions of Handsome Lake. Although these two Native leaders lives 200 years apart and worked independently of each other, the similarities between them represent independent inventions that have been triggered by parallel conditions.

Among Native Hawaiians and the Maori of New Zealand, furthermore, profound similarities also exist. Thus, as Salzman (2001) emphasizes:

> Old Hawaiian customs, previously bonded together by ancient Polynesian beliefs, now fractured by the overthrow of the traditional religion were collapsing at all levels. As a result of the understandably bewilderment, Hawaiians plunged to a new low. (p. 177)

The responses of Native Hawaiians to this trauma also parallel those of the Iroquois. Unprecedented stress resulted in a breakdown of society. Cultural disintegration, however, is currently being mitigated by an embrace and revitalization of the Native culture, on the one hand, while adjusting it to prevailing/unavoidable conditions on the other. As a result, a pattern of substance abuse and eventual recovery that is similar to that exhibited by the Iroquois has been noted.

The parallels between the nineteenth century Iroquois and the Maori of New Zealand are even more striking. As Gilgen (1996) observes:

> There are many similarities between (Native American and Maori) experiences.... A disproportionate over-representation in the prisons, abhorrent statistics regarding disease and health issues, dismal failure of the educations al system, and the highest ratio of unemployed people in the country. (p. 52)

Gilgen continues:

> My ancestors were traumatized by a great death, a period in which Maori culture was attacked physically, spiritually, and culturally through disease, land confiscation, inter-tribal warfare, and the introduction of alcohol and non-indigenous religions. To deal

> with the rape of our land and culture, we also used a range of coping mechanisms that included self-blame, alcohol abuse, violence among ourselves, depression, suicide, and denial. (p. 52)

These conditions and responses, of course, closely resemble the situation of the nineteenth century Iroquois. The independently invented means of overcoming such circumstances, furthermore, was a form of cultural renewal that parallels the suggestions of Handsome Lake.

Native people throughout the world need to recognize that, although they come from different cultural traditions, many individuals and Native societies are unified by negative impacts triggered by the dominant culture. The ways in which Native people have responded to these challenges, furthermore, have tended to include inappropriate and counterproductive responses (such as substance abuse.)

Different Native peoples can learn from each other regarding how to cope with the impacts of the outside world. In doing so, they can combine their experiences in order to formulate appropriate coping mechanisms and strategies of recovery. As a first step in this important process, the example of Handsome Lake's leadership among the nineteenth century Iroquois demonstrates how cultural renewal and personal recovery can coincide with each other.

It is hoped that the example of Handsome Lake will encourage substance abuse counselors who deal with Native people (as well as the clients themselves) to more effectively deal with the issue of cultural stress and its impact on substance abuse.

Appendix: A Note on Handsome Lake's Partisan Nature and its implication

While recalling the recovery of Handsome Lake and using it as a metaphor is useful, remembering that his life and his work also had a more circumscribed and controversial component is equally important. His teachings and vision, for example, led to the establishment of the "Long House" religion that combines long-established Iroquois traditions with socioeconomic strategies that meshed with the needs of the times. As is often the case, furthermore, the innovative strivings of one generation are apt to become the conservative force of stability in the next. Indeed, the Long House tradition of today (the lengthened shadow of Handsome Lake's vision) tends to be embraced by the more traditional or orthodox element of Iroquois society. Thus, in the contemporary world, Handsome Lake's Long House religion represents a specific set of circumscribed principles embraced by the socially conservative Iroquois, while the more "liberal" or "progressive" segments of Iroquois society are often at odds with those who hold such beliefs.

Here, of course, I have no interest in entering into any debate regarding the pros and cons of the contemporary Long House religion and its vision for the future of Iroquois society. Ultimately, the Long House religion has been established for almost 200 years and it has evolved on its own since the death of Handsome Lake. My goal is merely to emphasize that in the early nineteenth century Handsome Lake recognized that his culture was under profound attack. Faced with these attacks, he forged a way to preserve his traditions, on the one hand, while adjusting them to prevailing circumstances on the other. Handsome Lake, furthermore, clearly saw a link between a healthy society and personal sobriety.

Faced with rampant alcoholism among his people, he called for tight restrictions on alcohol and he was personally able to live a model life of recovery. Largely through his efforts, the Iroquois people reversed their downward plunge and reaffirmed their place as a proud Native nation.

References

Christopher, J. (1992) *How to stay sober: Recovery without religion.* Buffalo, New York: Promethus.

Christopher, J. (1997). Secular organizations for sobriety. In J. H. Lowinson, R. B. Ruiz, R. B. Milman, & J. G. Langrod (Eds.), *Substance abuse: A comprehensive textbook.* Baltimore: Williams and Williams.

Cloward, R. A., & Ohlin, L. E. (1960). *Delinquency and opportunity: A theory of delinquent gangs.* Glencoe, IL: Free Press.

Dodes, L. (2002). *The heart of addiction: A new approach for understanding and managing alcoholism and other addictive behaviors.* New York: Harper Collins.

Dressler, D. (1969). *Sociology: The study of human interaction.* New York: Alfred A. Knopf.

Erikson, K. T. (1966). *Wayward puritans: A study in the sociology of deviance.* New York: Wiley.

Fenton, W., & Tooker, E. (1951). On the development of the Handsome Lake religion. In W. N. Fenton (Ed.), *Symposium on local diversity in Iroquois culture.* Washington, DC: Bureau of American Ethnology.

Hovarth, A. T. (1997). Alternative support groups. In J. H. Lowinson, P. Ruiz, R. B. Millman, & J. G. Langrod (Eds.), *Substance abuse: A comprehensive textbook* (pp. 390–396). Baltimore: Williams and Wilkins.

Jankowski, M. S. (1991). *Islands in the street: Gangs and American urban society.* Berkeley: University of California Press.

Jenkins, P. (1992). *Intimate enemies: Moral panics in contemporary Great Britain.* New York: Aldine de Gruyter.

Kirkpatrick, J. (1978). *Turnabout: Help for a new life.* New York: Doubleday.

Kirkpatrick, J. (1990). *Stages of the new life program.* Quakertown, PA: Women for Sobriety.

MacIver, R. M. (1950). *The ramparts we guard.* New York: Macmillan.

Merton, R. (1957). *Social theory and social structure.* New York: The Free Press.

Napoleon, H. (1996). *Yunaraq: The way of being human.* Fair-banks: Alaska Native Knowledge Network.

Parker, A. C. (1913). *The code of Handsome Lake.* New York: State Education Department.

Peele, S. (1992). *Truth about addiction and recovery.* New York: Simon & Schuster.

Salzman, M. (2001). Cultural trauma and recovery: Perspectives from terror management theory. *Trauma, Violence and Abuse, 2*(2), 172–191.

Trimpey, J. (1989). *Rational recovery from alcoholism: The small book.* New York: Delacorte.

Wallace, A. F. C. (1952). Halliday Jackson's Journal to the Seneca Indians. *Pennsylvania History, 19,* 117–147, 325–349.

Wallace, A. F. C. (1970). *The death and rebirth of the Seneca.* New York: Knopf.

Walle, A. H. (1998). *Cultural tourism: A strategic focus.* Boulder CO: Westview Press.

Walle, A. H. (2004). *The path of Handsome Lake: A model of recovery for Native people.* Greenwich, CT: Information Age.

Questions

1. What are the similarities/differences between the Handsome Lake method and AA's twelve steps?
2. How is the Handsome Lake method tailored to the specific needs of Indigenous persons given the extreme pressures (and threat of disintegration) that their cultures face?

End-of-Unit Questions

1. We learned about the shadow of race/ism and the ocean of white supremacy as well as about the long history of injustice by the medical establishment that people of color and Indigenous persons have faced in Eurocolonial societies. How does this affect the way we should conduct human research and think about the attitudes that marginalized racialized, ethnic, and Indigenous groups hold toward the medical establishment? What are some ways to contend with the race/ist history of our institutions of healthcare and medicine in order to build more just, inclusive, and humane institutions?
2. Would it be possible to improve your preferred moral theory by applying the lessons from this unit concerning the problems faced by persons marginalized because of their race, Indigeneity, and ethnicity? If yes, how can you refine your preferred moral theory to incorporate these lessons? If no, explain why not. (For example, if you're attracted to consequentialism, how can you develop a consequentialist approach to solving bioethical problems that effectively produces better consequences for marginalized racial, Indigenous, and ethnic groups?)

Unit II

The Specter of Ableism in Healthcare and Medicine

Introduction to the Unit

In this unit, we explore how bioethical issues are complicated when we center the perspectives/experiences of disabled persons. It aims to

- educate readers as to the meaning and significance of the concept of disability,
- give readers a sense of the systemic oppression that disabled persons face, and
- acquaint readers with some insightful solutions to the problems of healthcare and medicine that emerge from centering the perspectives/experiences of disabled persons.

The Varied and Holistic Nature of Disability

Disability is ethically important in part because there is no default way that humans move, understand, communicate, process, or exist (Imani, 2021, p. 77) and because disabled people form the world's largest minority (Ladau, 2021, p.

1).[1] Disabled people are not a monolith. There is great diversity in how disability is experienced and discussed both within and outside the disability community.[2]

As disability rights and inclusion activist and speaker Imani Barbarin explains, disability is "a holistic experience, so it must have a holistic definition." It is not merely a physical diagnosis, "but a lived experience in which parameters and barriers are placed upon our lives because of a physical diagnosis" (cited in Ladau, p. 9). Accordingly, disability activist and speaker Rebecca Cokley defines **disability** in an expansive and empowering way as "a lens that crosses all communities and centers on the health implications and infinite creativity of a people subjected to ableism" (cited in Imani, 2021, p. 78). Here, ableism is an interpersonal and structural form of discrimination faced by disabled persons that we will unpack below. Disability then can be understood both

- as a relationship to the conditions of ableist oppression, and
- as a lived experience that consists of surviving within and navigating that oppressive system.

It is important to keep in mind that this definition is one that comes from disabled persons themselves. As Imani notes, this stands in contrast to many institutional definitions, such as the one from the CDC (2020): "Any condition of the body or mind (impairment) that makes it more difficult for the person with the condition to do certain activities (activity limitation) and interact with the world around them (participation restrictions)." By centering the perspective of disabled people, we see that this definition gets things backward: disabled people are restricted *not* by their disabilities but rather by an ableist society (one that is designed to accommodate only abled people). Abled people are ones who are already accommodated within the oppressive system of ableism. That is why they are seen as those who "move, communicate, process, and exist in ways that society views as acceptable or even as the default" (Imani, 2021, p. 78).

We can flesh out our comprehension of disability by surveying different models/understandings of disability.

Models of Disability

Tragedy Model

Disability—impairment that is tragic and inherently involves loss

This common ableist model[3] sees disabled people as objects of pity from internalized ableism. It can

1. As of 2021, Ladau notes that there are more than one billion disabled people around the world (2021).
2. This variety is embodied in there being no one right way but rather two main ways of referring to disability: person-first language (persons with disabilities) and identity-first language (disabled persons), usage of which varies between and across different communities (Imani, 2021, pp. 84–85).
3. I owe these models to Imani (2021, Chapter 4), who gives a more complete treatment.

be seen at play when disabled people are treated as inspirational or heroic because they "overcome" their disability (e.g., Stephen Hawking).

Economic Model

Disability—impairment that affects productivity

This is an ableist and classist model that equates human value with economic productivity and fails to recognize that

- everyone inherently has value and deserves respect, and
- *productivity* and *functionality* are relative terms (people are productive in different ways, e.g., helping manage emotions vs. generating more raw materials vs. effectively communicating information).

Individual Model

Disability—impairment that the individual is to deal with

Although this model can positively emphasize the autonomy of disabled persons, it is often used to perpetuate ableism by measuring disabled people against each other (on the basis of how much they sacrifice) and trying to show that other disabled persons can "make it" if they try hard enough.

Medical Model

Disability—biological impairment to be diagnosed and treated or "cured"

This common model can be helpful in providing a way forward with diagnoses and/or treatments of disability if available (e.g., diagnosing ADHD or developing prosthetics), but its inherent treatment of disabled persons as needing to be fixed or cured has dehumanizing implications. In biomedical contexts, people tend to default to this model. However, it is essential to remember that it is not the only model available.

This model has been used by **eugenics**, a violent ideology that holds that there are "good genes" and "bad genes" in the human species, and that the "bad genes" should be eradicated. Unfortunately, eugenicist ideology has been historically influential and has been used to harm many marginalized groups, including, marginalized racialized and ethnic groups, and disabled and LGBTQ+ people. Although it has been shown to be unscientific and harmful, eugenicist ideology recurs, is prevalent today, and needs to be combatted.

Social Model

Disability—biological (mental/physical) variation[4] + ableist nonaccommodation by social environment

4. Following Rashed's (2019) development and application of the social model of disability to madness.

This model (developed by disability scholars) stresses the interaction between social environment and the expectations of nonvariation in certain traits, explaining that disabled persons are not primarily disadvantaged by their bodies or physical diagnoses but by ableist ideologies and social and literal constructions within society (Imani, 2021, p. 81). The social model of disability should be front and center in our minds as we seek to cultivate more just institutions, ones that are less subject to the pernicious influence of ableism. Moreover, given the prevalence of the medical model in biomedical contexts, focusing on the social model can help us keep in mind a more inclusive alternative and thus can be an effective way of cultivating less ableist institutions of medicine and healthcare.

The Omnipresent Specter of Ableism

Ableism "is the systematic prioritization of abled people over disabled people and the resulting marginalization of disabled people" (Imani, 2021, 91). Ableism is a system of oppression that affects people's beliefs, sense of self, and the way we talk, and it is reinforced through the media, policy, and interpersonal and institutional contexts. As disability theorists and activists emphasize, *all* abled persons are (and should see ourselves as) merely temporarily abled. We were not abled when we were young, and we will not be abled at some point in the natural course of our lives. However, ableism erases this fact and leads to abled people forming their sense of self based on their abled status. This form of discrimination (which, like race/ism, comes in individual, institutional, and cultural forms) is pervasive in Eurocolonial capitalist societies. Some examples:

- Ableism manifests itself when disabled people are seen as "contributing less" and therefore as less worthy of respect and dignity, even though ableism itself restricts the ways that disabled people can contribute to society.
- Ableism is woven into negative figures of speech that most people don't even think about when they use them, such as "being blind to" or "falling on deaf ears."

If race/ism is a shadow cast by our Eurocolonial history that darkens every aspect of our social world, ableism is an ever-present (often invisible to abled persons) specter[5] that haunts every aspect of our social world, disproportionately harming disabled persons. This specter is an antagonistic organic unity over our social world, including the institutions of healthcare and medicine, that makes these institutions less valuable than the sum of their parts. It consists of ableist ideologies, institutions, and structures that unfairly accommodate and privilege (and thus create synergies in the lives of) abled persons and unfairly disadvantage (and thus create antagonisms in the lives of) disabled persons. This unjust distribution of synergies and antagonisms across dis/ability lines itself yields overall antagonisms in society because of the injustice and inefficiency of this unequal distribution of synergies and antagonisms. Much more can be, should be, and has been said (by disability scholars and activists) to articulate the aspects to this specter

5. This analogy can be found in the work of disability scholars (e.g., Campbell, 2009; Wiener, 2018).

and the myriad ways it harms everyone and disproportionately harms disabled persons.[6] But this initial discussion provides a critical lens for tackling social and bioethical problems, a lens that can be further articulated.

The Invisibility of Privilege

The invisibility of the specter of ableism and the systemic accommodation of abled persons to the exclusion of disabled persons make vivid an essential point about the nature of social privilege highlighted by Professor Peggy McIntosh: It is experienced as invisible, not as a privilege, but as the default, as just the way things are (2009).[7] As she eloquently puts it, privilege is "like an invisible weightless knapsack of special provisions, assurances, tools, maps, guides, codebooks, passports, visas, clothes, compass, emergency gear, and blank checks" (2009, p. 91). This point generalizes to all forms of social privilege, including heterosexual, cisgender, and abled privilege. Award-winning educator and philosopher Maureen Linker helpfully observes that we can help make sense of privilege/disadvantage using the metaphor of an E-ZPass (2015, pp. 68–70). Privilege is a social E-ZPass on the road to social rights and goods (e.g., environmental accommodation or the acceptance of your romantic partner). Disadvantage, in turn, is the lack of such a pass, which leads to experiencing expected and unexpected obstacles on the way to those same social rights and goods.

Our intersectional approach recognizes that privilege and disadvantage, like identity, are not additive or monolithic. We must accordingly recognize that different forms of social privilege and disadvantage can interact in complex ways in different contexts, given people's intersectional identities, in ways that produce complex experiences of privilege and disadvantage for them.

Intersectionality and Disability Justice

Our intersectional approach to bioethics requires us to emphasize the disability justice movement. As Sins Invalid[8] cofounder and executive director Patty Berne notes, "While a concrete and radical move

6. For example, ableism underpins other forms of discrimination, like race/ism and sexism, serving as an "organizing grounding principle" in the construction of asymmetric social categories like gender, race, class, and sexuality (Erevelles, 1996, p. 526). It erases much of the violence that disabled persons face, and it makes the visible violence they face seem justifiable (Mingus, 2018); it forces disabled people to navigate systems in isolation (Milbern, 2017); it infuses eugenics-laden sentiments—such as that disabled people create suffering—into our culture (Kurisato, 2018); it leads nondisabled activists of color to exclude or stop supporting disabled persons (Lakshmi Piepzna-Samarasinha, 2019, pp. 254–255).
7. This is arguably both because of how a lack of impediment is experienced but also, as Linker (2015) points out, because of what Professor Sarah Ahmed calls the "systemic unseeing" of social identity, in which the complex realities of social identity and inequality are "flattened into a narrative about individuals (not social systems) with good or bad attitudes (not systemic advantages and disadvantages)" (cited in Linker, 2015, p. 4).
8. Sins Invalid (https://www.sinsinvalid.org/) is a disability justice performance project that centers disabled persons facing multiple

forward, the Disability Rights Movement simultaneously invisibilized the lives of peoples who lived at the intersection of junctures of oppression—disabled people of color, immigrants with disabilities, queers with disabilities, people with disabilities who are houseless, people with disabilities who are incarcerated, people with disabilities who have had their ancestral lands stolen among others" (Berne, 2017). Berne rightly notes that the shadow of race/ism (and ocean of white supremacy) and the specter of ableism "are inextricably entwined," since they were "forged in the crucible of colonial conquest and capitalist domination" (Berne, 2017). Centering the experiences/perspectives of those who face multiple forms of oppression requires adopting not just a disability rights framework, but a **disability justice** framework. As writer, organizer, performance artist, and educator Leah Lakshmi Piepzsna-Samarasinha explains, "Disability justice centers sick and disabled people of color, queer and trans disabled folks of color, and everyone who is marginalized in mainstream disability organizing" (2019, p. 22). This approach reveals how ableism helps make other systems of oppression possible and how dismantling ableism "is part of social justice" (Lakshmi Piepzsna-Samarasinha, 2019, p. 22). Disability justice thus constitutes an intersectional framework for tackling ableism *together with* other systems of oppression, a framework that understands the interrelations between these systems and how they all "benefit from extracting profits and status from the subjugated 'other'" (Berne, 2017). We must therefore look out for the ways in which the shadow of race/ism, the specter of ableism, and other systems of oppression interact to harm people in layered, complex ways.

This unit's readings flesh out this intersectional approach and further articulate our critical lens for tackling bioethical problems faced by disabled persons in more informed and nuanced ways.

Unit Readings

The first reading nuances the bioethical issue of the physician–patient relationship by centering the lived experience of disabled patients. S. Kay Toombs (2004) reflects on her own experience as someone with chronic disability. She argues that the experience of chronic disability provides a significant opportunity for this relationship but that adequately negotiating it requires a shift from bodily well-being to personal well-being and that physicians regard patients as experts concerning what is "normal" in their own bodily experience.

The second reading examines the cultural labor and activism of the "Not Dead Yet" disability rights group (Ginsburg & Rapp, 2015) and how the group has shaped the way disabled persons imagine their social group as a whole. This arms the reader with a better understanding of how disabled persons experience their sociality. The authors build on their ethnographic work to argue that disability should be recognized as central to the human condition, spelling out lessons concerning the emergence and suppression of disability consciousness, the constant reinvention of the medical model of disability in

forms of marginalization. The organization challenge paradigms of normalcy and beauty and offer a vision of beauty and sexuality inclusive of all bodies and communities.

biomedical contexts, and the enormous implications of shifting disability demographics for the political economy of caretaking.

The third reading fleshes out this book's intersectional approach by centering the perspective of individuals who are marginalized because of the intersection of their race, disability, class, and gender. The authors' in-depth approach draws key lessons concerning

- the way people facing multiple forms of marginalization experience multiplicative oppression that puts them in danger of what critical race feminist scholar Patricia Williams calls "spirit murder" (cited in Erevelles & Minear, 2010, p. 143) because they are seen as having so little social and economic value to contribute to society and
- the role that disability ideology plays in oppressively organizing society throughout our Eurocolonial history and in today's capitalist society.

These readings all consider how centering the perspectives/experiences of disabled persons can help us better understand the problems faced by marginalized persons, as well as how doing so can help provide more nuanced approaches and solutions to social and biomedical problems.

References

Berne, P. (2017). Skin, tooth and bone—The basis of our movement is people: A disability justice primer. *Reproductive Health Matters, 25*(50), 149–150.

Campbell, F. A. K. (2009). *Contours of ableism: The production of disability and abledness*. Springer.

Centers for Disease Control and Prevention. (2020, September 12). *Disability and health overview: Impairments, activity limitations, and participation restrictions*. U.S. Department of Health and Human Services. Retrieved August 29, 2022, from https://www.cdc.gov/ncbddd/disabilityandhealth/disability.html

Erevelles, N. (1996). Disability and the dialectics of difference. *Disability & Society, 11*(4), 519–538.

Erevelles, N., & Minear, A. (2010). Unspeakable offenses: Untangling race and disability in discourses of intersectionality. *Journal of Literary & Cultural Disability Studies, 4*(2), 127–146.

Ginsburg, F., & Rapp, R. (2015). "Not Dead Yet": Changing disability imaginaries in the twenty-first century. In V. Das & C. Han (Eds.), *Living and Dying in the Contemporary World* (pp. 525–541). University of California Press.

Imani, B. (2021). *Read this to get smarter: About race, class, gender, disability & more*. Ten Speed Press.

Kurisato, M. (2018). They had names. In A. Wong (Ed.), *Resistance and hope: Essays by disabled people: Crip wisdom for the people*. Alice Wong.

Ladau, E. (2021). *Demystifying disability: What to know, what to say, and how to be an ally*. Ten Speed Press.

Lakshmi Piepzsna-Samarasinha, L. (2019). *Care work: Dreaming disability justice*. Arsenal Pulp Press.

Linker, M. (2015). Intellectual empathy: Critical thinking for social justice. University of Michigan Press.

McIntosh, P. (2009). White privilege and male privilege: A personal account of coming to see correspondences through work in women's studies. In S. Shaw and J. Lee (Eds.), *Women's voices, feminist visions: Classic and contemporary readings* (4th ed., pp. 91–98). McGraw-Hill.

Milbern, S. (2017). Reflections as Congress debates our futures. In A. Wong (Ed.), *Resistance and hope: Essays by disabled people: Crip wisdom for the people*. Alice Wong.

Mingus, M. (2018). Building back belonging, hope and possibility. In A. Wong (Ed.), *Resistance and hope: Essays by disabled people: Crip wisdom for the people*. Alice Wong.

Rashed, M. A. (2019). In defense of madness: The problem of disability. *The Journal of Medicine and Philosophy: A Forum for Bioethics and Philosophy of Medicine, 44*(2), 150–174.

Sins Invalid. (2022). *Sins Invalid*. Retrieved August 29, 2022, from https://www.sinsinvalid.org/

Toombs, S. K. (2004). "Is she experiencing any pain?": Disability and the physician–patient relationship. *Internal Medicine Journal, 34*(11), 645–647.

Wiener, D. (2018). Review of the book *Resistance and hope: Essays by disabled people: Crip wisdom for the people*, edited by A. Wong. *Wordgathering: A journal of disability poetry and literature*. https://wordgathering.syr.edu/past_issues/issue48/reviews/wong.html

"Is She Experiencing Any Pain?"

Disability and the Physician-Patient Relationship

S. K. Toombs

S. K. Toombs, "'Is She Experiencing Any Pain?': Disability and the Physician-Patient Relationship," *Internal Medicine Journal*, vol. 34, no. 11, pp. 645–647.

Editor's Introduction

In this reading, S. Kay Toombs provides nuance to our understanding of the ethics of the physician-patient relationship by centering the lived experience of disability. The author's experience as a chronic progressive multiple sclerosis patient with significant disability informs her reflection on these issues, allowing her to discuss unique challenges and lessons for the ethics of the physician-patient relationship. S. Kay Toombs, PhD is professor of philosophy emeritus at the Philosophy Department of Baylor University in Waco, Texas. She is the editor of the *Handbook of Phenomenology and Medicine*, an interdisciplinary handbook that explores the intersection of the philosophy of medicine, bioethics, and phenomenology (the study of the structures of consciousness and lived experience).

As a person who lives with chronic progressive neurological disease (multiple sclerosis) and significant disability, I have an intimate knowledge of the physician-patient relationship from the perspective of the patient. Over the years, I have become aware that chronic disability poses unique challenges in the clinical context—challenges that, if unrecognized, can unwittingly undermine even the most well-intentioned efforts to provide optimal care.

In reflecting on these challenges, I want to begin by stressing that chronic disability means much more to the patient than simply a mechanical dysfunction or discrete disease pro cess. Living with permanent incapacity represents a distinct way of being-in-the-world, a way of being that affects one's sense of self, one's relationships with others, one's ability to interact in (and with) the surrounding world, one's family and professional life, one's ability to exercise control and to be autonomous, and one's relationship with one's body.[1] Given the chronic nature of such bodily disorder, it is not possible to restore the patient to a former state of health characterized by the absence of bodily malfunction. Consequently, the clinical goal must be broadened to encompass not only the cure of disease but, as importantly, the project of assisting patients to live well in the face of ongoing bodily limitation. An important way to conceive this project is to focus on personal (and not simply bodily) well-being. By functioning well at the personal level, I have in mind such things as being able to engage in activities that are meaningful, sustaining important relationships, and retaining a sense of personal integrity.

In stressing personal, as opposed to bodily, well-being, it is important to make a sharp distinction between the functioning of the body and the functioning of the person. The prevailing biomedical model of illness and the overriding focus on physical pathology gives priority to the well functioning of the physical organism—with the assumption that if the body functions well so does the person. In the case of chronic disability, this assumption is deeply problematic. For example, quantitative measurements of disability, in and of themselves, do not convey whether a patient can function well at the personal level. In my own case, functioning well at the personal level does not depend on whether I can walk, although it does relate to my ability to manage my illness in such a way that I can pursue those projects that are meaningful to me.

Focusing primarily on assessments of physical functioning as the most accurate measure of wellness can paradoxically disrupt the task of functioning well at the personal level. Patients and medical professionals alike might be tempted to pursue medical interventions that are extremely disruptive of the patient's life and that result in minimal improvement in bodily function. I learned this lesson personally when undergoing a course of chemotherapy in an attempt to slow down the progression of my disease. The treatment was worse than the illness. Monthly infusions of Cytoxan (cyclophospamide; Bristol-Myers Squibbs, New York, NY) caused nausea, vomiting and prostrating weakness for three of every four weeks. After four months, I chose to discontinue the treatment on the grounds that it totally disrupted my life. Although my neurologist supported my decision, he voiced disappointment and pointed out that tests

1. Toombs SK. Reflections on bodily change: the lived experience of disability. In: Toombs SK, ed. *Handbook of Phenomenology and Medicine.* Dordrecht, The Netherlands: Kluwer Academic Publications; 2001:247–261.

indicated a slight improvement in my ability to lift my right leg. However, for me, this minimal gain in physical function was not worth the erosion in my quality of life.

Weighing the harms and benefits of treatment is more difficult for those living with chronic disability. If one has an acute disease, one knows that the disruption of treatment will be short lived, with an end result of cure. Consequently, the certainty of future benefit enables one to "put up with" temporary discomfort, even if it is extreme. However, when future benefit is uncertain and disruption is ongoing, patients and physicians must take seriously the impact of therapy on the patient's quality of life. Even noninvasive tests can be particularly difficult for people with disabilities. As an example, for someone like myself with compromised bladder and bowel control, tests that involve drinking large amounts of fluids (or cleansing the gastrointestinal tract) can be especially burdensome.

Physical barriers also make testing difficult for people with disabilities. A survey in the United States showed that women with severe disabilities are less likely to receive annual pelvic exams than able-bodied women, and 23 percent of women with spinal cord injuries reported that it was impossible to have a mammogram, either because the equipment could not be positioned for them or because there was no accessible room for mammograms.[2] Indeed, very few doctors' offices have accessible examining tables, which makes even a routine physical examination problematic for someone who uses a wheelchair.

One of the most debilitating aspects of chronic disability is the loss of bodily control. An important task for clinicians is that of assisting patients to develop concrete strategies to compensate for bodily limitation. It is vitally important that patients recognize there is always some level of control that one can exercise, even in the face of increasingly disruptive symptoms. This task is not limited to instituting medical treatment. Rather, it involves exploring with the individual patient the specific manner in which bodily malfunction disrupts his or her life at the personal level. In this connection, it is helpful not simply to ask patients specific questions, such as "Are you experiencing increased spasticity?," but to include more global inquiries, such as "What is the most difficult thing for you to deal with in your daily life?" Sometimes even simple strategies, such as controlling intake of fluids to minimize the risk of incontinence in social situations, learning to adjust daily schedules to compensate for fatigue, or acquiring mobility aids to counteract weakening muscles, can significantly improve a patient's quality of life. For example, if a patient is greatly fatigued by the effort of walking, using a wheelchair might conserve energy and permit increased social interaction, resulting in a much fuller personal and social life. In this respect, choosing to use a wheelchair is not to be equated with "giving in" to the disease. Rather, "giving up" in one area might well free the patient to embrace other important areas of life.

Of course, it is vital that physicians recognize the extent to which negative cultural attitudes make it extraordinarily difficult for people with disabilities to retain a sense of personal well-being in the face of permanent physical incapacity. We live in a culture that places inordinate value on independence, beauty, health, and physical fitness. People with disabilities are far from the ideal. In the eyes of the able-bodied, there is a widespread assumption that disability is incompatible with living a meaningful life. When others

2. Nosek MA, Howland CA. Breast and cervical cancer screening among women with physical disabilities. *Arch Phys Med Rehabil.* 1997;78(Suppl 5):S39–44.

observe I am in a wheelchair, they make the immediate judgement that my situation is an essentially negative one, that I am unable to engage in professional activities, and that I am wholly dependent on others. On many occasions strangers have said to me "Aren't you *lucky* to have your husband?" This is not so much a comment about my husband's character as it is a perception that my relationship with him is purely one of burdensome dependence. In observing my physical incapacities, people assume that my intellect is likewise affected. Strangers invariably address questions to my companion and refer to me in the third person: "Where would *she* like to sit?," "Would *she* like us to move this chair?" Such negative responses from others are demeaning and reinforce the sense that disability reduces personal and social worth. Unfortunately, such attitudes also exist in the clinical context. In a national survey, women with severe disabilities reported that if they were accompanied by another person, more often than not the doctor addressed questions to their companion rather than speaking to them directly (Nosek *et al.* unpubl. data 1992, 1995): "Is *she* experiencing any pain?"

An important way for physicians to promote personal well-being is to consciously reject such stereotypical attitudes about persons with disabilities. Indeed, patients with chronic disabilities have an especially important role to play in the physician-patient relationship. Those of us who live with permanent bodily disorder have an intimate knowledge of our bodies as we must constantly pay attention to them. Thus, we are often aware of even minute changes in function and sensation (changes that might not be readily apparent to the physician). Although physicians have the expert medical knowledge to comprehend and assess the disease pro cess, patients with chronic disabilities have an equally expert knowledge of what is "normal" and "abnormal" with respect to their own bodily experience. Both types of knowledge are essential to the task of assessing and dealing with bodily disorder. People with disabilities are also experts at knowing how best to work with their recalcitrant bodies—a knowledge that is too often disregarded by medical professionals. As an example, Robillard (a quadriplegic) describes his frustration when trying to tell X-ray crews how to position his body to avoid muscle and coughing spasms, only to be ignored and informed erroneously that (as professionals) they "knew what they were doing."[3]

In conclusion, I would like to stress that, although chronic disability poses specific challenges, it also provides a significant opportunity in the doctor-patient relationship. The shift in focus from bodily to personal well-being (a shift that involves exploring with patients the multiplicity of ways in which ongoing disability impacts on their daily lives) and the necessity of including the patient as an active participant in the long-term management of a chronic condition provide an exceptional occasion for clinicians to forge close and rewarding partnerships with patients.

3. Robillard AB. *The Meaning of Disability: The Lived Experience of Paralysis.* Philadelphia: Temple University Press; 1999.

Question

1. Toombs discusses how the ethics of the physician-patient relationship is complicated by centering the experience of persons with disability in a way that requires a shift from bodily to overall well-being and centering the patient's expert knowledge of "normalcy" in their body/lived experience. What are some concrete ways in which a healthcare provider can focus on overall well-being and take seriously a patient's expert knowledge of their own body/experience?

"Not Dead Yet"

Changing Disability Imaginaries in the Twenty-First Century

Faye Ginsburg and Rayna Rapp

Editor's Introduction

This reading examines the Not Dead Yet disability rights group and how their cultural labor and activism have been crucial to changing people's imaginaries about disability (i.e., the values, symbols, institutions, and laws, through which disabled people interpret their social group as a whole). It draws on ethnographic work by the authors to examine the dynamics of disability imaginaries and relate them to the human life cycle, our evolving concept of "normal," and issues of social justice.

The authors' discussion builds on their ethnographic work on disability across the lifespan and considers the topic of disability in multiple domains and sectors of everyday life. Faye Ginsburg, PhD is director of the Center for Media, Culture, and History and Kriser professor of anthropology at New York

University. Her research interests include social anthropology, ethnography of media, social movements in the United States, and disability. Rayna Rapp, PhD is a professor and associate chair of anthropology at New York University whose research interests include gender and health, the politics of reproduction, and disability.

But I'm not dead yet!!

Monty Python and the Holy Grail

Not Dead Yet (NDY) is a U.S.-based disability rights group founded in 1996 that opposes euthanasia and assisted suicide. The group—establishing its credentials for ironic and deadpan humor—takes its name from the scene quoted above in the film *Monty Python and the Holy Grail,* in which plague victims are thrown onto a cart and hauled off to be buried. A man dumped on a pile of corpses protests that he is "not dead yet!!" but his cries are ignored as the tumbrel rolls on in a Pythonesque moment of gallows humor. Not Dead Yet offers noisy opposition to "deadly forms of discrimination against old, ill and disabled people... [and] demands the equal protection of the law for the targets of so called 'mercy killing' whose lives are seen as worthless" (Drake 2013).

We start our [reading] with the case of NDY to highlight the cultural labor and activism that have been crucial to changing the disability imaginary in America (and elsewhere) beginning in the late twentieth century, when the presence of disability in public life became increasingly visible. A central part of these conversations has to do with who is entitled not only to the rights of citizenship, a watershed accomplishment of legislation in the United States and elsewhere, but to life itself, whatever supports that might require.

Not Dead Yet is one of many social formations that make up the evolving American "disability world" that we have been studying over the last decade, starting with questions about how knowledge (or ignorance) of disability enters into prenatal diagnosis decisions (R. Rapp 2000; Ginsburg and Rapp 1999). Later, as parents of children with disabilities, we began an exploration of how children have come to be classified for special educational services. They currently represent 13%–15% of the nation's students; in New York City, where we focus our work, the number is 17%. We became particularly interested in how families, schools, clinicians, scientists, media makers, and activists have all been reimagining both domestic and public life around that social fact. As we follow children, families, and projects over time, we have expanded our framework to encompass questions of disability as they are imagined and organized over the life cycle (R. Rapp and Ginsburg 2011, 2012; Ginsburg 2012).

In 1999, Not Dead Yet made headlines through its demonstrations against Peter Singer, an Australian philosopher hired by Princeton University, whose writings support infanticide of disabled newborns. Not inclined to pull punches, NDY labeled him "the most dangerous man on earth" (Hari 2004). In the twenty-first century, NDY activists amplified their dissent, becoming increasingly visible during high-profile controversies about living and dying with disabilities. In 2004, for example, the group protested the removal of Terri Schiavo's feeding tube,[1] as well as the message of the movie *Million Dollar Baby,* in which the injection of an overdose of adrenalin to euthanize a suicidal woman rendered quadriplegic from a boxing accident is depicted as a compassionate act. Not Dead Yet's unruly and disruptive protests underscore the dark edge of the current zeitgeist, illuminated by their activism on behalf of people with disabilities. The questions of life and death that these eruptions pose—infanticide for profoundly disabled newborns, the complex issues raised by long-term life support, the popular cinematic portrayal of a "preference" for death over living with disability—are unquestionably part of contemporary social life. Yet they build on a history in which assumptions about the appropriateness of ending the lives of those with what were then considered severe disabilities were widely accepted as part of the heritage of eugenic thinking.

The Long Shadow of Eugenics: The Doubled Telos of Modernity

Our opening examples emphasize that issues of living and dying related to disability are "not dead yet"—always in conversation with a long trajectory of debate on vexed issues of medical intervention, stigma, and social isolation. Indeed, the present-day disability rights movement is haunted by—and protesting against—the legacy of eugenic ideas and resulting social policies that in the early twentieth century made their way from the United Kingdom to the United States to Germany and then resonated across the globe. These clashing perspectives—of eugenics and disability rights—represent what we have elsewhere labeled the doubled telos of modernity (R. Rapp and Ginsburg 2001). By this we mean that the democratizing impulse toward the inclusion of disability is inevitably in tension with what may be considered its opposite: the drive toward perfectibility that fuels much recent culturally seductive neoeugenic medical innovation and intervention. These seeming antinomies, we argue, are foundational to the complex biopolitics that shape living and dying in the current era. We suggest that the intensity and salience of disability in contemporary public discourse, whether repressed or embraced, flows from the fact that disability is a category that any of us might enter in a heartbeat, or over the slower course of the debility that comes if we are lucky enough to live on into old age. As disability activists frame it, we are all only "TAB": temporarily able-bodied. Whether Foucauldian, Freudian, or Freirian, this [reading] is deeply indebted to that perspective and the recognition it demands of the existential fragility of all bodily states and the consequent deep need for human interdependence across the life course. The "disability world" profoundly rejects the reduction of impairments to a medical model. Our perspective is in harmony with our editors' concerns to show how life and death are not "polar opposites but intensities that wax and wane and are co-present in all life events."

1. Terri Schiavo was a young woman who at age twenty-seven, in 1990, suffered a cardiac arrest resulting in massive brain damage. She was put on prolonged life support and continued to live in a persistent vegetative state. Her husband's wish to terminate life support for her was challenged by Schiavo's parents; she stayed on life support due to state and federal legislative intervention until 2005, when life support finally was terminated. The controversial case became a public social drama attracting strong opinions and extensive multimedia coverage in support of both sides.

Indeed, as some of our subjects "aged out" of the school system into young adulthood, our own fieldwork expanded to encompass what has come to be understood as the crisis in transition. Schools have been compelled by federal and state law to meet the needs of all children, however imperfectly, regardless of disability. Once people with disabilities (PWDs) enter the world beyond the educational system, access to services, higher education, meaningful work, independent living, and caretaking needs is far less available, particularly for those at the lower ends of the socioeconomic spectrum. If demographic trends increase as projected—a point we address below—this situation will only intensify: the number of disabled citizens in the total U.S. population, currently estimated at 19%, will undoubtedly increase significantly over the next decade (Administration on Aging 2013).

As we have learned repeatedly in our research, the concept and experience of disability are always deeply entangled with changing family and kinship formations, state policies, caretaking economies, and forms of public culture that literally can shape life and death in North America and around the globe. Historians have played an important role in showing us how quickly attitudes toward disability can change from life enhancing to deeply discriminatory and even eugenic. Their scholarship reminds us, for example, that people with disabilities were proscribed from civic space across much of the twentieth century. Such practices were reinforced in the United States beginning in the 1860s, when the so-called Ugly Laws prohibited citizens with disabilities from appearing in public space, enduring in some states until the 1970s (Schweik 2009). Such prejudice against disability included the encouragement of passive infanticide and other eugenic ideologies in early-twentieth-century America that migrated to Nazi Germany, where murderous policies against people with disabilities (among other populations) escalated to genocide (Pernick 1996; Longmore and Umansky 2001). In much of the developed West, more mundane forms of institutionalized bias against disability persisted well after World War II, as families were regularly encouraged to institutionalize their disabled children "for their own good," despite the fact that in such settings, people suffered from neglect and abuse and were at times used as captive experimental subjects for medical trials (Stern 2005). Such practices and their life-threatening consequences were accepted as normative aspects of living and dying until the rising disability rights movement and other allied forces scrutinized and protested this kind of dehumanization that was being muffled by the language of medical expertise.

This kind of eugenic thinking, we argue, is "not dead yet" and continues to shadow the status of disability in the present in what we would call its neoeugenic form, over the life cycle from birth to death. As noted above, the philosopher Peter Singer's utilitarian argument that families should have the choice to euthanize severely disabled newborn infants is based on the hypothetical burden such children might place on parents' "preferences for happiness" (Singer 1993, 1995). His position has been widely challenged by disability rights activists as with the aforementioned case of the 1996 Not Dead Yet protests. In 2002, he engaged in a public debate with the late Harriet MacBryde Johnson, the high-profile disability rights activist and lawyer who lived until 2008 with a congenital degenerative neuromuscular disease. Their debate became the subject of a subsequent widely circulated *New York Times Magazine* cover story, "Unspeakable Conversations" (Johnson 2003). Johnson began her critique by sketching a primal family drama about living and dying imagined from Singer's philosophical perspective:

> He simply thinks it would have been better, all things considered, to have given my parents the option of killing the baby I once was, and to let other parents kill similar babies as they come along and thereby avoid the suffering that comes with lives like mine and satisfy the reasonable preferences of parents for a different kind of child.... As a shield from the terrible purity of Singer's vision, I'll look to the corruption that comes from interconnectedness. To justify my hopes that Singer's theoretical world—and its entirely logical extensions—won't become real, I'll invoke the muck and mess and undeniable reality of disabled lives well lived. That's the best I can do. (Johnson 2003)

Anthropologist Gail Landsman, drawing on her work on maternal care of disabled infants, offers another critique of the instrumentalism that Singer brings to the evaluation of the worth of human life when disability is involved. In contradistinction to Singer's assertion that "killing a disabled infant is not morally equivalent to killing a person" (Singer 1993, 161), Landsman takes his position as a point of entry "for analyzing the relationship among concepts of personhood, the transformative experience of mothering infants with disabilities, and the commodification of babies in North American culture" (Landsman 2004, 101). In her 2009 ethnography, *Reconstructing Motherhood and Disability in the Age of "Perfect" Babies,* Landsman analyzes changes in maternal narratives of sixty mothers with babies newly diagnosed with congenital disabilities over their first several years of adjustment. She shows how this group of mothers, using medical services in upstate New York, have struggled to transform the medical model that initially defined their children into a counternarrative of maternal and familial incorporation (Landsman 2009). In our own research among families in the New York City area with children with disabilities, we constantly encounter the construction of such "new kinship imaginaries." We use this term to describe the substantial sociocultural work that parents and especially mothers engage in to create alternative models of family life that creatively encompass life with a difference (R. Rapp and Ginsburg 2011). We note that these parental narratives are the foundation for more-public disability imaginaries as they emerge from the intimacies and injuries of familial life and into a range of media, from books and blogs to curricular innovation. They speak to the concerns of the editors of this volume to "capture the texture of contemporary life by showing how one becomes vulnerable to disease, accident, death, but also forms of institutional creativity and attentiveness to others in one's world, the formations and deformations of life and death."

Narratives of difference and their place in family life cycles can have profound and contested consequences. This is evident in cases that have emerged as public social dramas—notably, the case of so-called pillow angel "Ashley X," born in 1997 with static encephalopathy, a condition in which her brain does not develop. In 2004, anticipating the complexities of puberty for a vulnerable child, her parents requested and received permission from the bioethics board at their hospital for radical surgery that excised Ashley's breast buds and reproductive organs in order to control her growth. Their goal was to more easily manage her care at home as she grew older and larger. When this story became public in 2006 in an article in the *Archives of Pediatrics & Adolescent Medicine* (Gunther and Diekema 2006), this decision was subject to considerable scrutiny and critique by disability activists, medical professionals, and scholars alike (Battles and Manderson 2008; Kittay 1999, 2011). For example, bioethicist Arthur Caplan criticized what has come to be called the Ashley Treatment on national television, where it was discussed widely. His argument succinctly summarized the disability rights position: it is "a pharmacological solution for a social failure—the fact that American society does not do what it should to help severely disabled children and their families" (Caplan 2007). Others weighed in with more emotionally laden language: Not Dead Yet, together with Feminist Response in Disability (FRIDA), spoke of the treatment as a violation of Ashley's human rights, labeling it "invasive medical experimentation," "mutilation" and "desexualization." The Disability Rights Education and Defense Fund (DREDF) declared, "[W]e hold as non-negotiable the principle that personal and physical autonomy of all people with disabilities be regarded as sacrosanct" ("Ashley Treatment" 2013).

As the Ashley X debate renders evident, medical technologies are frequently embroiled in questions regarding living and dying with disability. Complex ethical questions are often framed in medical terms as they emerge in a variety of situations across the life cycle. Yet, this social drama and our research demonstrate that such a frame is too narrow: they need to be understood in the context of kin and community, the often substantial demands of caretaking, and the perspectives brought into view by disability rights activism.

Life, Death, and Assistive Reproductive Technologies

Of the many recently developed medical technologies, assistive reproductive technologies (ARTs) play one of the most prominent roles in discussions of living and dying in the context of disability, resurrecting older eugenic questions in new form. Since the 1970s, a burgeoning popular and scholarly literature has emerged, responding to the escalating panoply of genetic tests increasingly being used for "quality control" of anomalies present in both parents and fetuses (Adams 2012; Parens and Asch 2000). Such ideas have a complex resonance with the selective but worldwide uptake of ARTs and the choices placed upon pregnant women and their supporters as knowledge of fetal anomalies expands. Feminist disability scholars in particular have raised ethical issues about the cultural values that discourage the continuation of pregnancies when embryos or fetuses are diagnosed with genetic variances (Asch 2000; Kittay and Kittay 2000; Saxton 2000).

The growing need to incorporate disability inclusion perspectives—what we call the social fund of knowledge about what might be required to live with impairment—as a necessary part of reproductive testing (and consequently, potential abortion decisions) is more acute than ever. The case of a recently introduced ART, noninvasive prenatal testing (NIPT), is exemplary. This test, first used in 2011 and increasingly available, promises earlier diagnostic first-trimester information regarding "fetal anomalies" with a simple blood test that might lead directly to the choice to terminate a pregnancy. Right now, for the 75% of American women with access to standard prenatal care, routine screening blood tests in both the first and second trimesters tell a pregnant woman that she is at heightened or lower-than-average risk for carrying a fetus with a known impairment, but they do not provide a direct diagnosis. Those promoting NIPT tests claim that they can perform a direct diagnosis of fetal abnormalities significantly earlier and more accurately than can older forms of blood screening. Right now, however, NIPT can pick up only chromosomal conditions such as Down syndrome. Its capacity to diagnose a wider range of disorders at the level of DNA analysis, with consequences we may not yet clinically understand, is under investigation. As a result of its potential diagnostic strength, ease of delivery, and capacity to reach a much wider demographic, those working on NIPT make powerful, and potentially lucrative, claims to replace older forms of prenatal screening. With prior screening technologies, only women considered to be "at risk" went on to have their fetuses directly diagnosed. Now, as NIPT is becoming routinized as a replacement for prior screening systems, the goal of having *all* pregnant women tested relatively quickly radically expands the likelihood that many more women will encounter a diagnosis of fetal impairment and be faced with an abortion decision (Lo et al. 1998).[2]

The molecular science behind these new technologies is commercializing at a rapid rate. Moreover, new tests now pick up some anomalies that have unknown clinical significance. In such cases, women and their supporters will be faced with a decision to end or continue a pregnancy without understanding how a fetus with atypical genetic sequences might actually develop. Early studies suggest that virtually all who are involved, from medical staff to the women who receive the test, have very little comprehension of the serious consequences that this "simple blood test" may entail, even if the diagnosis is clear (Bernhardt et al. 2013; Sayres et al. 2012). Yet current market-driven techno-innovation threatens to muffle a necessary conversation about the ways that neoeugenic thinking is proliferating in routinized prenatal care, with abortion as the likely outcome of a "positive diagnosis." In other words, the range of conditions available for testing is increasing geometrically under market-driven conditions, but the fund of social knowledge accompanying such decision making—what it might be like to live with a particular disability—is woefully inadequate for a generation of women and their partners who face the dilemma of being "moral pioneers" in these intimate matters of life and death (Dollar 2012; Franklin and Roberts 2006; R. Rapp 2000; R. Rapp and Ginsburg 2007, 2012). The "choice" regarding who is admitted to the human community—with or without a disability—is officially placed on the shoulders of the family, assisted by emergent Foucauldian pastoral professions such as genetic counseling (Roberts 2009; Samerski 2009). Despite the fact that genetic counselors are trained to be "value neutral," some argue that the very existence of this technology and its routinized use assume that potentially disabled fetuses will be aborted, and thus suggest the need for more public awareness around these practices (Parens and Asch 2000).

Additionally, the aura of scientific expertise surrounding such testing obscures the limitations built into virtually all medical technology and procedures. As a result, people are particularly unprepared when they unexpectedly fall into the very small minority who receive a false negative diagnosis. This was the case of author Emily Rapp, whose child was born with an anomalous and fatal form of Tay-Sachs disease. As she explained in a blog post: "The prenatal test I took for Tay-Sachs was negative; our genetic counselor didn't think I needed the test, since I'm not Jewish and Tay-Sachs is thought to be a greater risk among Ashkenazi Jews. Being somewhat obsessive about such matters, I had it done anyway, twice. Both times the results were negative" (E. Rapp 2011).

Despite the rarity of her situation, the resulting ethnographic reality that Emily Rapp provides in her compelling account of parenting a child with Tay-Sachs is nonetheless instructive. Such cases are

2. The rollout of NIPT has already begun, with twenty-seven academic medical centers in the United States and several national health ministries in Western Europe testing these new diagnostic technologies on women deemed high risk who also receive amniocentesis and/or sonograms so that results can be compared.

particularly challenging for the creation of a "new kinship imaginary" in the face of a severely foreshortened life. In her influential 2013 memoir, *The Still Point of the Turning World,* Rapp writes movingly of what it's like to live with so truncated a horizon as a parent, and how that shifts her understanding of the deep humanity of caretaking: "How do you parent without a net, without a future, knowing that you will lose your child, bit by torturous bit? Depressing? Sure. But not without wisdom, not without a profound understanding of the human experience or without hard-won lessons, forged through grief and helplessness and deeply committed love, about how to be not just a mother or a father but how to be human" (2013, 11).

Although books chronicling parental grief over the loss of a child are a well-known genre, we single this one out because it serves as a cautionary tale regarding the imperfections of medical technology, and the entanglement of expectations of life and death that ensue when it fails. When books such as this are widely reviewed and subject to commentary (as was the case with Rapp's acclaimed account of a "genetic mistake"), they enter into our "cultural DNA," stimulating a renewed public conversation about life, death, and disability. Indeed, she chronicles the problematic consequences of the muting of such discussions. She writes about bristling "at the lack of information and resources for parents... involved in the daily grind of making the short lives of their children as full as possible for two, three, maybe six years at the outward reach" (2013, 12). Her words remind us that attention to medical and scientific arenas too often masks an important site of social significance: the creation of new cultural imaginaries that address the daily challenges of caretaking that some disabilities can require.

This is not to deny that medical technologies often offer life-enhancing possibilities, enabling the survival and inclusion of many people with disabilities who in the past might have died or lived under far more limited circumstances. These range from neonatal intensive care units (NICUs) to feeding tubes to breathing technologies and even antibiotics and antiseizure meds. Of course, the question of disability, its cultural location, and technological supports in resource-poor contexts where such interventions are rarely available raises other questions that we address elsewhere (Ginsburg and Rapp 2013).

In the developed world, for example, such interventions help sustain the lives of compromised infants, those with spinal-cord injuries, wounded soldiers, the frail elderly, and many others who have benefited from a range of techno-possibilities. Furthermore, turning eugenics on its head, the spread of disability consciousness has given greater support to couples with disabilities who choose to create families of their own, enhancing what the experience of disability means in both the contemporary moment and an imagined future (Finger 1999; O'Toole and Doe 2002).

Kinship, Caretaking, and the New Normal

As our [reading] thus far makes clear, the category of disability frequently escapes the confines of the medical, establishing the grounds for a "new normal." Disability imaginaries are constantly reinvented. They reverberate across multiple arenas, from the most intimate realms of sociality shaped by religion, kinship, and family life to schools, to housing, and to community-based forms of recognition. Other arenas in which disability issues are being reframed include a remarkably wide range of arts and letters, along with national legislative and juridical bodies, and international arenas such as the United Nations. These emerging cultural claims on inclusion, from pregnancy decisions to care for those dealing with extreme old age, bring new challenges to families and other intimates whose experiences of living and dying are necessarily shaped by the fact of disability, and the daily life adjustments it entails. In addition to the medical innovations discussed above, a range of seemingly mundane material alterations contribute to a sense of the "new normal" as incorporative of disability. These might include (among other things) the routinization of universal design in the built environment, the incorporation of service dogs, closed captioning and audio description for media, and a variety of other creative accommodations (Becker 1980; Cohen 1998; Layne 1996; Leibing and Cohen 2006: Livingston 2005; MacMakin 2011).

Such cultural shifts in thinking about living with disability—from kinship imaginaries and daily practices to legislative and judicial interventions—have taken place over the last half century. In particular, the relationship of people with disabilities to their natal families was redefined dramatically in the wake of the movement for deinstitutionalization in the 1970s that required households and families to accommodate unanticipated "returning" members. As a result, caretaking responsibilities in the household and the production of family narratives embracing rather than excluding the fact of disability have required continual creativity, and have moved cultural circuits beyond the intimacy of family life. This sort of "public storytelling" has worked its way into media of all sorts and in many parts of the world, ranging from personal memoirs and television shows to scholarly works that offer compelling perspectives on the "new normal" established by living life with a difference (Bérubé 1996; Frank 2000; Grinker 2007; Phillips 2009; R. Rapp and Ginsburg 2001).

A recent exemplary case of such cultural activism, Andrew Solomon's 2012 book *Far From the Tree: Parents, Children and the Search for Identity,* tells the collective story of over three hundred families whose children have a range of disabilities and differences such that they "fell far from the family tree" as it was once imagined. Solomon interviewed these parents over a period of ten years in order to understand their experiences of creating family life with children whose differences include deafness, Down syndrome, autism, dwarfism, schizophrenia, multiple congenital disabilities, criminality, transgender identity, being prodigies, and being children of rape. While these categories do not fit together seamlessly, collectively the stories enable Solomon to claim that such families are "united in our differences." As he writes on his book jacket, "Many families grow closer through caring for a challenging child; most discover supportive communities of others similarly affected; some are inspired to become advocates and activists, celebrating the very conditions they once feared." Although he doesn't name these activities as a dimension of caretaking, learning to enact a supportive kinship imaginary makes these cases compelling evidence of the possibilities of living life with a difference. The broad range of families that appear in his book, along with its enthusiastic public reception, illustrate a pervasive hunger for narratives that reflect the evidence of experience of "the new normal" as widespread.

A prominent theme in all these works is the significance and life-changing intensity of caretaking as an activity that frequently underscores the particular kind of interdependence that shapes the circumstances of life with a disability. Influential feminist philosophers Eva Kittay and Martha Nussbaum have taken an analytic approach to this topic, using it as an optic to examine the fundamental interdependence of social life. They argue that a recognition of caretaking—in its mundane as well as more extreme forms—is an often unarticulated requirement of real social justice. For example, Kittay attends to "love's labor" (also the title of her book); by this she means the often unrecognized, mostly unremunerated, and deeply gendered work of caring for family members whose disabilities render them profoundly dependent. Kittay's work was inspired by her experiences providing constant care for her daughter Sesha, born with severe cognitive impairment (Kittay 1999). She develops a sophisticated analysis of the gendered assumptions built into our kinship imaginary via a "dependency critique" of equality: "A conception of society viewed as an association of equals masks inequitable dependencies, those of infancy, childhood, old age, illness and disability" (xi). She champions the political and economic recognition of caretaking labor that human dependency requires and the particular nexus of interdependence that characterizes all family life. Her fellow feminist philosopher Martha Nussbaum (2006) also critiques theories of social justice built on notions of rational autonomous subjects. Speaking as a scholar and devoted aunt to a nephew diagnosed with both Asperger's and Tourette's syndromes, she advocates a legal philosophy that accounts for unequal capacity as well as human dignity. Nussbaum asks how we can best extend recognition and the rights of citizenship to those with profound mental and physical disabilities, appreciating that these capacities vary significantly for individuals across the life course. She writes of these instances with an exquisite sensitivity to the ways that legal theory and policy have consequences in daily life:

> Extreme dependency comes in many forms.... Washing the body of a child with Down Syndrome seems vastly easier to contemplate than washing the incapacitated and incontinent body of a parent who hates being in such a condition, especially when both the washer and the washed remember the parent's prime. So the way we think about the needs of children and adults with disabilities is not a special department of life, easily cordoned off from the "average case." It also has implications for the way we think about our parents as they age—and about the needs we ourselves are likely to have if we live long enough. As the life span increases, the relative independence many of us enjoy looks more and more like a temporary condition, a phase of life that we move into gradually, and which we all too quickly begin to leave. Even in our prime, many of us encounter shorter or longer periods of extreme dependency on others—after surgery or a severe injury, or during a period of depression or acute mental stress. (Nussbaum 2001)

The implication of Nussbaum's prescient discussion of not only everyday life but the vagaries of dependency over the life cycle helps "scale up" our analysis.

The eruption of disability into public consciousness in places like North America is linked to a transforming demographic reality that we ignore at our peril. A growing number of people are surviving who might not have in the past, from those diagnosed with life-threatening conditions as infants, to people of all ages living with disabilities however they were acquired, to the increasing longevity of people into extreme old age, with all the frailties that might entail. These social facts not only broaden the range of disability awareness but also raise difficult questions regarding both the daily life experience and political economy of care. Indeed, more and more adults with and without disabilities find themselves in the center of what we have come to call the "Intergenerational Vortex of Caretaking" (or IVoC) as kin demands extend across households and life cycles. The immediate recognition of this term as accurate, humorous, and dismaying among many of our respondents (who find popular terms such as *the sandwich generation* too anemic) suggests its resonance with the complexity of their lives as caretakers. A glance at national statistics makes clear that their domestic experiences are very much part of a broader social reality.

Disability and Demographics

In the demographic projections from the U.S. Census and accompanying studies, it is evident that the percentage of Americans with disabilities is both an expanding portion of the population and a growing absolute number. To give a rough sense of the scale, as of 2010, the U.S. Census estimates that there were fifty-seven million people with disabilities in the civilian noninstitutionalized population; they constitute 19% of the population. Approximately 15% of these are of school age (between four and twenty-one years of age) while 50% of adults over sixty-five (currently 12.4% of the population) are living with some form of disability, whether or not they comfortably embrace that label (U.S. Census Bureau 2012). By 2030, the elderly population of the United States is expected to grow to 19% of the total population, with significant consequences for the total number of disabled citizens potentially requiring care (Administration on Aging 2013; Knickman and Snell 2002).

The implications for the rapid growth of disability as a social category and its attendant consequences in terms of services and caretaking are clearly visible, for example, in the data on two conditions that emerge at different positions in the life cycle. Both have gained considerable public attention in twenty-first-century America: autism spectrum disorders (ASDs) and age-related dementia, particularly with the rise of "the new old age"—the issues that have emerged as many more of our elderly live beyond eighty-five years of age, and some well into their nineties. Together the numbers associated with these diagnoses indicate an escalating presence of disability in daily life, raising questions of caretaking and incorporation of difference into the body politic. A 2008 Centers for Disease Control and Prevention (CDC) study, based on school records, noted the increasing prevalence of ASDs since 2000; the numbers have almost doubled in less than a decade. This research estimates that one in eighty-eight children (aged one through eight) has been diagnosed with an ASD, one that generally requires considerable support (Hoffman 2013).

A more recent, 2011 survey by the CDC based on random telephone interviews shows an even higher incidence, "with parents describing 1 in 50 children as having significant social or other challenges" (CDC 2011). Whatever the correct number (and these are constantly contested figures), the implications for social support are clear. As autism expert Deborah A. Fein explained in response to the latter study: "We need to find ways of funding and providing help to these children" (quoted in Hoffman 2013). At the other end of the age spectrum, a recent report suggests that the number of people over sixty-five diagnosed with dementia will double by 2040, "skyrocketing at a rate that rarely occurs with a chronic disease" (Hurd et al. 2013). As Donald Moulds, acting assistant secretary for planning and evaluation at the federal Department of Health and Human Services, commented, "The long-term care costs associated with people with dementia are particularly high because of the nature of the disease. People eventually become incapable of caring for themselves, and then in the vast majority of cases, their loved ones become incapable of caring for them" (quoted in Belluck 2013). Dr. Michael Hurd (an economist and lead author of the study), speaking to the implications of this research, made clear that the costs go beyond the numbers, which, he explained "could not capture the full toll of the disease." In a refreshingly candid if sobering moment on the limits of disciplinary knowledge, Hurd offered an existential reflection on the implications of this study: "'One thing we haven't talked about, and it's not in the paper, is the tremendous emotional cost,' he said. 'Economists are coldhearted, but they're not that coldhearted'" (quoted in Belluck 2013).

Thinking Forward

These numbers provide powerful evidence of the significance of the study of disability for anthropologists and others. Despite the social and political progress that has been made toward recognizing full citizenship of people with disabilities in North America and beyond, for many this topic evokes the problems of marginalized identities. On the contrary, we argue that disability should be recognized as central to the human condition and also part of a tectonic shift in our overall social structure, with enormous implications for the political economy of caretaking.

Our ethnographic work on disability across cycles of living and dying is helping us to understand how new cultural imaginaries are emerging in many sectors of everyday life. Disability consciousness both erupts and is suppressed continually in many dispersed social locations in which questions of living and dying are never far from the surface. These include but are not limited to in vitro fertilization (IVF) clinics, mothers' groups, special-education classrooms, activist initiatives, and the popular realm of books, film festivals, television shows, and a mushrooming digital presence (Ginsburg 2012), not to mention the long-standing sites of doctors' offices and scientific laboratories, where the medical model of disability is constantly reinvented. While their connections are not always evident, collectively they demonstrate the complexity of the doubled telos of modernity we have identified in the cases we discuss in this [reading]. As we have followed our subjects and our topic across such multisited domains, we as anthropologists have come to appreciate how ubiquitous disability is as a social fact. The demographic statistics we cite are an instantiation in another register of this recognition. The numbers underscore what our ethnographic allies have been teaching us about their quotidian experiences with the differences that disabilities make.

In order to comprehend the impact of the upturn in numbers of Americans with disabilities throughout the life cycle, we have had to tack back and forth between the intimacy of qualitative interviews and observations that offer insight into their experiential reality, and the abstractions of population trends. Social policy needs to take both these levels of concern into account, yet qualitative knowledge drawn from the daily life is too frequently sidelined. As we carry out research that attends closely to living, dying, and disability, we feel compelled to pose questions that we hope anthropology can illuminate. Why is it that we rarely hear of disability in political debate, even when a vice-presidential candidate is carrying around a child with Down syndrome? What kinds of resources are implicated if we are committed to a world that embraces inclusion and the necessary supports for people with disabilities to live as fully as possible in their communities? This is a particularly complicated question to address in an increasingly neoliberal zeitgeist where public expenditures are constantly at risk. For example, day programs for the elderly with dementia are under siege coast-to-coast, while school systems are struggling to provide basic related services for children with newly diagnosed disabilities. At the same time, the initiatives of people with disabilities and their supporters are changing the face of both public and private culture, slowly but surely. Beyond accessibility ramps (Russell 2002), we now have many accommodations that were unimaginable even two decades ago: closed captioning on television, service dogs on buses and in courtrooms and department stores, programs for those with autism and Alzheimer's in museums, and adaptive technologies built into digital tablets—to mention a few relatively recent innovations. Given the inevitable increase in disability across the life cycle sketched in the demographic profiles above, we predict that the shape of the "new normal" will continuously be under constant negotiation. As the disability rights activists with whom we work have taught us, we all have skin in this game. The lessons we learn from embodied difference are certainly not dead yet.

Note

We thank Veena Das and Clara Han for calling this [reading] into existence and for their patience with delays resulting from our own adventures in disability worlds. We are grateful to the Spencer Foundation and the NYU Institute for Human Development and Social Change for their support of this work, as well as to the many people who generously shared their stories with us. We also want to acknowledge with gratitude the excellent bibliographic assistance of Dr. Alison Cool.

References

Adams, Rachel. 2012. "Looking for Suffering in All the Wrong Places." *Huffington Post,* May 9. Accessed September 25, 2012. www.huffingtonpost.com/rachel-adams/looking-for-suffering-in-all-the-wrong-places_b_1503069.html.

Administration on Aging. 2013. "Aging Statistics: Dept. of Health and Human Services." Accessed June 20, 2013. www.aoa.gov/Aging_Statistics/.

Asch, Adrienne. 2000. "Why I Haven't Changed My Mind about Prenatal Diagnosis: Reflections and Refinements." In *Prenatal Testing and Disability Rights,* edited by Erik Parens and Adrienne Asch, 234–60. Washington: Georgetown University Press.

"Ashley Treatment." 2013. Wikipedia. Accessed June 20, 2013. http://en.wikipedia.org/w/index.php?title=Ashley_Treatment&oldid=553142604.

Battles, Heather T., and Lenore Manderson. 2008. "The Ashley Treatment: Furthering the Anthropology of/on Disability." *Medical Anthropology* 27 (3): 219–26.

Becker, Gaylene. 1980. *Growing Old in Silence.* Berkeley: University of California Press.

Belluck, Pam. 2013. "Dementia Care Costs Are Soaring, Study Finds." *New York Times,* April 3. Accessed June 20, 2013. www.nytimes.com/2013/04/04/health/dementia-care-costs-are-soaring-study-finds.html.

Bernhardt, Barbara A., Danielle Soucier, Karen Hanson, M. S. Savage, L. Jackson, and R. J. Wapner. 2013. "Women's Experiences Receiving Abnormal Prenatal Chromosomal Micro-array Testing Results." *Genetics in Medicine* 15 (2): 139–45.

Bérubé, Michael. 1996. *Life As We Know It: A Father, a Family, and an Exceptional Child.* New York: Pantheon Books.

Caplan, Arthur. 2007. "Is 'Peter Pan' Treatment a Moral Choice?" Msnbc.com. Accessed June 20, 2013. www.nbcnews.com/id/16472931/ns/health-health_care/t/peter-pan-treatment-moral-choice/.

CDC (Centers for Disease Control and Prevention). 2011. "New Data on Autism Spectrum Disorders." Accessed March 4, 2015. http://www.autism.org.sg/resources/articles/CDC-Features-New-Data-on-ASD.pdf.

Cohen, Lawrence. 1998. *No Aging in India: Alzheimer's, the Bad Family, and Other Modern Thing*s. Berkeley: University of California Press.

Dollar, Ellen Painter. 2012. *No Easy Choice: A Story of Disability, Parenthood, and Faith in an Age of Advanced Reproduction.* Louisville, KY: Westminster John Knox Press.

Drake, Stephen. 2013. "Rochester Disability Community Remembers Disabled Victims of Domestic Violence, Deaf Victims of Euthanasia as Part of National Disability Mourning Day." February 27. Accessed March 3, 2015. http://www.notdeadyet.org/2013/02/rochester-disability-community-remembers-disabled-victims-of-domestic-violence-deaf-victims-of-euthanasia-as-part-of-national-disability-mourning-day.html.

Finger, Anne. 1990. Past Due: A Story of Disability, Pregnancy and Birth. Berkeley, CA: Seal Press.

Frank, Gelya. 2000. *Venus on Wheels: Two Decades of Dialogue on Disability, Biography, and Being Female in America.* Berkeley: University of California Press.

Franklin, Sarah, and Celia Roberts. 2006. *Born and Made: An Ethnography of Preimplantation Genetic Diagnosis.* Princeton, NJ: Princeton University Press.

Ginsburg, Faye. 2012. "Disability in the Digital Age." In *Digital Anthropology,* edited by Heather A. Horst and Daniel Miller, 101–26. London and New York: Berg Publishers.
Ginsburg, Faye, and Rayna Rapp. 1999. "Fetal Reflections: Confessions of Two Feminist Anthropologists as Mutual Informants." In *Fetal Subjects, Feminist Positions,* edited by Lynn M. Morgan and Meredith W. Michaels, 279–95. Philadelphia: University of Pennsylvania Press.
———. 2013. "Disability Worlds." *Annual Review of Anthropology* 42:53–68. Accessed March 3, 2015. http://www.annualreviews.org/doi/abs/10.1146/annurev-anthro-092412-155502.
Grinker, Roy Richard. 2007. *Unstrange Minds: Remapping the World of Autism.* New York: Basic Books.
Gunther Daniel F., and Douglas S. Diekema. 2006. "Attenuating Growth in Children with Profound Developmental Disability: A New Approach to an Old Dilemma." *Archives of Pediatrics & Adolescent Medicine* 160 (10): 1013–17.
Hari, Johann. 2004. "Peter Singer: Some People Are More Equal Than Others." The Independent. Accessed June 18, 2013. www.independent.co.uk/news/people/profiles/peter-singer-some-people-are-more-equal-than-others-6166342.html.
Hoffman, Jan. 2013. "Parental Study Shows Rise in Autism Spectrum Cases." *New York Times,* March 20. Accessed June 20, 2013. www.nytimes.com/2013/03/21/health/parental-study-shows-rise-in-autism-spectrum-cases.html.
Hurd, Michael D., Paco Martorell, Adeline Delavande, Kathleen J. Mullen, and Kenneth M. Langa. 2013. "Monetary Costs of Dementia in the United States." *New England Journal of Medicine* 368 (14): 1326–34.
Johnson, H. M. B. 2003. "Unspeakable Conversations." *New York Times,* February 16. Accessed June 20, 2013. www.nytimes.com/2003/02/16/magazine/unspeakable-conversations.html?pagewanted=all&src=pm.
Kittay, Eva Feder. 1999. *Love's Labor: Essays on Women, Equality, and Dependency.* New York: Routledge.
———. 2011. "Forever Small: The Strange Case of Ashley X." *Hypatia* 26 (3): 610–31.
Kittay, Eva Feder, and Leo Kittay. 2000. "On the Expressivity and Ethics of Selective Abortion for Disability: A Conversation with My Son." In *Prenatal Testing and Disability Rights,* edited by Erik Parens and Adrienne Asch, 165–95. Washington: Georgetown University Press.
Knickman, James R., and Emily K. Snell. 2002. "The 2030 Problem: Caring for Aging Baby Boomers." *Health Services Research* 37 (4): 849–84.
Landsman, Gail. 2004. "'Too Bad You Got a Lemon': Peter Singer, Mothers of Children with Disabilities, and the Critique of Consumer Culture." In *Consuming Motherhood,* edited by Janelle S. Taylor, Linda L. Layne, and Danielle F. Wozniak, 100–121. New Brunswick, NJ: Rutgers University Press.
———. 2009. *Reconstructing Motherhood and Disability in the Age of "Perfect" Babies.* New York: Routledge.
Layne, Linda L. 1996. "'How's the Baby Doing?' Struggling with Narratives of Progress in a Neonatal Intensive Care Unit." *Medical Anthropology Quarterly* 10 (4): 624–56.
Leibing, Annette, and Lawrence Cohen, eds. 2006. *Thinking about Dementia: Culture, Loss, and the Anthropology of Senility.* New Brunswick, NJ: Rutgers University Press.
Livingston, Julie. 2005. *Debility and the Moral Imagination in Botswana.* Bloomington: Indiana University Press.
Lo, Y. M., N. M. Hjelm, C. Fidler, I. L Sargent, M. F. Murphy, P. F. Chamberlain, P. M. Poon, C. W. Redman, and J. S. Wainscoat. 1998. "Prenatal Diagnosis of Fetal RhD Status by Molecular Analysis of Maternal Plasma." *New England Journal of Medicine* 339 (24): 1734–38.
Longmore, Paul K., and Lauri Umansky. 2001. *The New Disability History: American Perspectives.* New York: New York University Press.
MacMakin, Mary. 2011. "Women with Disabilities." In *Land of the Unconquerable: The Lives of Contemporary Afghan Women,* edited by Jennifer Heath and Ashraf Zahedi, 200–211. Berkeley: University of California Press.
Not Dead Yet. N.d. "About Not Dead Yet." www.notdeadyet.org. Accessed June 15, 2012
Nussbaum, Martha C. 2001. "Disabled Lives: Who Cares?" *New York Review of Books,* January 11. Accessed September 24, 2012. www.nybooks.com/articles/archives/2001/jan/11/disabled-lives-who-cares/.
———. 2006. *Frontiers of Justice: Disability, Nationality, Species Membership.* Cambridge, MA: Belknap Press; Harvard University Press.
O'Toole, Corbett Joan, and Tanis Doe. 2002. "Sexuality and Disabled Parents with Disabled Children." *Sexuality and Disability* 20 (1): 89–101.
Parens, Erik, and Adrienne Asch, eds. 2000. *Prenatal Testing and Disability Rights.* Washington: Georgetown University Press.
Pernick, Martin S. 1996. *The Black Stork: Eugenics and the Death of "Defective" Babies in American Medicine and Motion Pictures since 1915.* New York: Oxford University Press.
Phillips, S. D. 2009. "Civil Society and Disability Rights in Post-Soviet Ukraine: NGOs and Prospects for Change." *Indiana Journal of Global Legal Studies* 16 (1): 275–91.
Rapp, Emily. 2011. "Notes from a Dragon Mom." *New York Times,* October 15. Accessed June 20, 2013. www.nytimes.com/2011/10/16/opinion/sunday/notes-from-a-dragon-mom.html.
———. 2013. *The Still Point of the Turning World.* New York: Penguin Press.
Rapp, Rayna. 2000. *Testing Women, Testing the Fetus: The Social Impact of Amniocentesis in America.* New York: Routledge.
Rapp, Rayna, and Faye Ginsburg. 2001. "Enabling Disability: Rewriting Kinship, Reimagining Citizenship." *Public Culture* 13 (3): 533–56.
———. 2007. "Enlarging Reproduction, Screening Disability." In *Reproductive Disruptions: Gender, Technology, and Biopolitics in the New Millennium,* edited by Marsha C. Inhorn, 98–121. New York: Berghahn Books.
———. 2011. "Reverberations: Disability and the New Kinship Imaginary." *Anthropological Quarterly* 84 (2): 379–410.
———. 2012. "The Paradox of Recognition: Success or Stigma for Children with Learning Disabilities." In *Contesting Recognition: Culture, Identity and Citizenship,* edited by Janice McLaughlin, Peter Phillimore, and Diane Richardson. London: Palgrave.

Roberts, Dorothy E. 2009. "Race, Gender, and Genetic Technologies: A New Reproductive Dystopia?" *Signs* 34 (4): 783–804.
Russell, Marta. 2002. *Beyond Ramps: Disability at the End of the Social Contract.* Monroe, ME: Common Courage Press.
Samerski, Silja. 2009. "Genetic Counseling and the Fiction of Choice: Taught Self Determination as a New Technique of Social Engineering." *Signs* 34 (4): 735–61.
Saxton, Marsha. 2000. "Why Members of the Disability Community Oppose Prenatal Testing and Abortion." In *Prenatal Testing and Disability Rights,* edited by Erik Parens and Adrienne Asch, 147–64. Washington: Georgetown University Press.
Sayres, Lauren C., Megan Allyse, Taylor A. Goodspeed, and Mildred K. Cho. 2012. "In the Public Interest?" *Science Translational Medicine* 4 (144): 144fs23.
Schweik, Susan M. 2009. *The Ugly Laws: Disability in Public.* New York: New York University.
Singer, Peter. 1993. *Practical Ethics.* Cambridge and New York: Cambridge University Press.
———. 1995. *Rethinking Life and Death: The Collapse of Our Traditional Ethics.* New York: St. Martin's Press.
Solomon, Andrew. 2012. *Far from the Tree: Parents, Children and the Search for Identity.* New York: Scribner.
Stern, Alexandra. 2005. *Eugenic Nation: Faults and Frontiers of Better Breeding in Modern America.* Berkeley: University of California Press.
U.S. Census Bureau. 2012. "Profile America Facts for Features: Anniversary of Americans with Disabilities Act: July 26." U.S. Census Bureau, July 25. Accessed June 20, 2013. www.census.gov/newsroom/releases/archives/facts_for_features_special_editions/cb12-ff16.html.

Questions

1. Do you agree or disagree with the authors' claim that modern society manifests a tension between the democratizing impulse toward inclusion and the drive toward perfectibility? Do you agree that this impulse and drive fuel, respectively, the disability rights movement and neoeugenic medical innovation? If so, what reasons can you give to support your answers?
2. Do you think that the drive to perfectibility is a harmful aspect of society? Can you give an example from real life (be it your own or that of someone you know) that supports your answer?

Reading 2.3

Unspeakable Offenses

Untangling Race and Disability in Discourses of Intersectionality

Nirmala Erevelles and Andrea Minear

Nirmala Erevelles and Andrea Minear, "Unspeakable Offenses: Untangling Race and Disability in Discourses of Intersectionality," *Journal of Literary and Cultural Disability Studies*, vol. 4, no. 2, pp. 127–145.

Editor's Introduction

In this article, Nirmala Erevelles and Andrea Minear center the perspective of individuals facing multiple forms of marginalization at the intersection of race, disability, class, and gender. Their discussion demonstrates how these multiple forms of marginalization concretely harm people at these intersections by drawing on Minear's experiences running a home school cooperative for students who did not seem to "fit" in public school. They also take an in-depth intersectional approach, building on Erevelles's theoretical background to draw key lessons for the role disability ideology plays in organizing society throughout history and in the present day. Nirmala Erevelles, PhD is a professor of social and cultural studies in the Department of Educational Leadership, Policy and Technology Studies at the University of Alabama. Her research interests include disability studies, Critical Race Theory, transnational feminism, postcolonial studies, and the sociology of education. Andrea Minear, PhD is a professor of elementary education at the Department of Curriculum and Instruction at the University of West Alabama, Livingston.

Content Warning: This reading contains descriptions of physical and sexual violence.

The Literature of Critical Race Feminist Theory approaches disability as an expression of intersectional identity wherein devalued social characteristics compound stigma resulting in so-called spirit murder.

Three diverging practices of intersectionality are identified as guiding scholarship on the constitutive features of multiply minoritizing identities: (1) anticategorical frameworks that insist on race, class, and gender as social constructs/fictions; (2) intracategorical frameworks that critique merely additive approaches to differences as layered stigmas; and (3) constitutive frameworks that describe the structural conditions within which social categories in the above models are constructed by (and intermeshed with) each other in specific historical contexts. In being true to Critical Race Feminist Theory approaches, the [reading] draws on two other narratives, one historical and one contemporary, to describe how individuals located perilously at the intersections of race, class, gender, *and* disability are constituted as non-citizens and (no)bodies by the very social institutions (legal, educational, and rehabilitational) that are designed to protect, nurture, and empower them.

> On October 29, 1984, Eleanor Bumpurs, a 270 pound, arthritic, sixty-seven year old woman was shot to death while resisting eviction from her apartment in the Bronx. She was $98.85, or one month, behind in her rent. New York City mayor Ed Koch and police commissioner Benjamin Ward described the struggle preceding her demise as involving two officers with plastic shields, one officer with a restraining hook, another officer with a shotgun, and at least one supervising officer. All the officers also carried service revolvers. According to Commissioner Ward, during the course of the attempted eviction Eleanor Bumpurs escaped from the restraining hook twice and wielded a knife that Commissioner Ward said was "bent" on one of the plastic shields. At some point, Officer Stephen Sullivan, the officer positioned furthest away from her aimed and fired his shotgun. It is alleged that the blast removed half of her hand so that, according to the Bronx district attorney's office, "it was anatomically impossible for her to hold the knife." The officer pumped his gun and shot again, making his mark completely the second time around. (Williams, 271)

In her essay, "Spirit Murdering the Messenger," Critical Race Feminist (CRF) Patricia Williams describes the brutal murder of a poor, elderly, overweight, disabled, black woman by several heavily armed police officers. Trapped at the intersections of multiple oppressive contexts, Eleanor Bumpurs's tattered body was quite literally torn apart by her multiple selves—being raced, classed, gendered, and disabled. In the essay, Williams reads this murder as an unambiguous example of "racism [experienced] as ... an offense so painful and assaultive as to constitute ... 'spirit murder'" (230). Toward the end of the essay Williams struggles to fathom why the officer who fired the fatal shots saw such an "'immediate threat and endangerment to life' .... [that he] could not allay his need to kill a sick old lady fighting off hallucinations with a knife" (234). In this quote, Williams recognizes Eleanor Bumpurs's disability when invoking her arthritis and possible mental illness. However, Williams deploys disability merely as a descriptor, a difference that is a matter of "magnitude" or "context," what another CRF scholar, Angela Harris, has described as "nuance theory" (14). According to Harris, "nuance theory constitutes black women's oppression as only an intensified example of (white) women's oppression" and is therefore used as the "ultimate example of how bad things [really] are" for all women (15).

While we agree with the critique of nuance theory in feminist analyses that ignore the real experiences of black women, we argue that CRF scholars deploy a similar analytical tactic through their unconscious non-analysis of disability as it intersects with race, class, and gender oppression. Disability, like race, offers not just a "nuance" to any analysis of difference. For example, one could argue that the outrage emanating from a heaving, black body wielding a knife sent a nervous (and racist) police officer into panic when confronted by his own racialized terror of otherness. But what about the other ideological terrors that loomed large in this encounter? Could the perception of Eleanor Bumpurs as a dangerous, obese, irrational, black woman also have contributed to her construction as criminally "insane" (disability) because her reaction to a "mere" legal matter of eviction (class) was murderous rage? And did our socially sanctioned fears of the mentally ill and our social devaluation of disabled (arthritic and elderly) bodies of color justify the volley of shots fired almost instinctively to protect the public from the deviant, the dangerous, and the disposable? We, therefore, argue that in the violent annihilation of Eleanor Bumpurs's being, disability as it intersects with race, class, and gender served more than just a "context" or "magnifier" to analyze the oppressive conditions that caused this murder.

In this [reading], we demonstrate how the omission of disability as a critical category in discussions of intersectionality has disastrous and sometimes deadly consequences for disabled people of color caught at the violent interstices of multiple differences. In the first section, we will theorize intersectionality as first proposed by Crenshaw and explore the different ways in which it can be utilized by both Critical Race Theory and Disability Studies to analyze the experiences of people located at the interstices of multiple differences. Next, true to CRT tradition, we draw on two other narratives, one historical and one contemporary, to describe how individuals located perilously at the interstices of race, class, gender, *and* disability are constituted as non-citizens and (no) bodies by the very social institutions (legal, educational, and rehabilitational) that are designed to protect, nurture, and empower them.

Intersectionality at the Crossroads: Theorizing Multiplicative Differences

With the deconstruction of essentialism, the challenge of how to theorize identity in all its complex multiplicity has preoccupied feminist scholars of color.[1] Kimberle Crenshaw, one of the key proponents of the theory of intersectionality, has argued that "many of the experiences black women face are not subsumed within the traditional boundaries of race or gender oppression as these boundaries are currently understood" (358). Part of the problem of "relying on a static and singular notion of being or of identity" (Pastrana, 75) is that the single characteristic that is fore-grounded (e.g. female or black) is expected to explain all of the other life experiences of the individual or the group. Additionally, Crenshaw points out that social movements based on a single identity politics (e.g. the Feminist Movement, Black Power Movement, GLBT and the Disability Rights Movement) have historically conflated or ignored intra-group differences and this has sometimes resulted in growing tensions between the social movements themselves.

Feminists of color have, therefore, had the difficult task of attempting to theorize oppression faced at the multiple fronts of race, class, gender, sexuality, and disability.[2] Thus, if one is poor, black, elderly, disabled, and lesbian, must these differences be organized into a hierarchy such that some differences gain prominence over others? What if some differences coalesce to create a more abject form of oppression (e.g. being poor, black, and disabled) or if some differences support both privilege/invisibility within the same oppressed community (e.g. being black, wealthy, and gay)? What happens if we use "race" as a stable register of oppression against which other discriminations gain validity through their similarity and difference from that register? (Arondekar)

In the face of this theoretical challenge, intersectionality has been set up as the most appropriate analytical intervention expected to accomplish the formidable task of mediating multiple differences. For example, Patricia Hill Collins writes that "[a]s opposed to examining gender, race, class, and nation as separate systems of oppression, intersectionality explores how these systems mutually construct one another ..." (63). CRF Adrien Wing writes:

> We, as black women, can no longer afford to think of ourselves as merely the sum of separate parts that can be added together or subtracted from, until a white male or female stands before you. The actuality of our experience is multiplicative. Multiply each of my parts together, WE X WE X WE X WE X I, and you have *one* indivisible being. If you divide one of these parts from one you still have *one*. (31)

But this is all much easier said than done. Attempts to deploy intersectionality as an analytical tool in academic research have taken on different forms with varying analytical outcomes—some more useful than others. McCall, in an overview of how intersectionality has been utilized in women studies' scholarship, has identified three different modes of theorizing intersectionality. The first mode uses an *anticategorical* framework based on the poststructuralist argument that social categories like race, gender, sexuality, and disability are merely social constructions/fictions. CRF scholars are, however, unwilling to completely do away with the social categories that constitute identity in the first place. As Crenshaw explains:

1. See e.g. bell hooks; Angela Davis; Audre Lorde; Gloria Anzaldúa; Gloria Hull, Patricia Bell Scott, and Barbara Smith.
2. For examples, consult Gloria Anzaldúa; Kimberlé Crenshaw; Angela Harris; Adrien Wing; and Audre Lorde.

> To say that a category such as race and gender is socially constructed is not to say that the category has no significance in our world. On the contrary, a large and continuing project for subordinated people ... is thinking about the way in which power is clustered around certain categories and is exercised against others. (375)

As a result, feminists of color are more apt to use an *intracategorical* framework that focuses on "particular social groups at neglected points of intersection of multiple master categories" (McCall, 1780). As Crenshaw explains:

> [I]ntersectionality provides a basis for reconceptualizing race as a coalition between men and women of color ... Intersectionality may provide the means for dealing with other marginalizations as well. For example, race can also be a coalition of straight and gay people of color, and thus serve as a basis for critique of churches and other cultural institutions that reproduce heterosexism. (377)

The intracategorical framework is especially promising to CRF scholars because it validates the reality of racism as it intersects with sexism and other social categories of difference (e.g. heterosexism; classism) in the everyday lives of women of color. However, Yuval-Davis, while producing a list of possible differences (potentially incomplete) that includes "'race'/skin color; ethnicity; nation/state; class, culture; ability; age; sedentariness/origin; wealth; North-South; religion, stage of social development" (202), asks if it is even conceivable to address all these possible social categories intersecting with a common master category (e.g. race or gender) at any given time? Do some differences acquire greater prominence than others (e.g. sexuality)? Are some "other" differences just added on to merely complicate and "nuance" this intersectional analysis (e.g. disability)?

If the intracategorical framework rejects merely tacking on another difference to its litany of categories (e.g. disability), it would have to, in effect, reject the additive approach to multiple differences and instead utilize what Yuval-Davis has described as the constitutive approach to multiple differences. This approach, while foregrounding the actual experiences of women of color at the intersection of multiple social categories, also describes the structural conditions within which these social categories are constructed by, and intermeshed with each other in specific historical contexts. McCall calls this third approach to theorizing intersectionality the *intercategorical* framework. Yuval-Davis explains:

> The point of intersectional analysis is not to find "several identities under one" .... This would reinscribe the fragmented, additive model of oppression and essentialize specific social identities. Instead the point is to analyse the differential ways by which social divisions are concretely enmeshed and constructed by each other and how they relate to political and subjective constructions of identities. (205)

Therefore, rather than merely adding disability to nuance an intersectional analysis, we will foreground the historical contexts and structural conditions within which the identity categories of race and disability intersect.

Points of Contact: At the Intersection of CRT and Disability Studies

In educational contexts, the association of race with disability has resulted in large numbers of students of color (particularly African American and Latino males) being subjected to segregation in so-called special-education classrooms through sorting practices such as tracking and/or through labels such as mild mental retardation and/or emotional disturbance.[3] The PBS film, *Beyond Brown: Pursuing the Promise* (Haddad, Readdean, & Valadez) substantiates these claims with the following statistics.

- Black children constitute 17 percent of the total school enrollment, but 33 percent of those labeled "mentally retarded".
- During the 1998–1999 school year more than 2.2 million children of color in U.S. schools were served by special education. Post-high school outcomes for these students were striking. Among high school youth with disabilities, about 75 percent of African Americans, compared to 39 percent of whites, are still not employed three to five years out of school. In this same time period, the arrest rate for African Americans with disabilities is 40 percent, compared to 27 percent for whites.
- States with a history of legal school segregation account for five of the seven states with the highest overrepresentation of African Americans labeled mentally retarded. They are Mississippi, South Carolina, North Carolina, Florida and Alabama.
- Among Latino students, identification for special education varies significantly from state to state. Large urban schools districts in California exhibit disproportionately large numbers of Latino English-language learners represented in special education classes in secondary schools.
- Some 20 percent of Latino students in grades 7 through 12 had been suspended from school according to statistics from 1999 compared with 15 percent of white students and 35 percent of African American students.

The association of race with disability has been extremely detrimental to people of color in the U.S.—not just in education, but also historically where associations of race with disability have been used to justify the brutality of slavery, colonialism, and neo-colonialism. Unfortunately, rather than nurturing an alliance between race and disability, CRT scholars (like other radical scholars) have mistakenly conceived of disability as a biological category, as an immutable and pathological abnormality rooted in the "medical language of symptoms and diagnostic categories" (Linton, 8). Disability studies scholars, on the other hand, have critiqued this "deficit" model of disability and have described disability as a socially constructed category that derives meaning and social (in)significance from the historical, cultural, political, and economic structures that frame social life.

Thus, at the first point of contact, both CRT and disability scholars begin with the critical assumption that race and disability are, in fact, social constructs. Thus, Haney Lopez explains "Biological race is an illusion .... Social race, however, is not .... Race has its genesis and maintains its vigorous strength in the realm of social beliefs" (172). Similarly, Garland-Thomson describes disability as "the attribution of corporeal deviance—not so much a property of bodies [but rather] ... a product of cultural rules about what

3. Artiles; Artiles, Harry, Reschly, and Chinn; Connor and Ferri; Reid and Knight; Watts and Erevelles.

bodies should be or do" (6). At their second point of contact, race and disability are both theorized as relational concepts. Thus, CRT scholars argue that "[r]aces are constructed relationally against one another, rather than in isolation" (Haney Lopez, 168) such that the privileges that Whites enjoy are linked to the subordination of people of color (Harris). Similarly, Lennard Davis points out that "our construction of the normal world is based on a radical repression of disability" (22) because "without the monstrous body to demarcate the borders of the generic … and without the pathological to give form to the normal, the taxonomies of bodily value that underlie political, social and economic arrangements would collapse" (Garland-Thomson, 20). Finally, at the third point of contact, both perspectives use stories and first-person accounts to foreground the perspectives of those who have experienced victimization by racism and ableism first-hand (Espinoza and Harris; Angela Harris; Ladson-Billings and Tate IV; Parker, Deyhle, and Villenas; Linton; Connor).

In building on these alliance possibilities, disability-studies scholars have argued that disability is, in fact, constitutive of most social differences, particularly race (Baynton; Erevelles 1996; James and Wu). One example to support the above claim lies in the historical narrative of eugenics as a program of selective breeding to prevent the degeneration of the human species. Colonial ideologies conceiving of the colonized races as intrinsically degenerate sought to bring these "bodies" under control via segregation and/or destruction. Such control was regarded as necessary for the public good. The association of degeneracy and disease with racial difference also translated into an attribution of diminished cognitive and rational capacities of non-white populations. Disability related labels such as feeble-mindedness and mental illness were often seen as synonymous with bodies marked oppressively by race (Baynton; Gould). Fearing that such characteristics could be passed down from generation to generation and further pose a threat to the dominant white race, "protective" practices such as forced sterilizations, rigid miscegenation laws, residential segregation in ghettoes, barrios, reservations and other state institutions and sometimes even genocide (e.g. the Holocaust) were brought to bear on non-white populations under the protected guise of eugenics. However, constructing the degenerate "other" was not just an ideological intervention to support colonialism. In the more contemporary context of transnational capitalism, Erevelles argues that:

> the 'ideology' of disability is essential to the capitalist enterprise because it is able to regulate and control the unequal distribution of surplus through invoking biological difference as the 'natural' cause of all inequality, thereby successfully justifying the social and economic inequality that maintains social hierarchies … [D]isability … is [therefore] the organizing grounding principle in the construction of the categories of gender, race, class, and sexual orientation. (526)

It is easy to dismiss eugenics as a relic of a bygone era, but the continued association of race and disability in debilitating ways necessitates that we examine how eugenic practices continue to reconstitute social hierarchies in contemporary contexts via the deployment of a hegemonic ideology of disability that have real material effects on people located at the intersections of difference. To illustrate the argument, we will now draw on the narratives of two protagonists, Junius Wilson and Cassie Smith.

The "Unspeakable" Life of Junius Wilson

The first narrative, the story of Junius Wilson, poignantly told in Susan Burch and Hannah Joyner's book, *Unspeakable: The Life of Junius Wilson*, occurred at the intersection of disability, race, gender, and class. Born in 1908 to Sidney and Mary Wilson in the predominantly African American community of Castle Hayne on the outskirts of Wilmington, North Carolina, Junius Wilson became deaf as a toddler. The tensions of raising a deaf child in poverty conditions within a political context of racial violence caused Sidney Wilson to desert his family, forcing his wife Mary to send the young Wilson to the residential North Carolina School for the Colored Blind and Deaf in Raleigh. In the segregated school in Raleigh, Wilson was initiated into a "black deaf community" and "Raleigh signs" that were specific to the school and that had almost no currency elsewhere—a fact that would later contribute to Wilson's social isolation in both the deaf and the black communities. Additionally, in line with racist ideologies of African American students' low mental capacities, the school encouraged vocational work over traditional classroom work, so while Wilson could write his name out, he was unable to read and write anything else. Then, in 1924, Wilson was expelled from the school because of a minor infraction and forced to return home.

Returning home from Raleigh, Wilson's habits of "touching or holding people, stamping feet and waving arms" (33) constructed him as a threatening figure in a society ruled by Jim Crow laws—habits that could compromise the safety of himself, his familiy, and his community. It was perhaps for all these reasons and in an effort to protect his family and his community that Arthur Smith, the family friend, accused the 17-year-old Junius Wilson of assaulting and attempting to rape his young wife, Lizzie. Thus, in August, 1925, Junius Wilson was arrested and taken to New Hanover County jail. Unable to communicate with Wilson, the court held a lunacy hearing where it was concluded that Wilson was both "feeble-minded" and dangerous, and was therefore committed to the criminal ward of the North Carolina State Hospital for the Colored Insane in Goldsboro that housed epileptics, "idiots," and other "mental defectives" and exerted institutional control rather than practices of healing.

With eugenics ideologies dominant in the early twentieth century, one means of social control was castration, the surgical removal of the testicles. Thus, in 1932, Wilson was castrated and henceforth was no longer perceived as a danger because he became "a submissive black man ... [with] eyes downcast, silent, and reserved ... a gentle childlike patient" (49). Seen now as a potentially useful worker, Wilson was sent to work in the Farm Colony (the farm attached to the hospital) and was leased to private farmers till his retirement in 1970, where he was transferred to a geriatric ward. Even though all charges against him were dropped by then, he continued to be incarcerated for another twenty years because it was conceived of as "the most benevolent course of action" (1).

In the 1970s, in response to the Civil Rights of Institutionalized Persons Act, Carolina Legal Assistance (CLA), a group of attorneys in Raleigh, found scores of African American men and women "dumped in hospitals, abandoned by communities, and otherwise mislabeled as feebleminded" (124), one of whom was Junius Wilson. After several years of lawsuits and the involvement of advocates and family members, Wilson was moved out to a cottage on the grounds of the hospital on February 4, 1994. He died on March 17, 2001. Hovering precipitously at the boundaries of race, class, gender, *and* disability, Wilson had been held in the isolating confines of the institution for more than three quarters of his life. Overwhelmed by the enormity of the crime committed against Wilson, Burch and Joyner (2007) ask, "How should a society—indeed, how can a society—make amends for past misdeeds?" (3).

But society seldom makes amends for past misdeeds. On the contrary, it is often apt to repeat them. Junius Wilson's story took place in the early twentieth century. Our second narrative, Cassie Smith's story, takes place in the present, almost a century later. The terrifying aspect of Cassie's story is that it continues Wilson's narrative, in effect becoming its sequel by once again foregrounding the violence that lies at the intersection of race, class, gender, *and* disability.

Her Time is up! Cassie Gotta Go!: Exclusion at the Intersections

One of the authors of this [reading], Andrea, had met Cassie two years ago at the home school cooperative, DAWN, which she ran for students like Cassie who did not seem to "fit" in public school. Cassie's mother, Aliya Smith, a single mother on disability for the last 15 years, lives in public housing with her daughter Cassie and her six-year-old son Charles in a small southern town. Cassie's father lives close by but has been mostly absent from her life. She had been very close to her grandmother who passed away a year ago.

On her first day at DAWN, Cassie tried desperately to fit in with the other eight adolescent girls at the school. She was dressed neatly. But she had severe eczema on her skin and was eyed suspiciously by the other girls as if her rash was contagious. Her hair was braided stylishly, but her braids were already loosening and falling out because she picked at her head continuously. Her big toothy grin gave way to raucous laughter, much louder than the children in the small school were used to. She tried so hard to be friendly, but she was met with wariness.

After barely less than a day of observation and evaluation, Andrea realized that Cassie could not read—a fact that she had successfully hidden from even her closest friends. When asked to write a journal entry, her sentences contained a string of three letter words that made little sense such as "pig as you as zoo cat by as no as dog pig as zoo no by you as zoo as cat red." Cassie "pretended" very well, opening her book, following along and even reading "along with" someone, saying a word immediately after the other person began the word. Because she did not read, she had limited knowledge of other subject areas. She could barely add and could not subtract. She recognized some coins, but could not figure money. Andrea realized with dismay that twelve-year-old Cassie was functionally illiterate.

When we interviewed Cassie and her mother, her turbulent and tragic educational history was slowly revealed. We learned to our horror that Cassie had been bounced around to a different school every year of her school life; two schools in some years. As a toddler, Cassie spent a lot of time with her grandmother because of Aliya's poor health. At age four, Cassie started out in a private preschool program at the Holy Trinity Baptist School. Without the benefit of records or first-hand knowledge, we wonder whether the fact that Cassie was an economically disadvantaged black child in an all-white school caused her to appear "behind" and uncontrollable. Aliya recalls, "She used to get temper tantrums and they told me if I couldn't get her straightened up, she gotta go!" Aliya moved Cassie to the Head Start program and then to her neighborhood school for kindergarten:

> And then they [the school personnel] said that she needed help (Cassie interjects: "No,

> I don't!"). So we had to go through evaluations, meetings, and stuff. They tried to say that she was mentally retarded. (Cassie interjects, "I am not MR!") ... [Aliya continues in response to Cassie] But she was then. So they sent her to Sally's Corner.

In this small southern town, Sally's Corner was touted as the haven for kids with severe emotional and behavioral problems. In its mission statement the school claimed to offer treatment based on "an interdisciplinary approach with psychology, education, nursing, psychiatry, social work and counseling comprising the professions that impact each client's treatment." The website also included several testimonials from parents and one child that described Sally's Corner very positively. Cassie's memories of Sally's Corner, however, were very dark:

> [*Sally's Corner*] is like a bad place. They put you there when you get in trouble. They restrain you. They put your arms like this ... sit on you kinda and put you in a room where no windows at and a little time out room by yourself .... And they come and look at you. And I say, "Let me out" and kick the door ....
>
> NE: What is it that that gets you really angry?
>
> Cassie: When somebody tries to fight with me and pull my hair
>
> NE: But the teachers don't try to fight with you, do they?
>
> Cassie: Oh I'll still fight you the big ole fat ole ... sit on me ... Half ton white folks.

By Cassie's own admission, we can understand that she was no easy client, and it is reasonable to assume that Cassie was in need of some kind of program that would help manage her fits of rage so she could also learn. And surely, they had all that expertise from the multi-disciplinary team to do something for her. But again, we do not really know what happened there except for this explanation from Aliya about why she wanted Cassie to leave Sally's Corner after only a couple of months there:

> They locked you up all the time. They had this jail cell. She had spit on the wall while she was in there. They called my mama [Cassie's grandmother]. I was sick at that time. My mama and my sister-in-law went. My mama was so mad when she went out there. She told them, "Open the door. Let that child outta there!" My mama did not understand. Actually she did not care. Like she [Cassie] was being treated like a dog or something ... And then they said that before she left she had to scrub the room. My mama said, "Get that child outta there!" And they said she could not leave before she did that. So my mom told Cassie what were the spots that she spit at. And to clean just them. They wanted her to clean the whole room! Then she got to get ready to go.... It was time for her to go.... Kept on trying to get her out.... They finally agreed and I got her to go to Woodberry Gardens.

Once again, while we acknowledge that we have only one side of the story, there are aspects that still puzzle us. Surely "a model treatment program" had more options for a small, angry five-year-old African

American girl with anger-management issues than being thrown into a "jail cell"? What was it about that tiny enraged black body that terrified the staff so much that they threw all their knowledge out of the window, opting instead for the behavioral strategy of "imprisonment"?

This was the educational legacy that Cassie would carry forward with her as she moved into the first grade at her new elementary school, Woodberry Gardens. After two good years she was inexplicably moved to Spartan elementary and once again to Nottingham. Each time, as Aliya put it, they told her that "It was time for her to leave there ... Her time was up."

Apparently, at this time, Cassie no longer held the label "mental retardation." Still, when asked, her mother just says, "She acted crazy!" She was now thrown into a regular program at Nottingham with no supports. Once again her academic and behavioral problems were exacerbated. Once again she was teased and called names by her peers. Once again she fought back—she cut a classmate's hair. And once again she suffered the consequences of her negative behavior. Less than two months before her graduation from elementary school, Cassie was transferred to her eighth school, Athena. Aliya was livid:

> You talking about somebody was mad. No! I could never understand why they sent her to Athena. I went over there and met with the teacher.... It had something to do with her learning. There was a month and half to graduate and they sent her to Athena. Then that teacher was up there ill-treating her.... They wanted her to graduate with her Athena [special education] class. And I said, "I didn't spend all that money and time at Nottingham for this. I was so mad. I told them that I would have her out of school if they would not let me take her out [of Athena]. Then they listened. When they figured out that I was not playing with them, they got those papers. Like they couldn't get them fast enough. They just moved them in the office. And I took her to Nottingham and she was there was for three days so that she could graduate with her class. And they did it [the graduation ceremomy] in such a way, that she had to be escorted. Like she was such a bad child. Like she was coming from prison. Her last two teachers had to walk with her side by side. She was the last one to walk.

Thus, after being in eight schools in eight years, Cassie came to DAWN, the home-school cooperative, as a sixth grader with a plethora of problems. In this supportive context, Cassie made great leaps in her social behavior and even made some academic headway. However, Andrea was forced to close DAWN at the end of the year for financial reasons, and so Cassie prepared to re-enter public school in the next fall.

Eager to learn, but receiving very little help in school, Cassie soon got frustrated and into fights again. She was sent to the Alternative School which ironically she actually liked because of the structure and individual attention. But then, even this realm of contentment vanished one day—the day of the "incident." One spring day, six students (four boys and two girls) were left without supervision in a classroom for a few minutes while one of the teachers walked a student to his car to speak to his mother. The boys teased and taunted the girls making rude, sometimes vulgar, suggestions and then laughing them off. One of the boys told Cassie, "So-and-so thinks you're pretty. He wants you to suck his dick." And so she went behind the cubbies and obliged.

By the next day, word spread all over the school. As the rumor gathered momentum, more and more people became aware, including the school counselor and the assistant principal. However, neither the classroom teacher, nor the parents of the perpetrators were notified for nearly two or three weeks. According to the Assistant Principal, there was an ongoing investigation and then a meeting was called with the Building Based Special Team (BBST) and the parent to discuss what they called a "manifestation determination." The question of the day: Was it Cassie's "learning disability" that caused her to have oral sex with a boy in her class or was this done on her own volition? Following "procedure" each member concurred that her "learning disability" could not have caused her to perform oral sex. She knew what she was doing. Therefore she was GUILTY. Under the zero-tolerance policy, this called for expulsion.

Not once did the committee even bother to look at Cassie's painful history of exclusion, segregation, incarceration, and negation. It was lucky that Andrea was there. Aliya was a poor advocate for her child. Intimidated, angry, confused, and defensive, she often ended up blaming her daughter for the "stupid thing she did." It was Andrea who saved the day. Drawing on her experiences as a former special education teacher, Andrea brought up Cassie's educational history of social isolation and low self-esteem that were the by-products of her "learning disability" and that may have influenced her decision to perform a sexual act that garnered her some form of warped recognition/respect/visibility among her peers. In addition, Andrea had to spell out the possible legal ramifications of leaving students unsupervised in a locked and isolated classroom for even a short period of time. We believe that it was the last statement that sealed the deal. It was not the history of educational abuse, but the threat of legal ramifications that made the committee decide that they would not recommend expulsion. Cassie would have another chance at school. But whether she would have the support that she needed to make it through another school year was still an open question.

The process of narrating Cassie's educational history during the interviews inadvertently produced an unpredictable benefit for Aliya. In a marked difference from the "professionals" who were reviewing Cassie's case, it was Aliya, confused, angry, troubled, and yet still hopeful, who was able to see how the different disruptive, demeaning, and punitive experiences that began early in Cassie's life were now responsible for the risky, sullen, and disorderly behaviors of her teenage daughter. Now with the gift of hindsight, and therefore conscious of her own disempowerment in the process, Aliya poignantly reflected:

> If I had known the system better, I would not have put her there [Sally's Corner]. But at that time I did not know the system. It seemed that they were trying to hurt me, rather than help me.

"Unspeakable Offenses": An Intercategorical Analysis of Intersectionality

Just like Junius Wilson, Cassie is also located at the boundaries of race, class, gender, *and* disability. Each of their stories brings to the forefront several questions: How does racism in its interaction with the inauspicious combination of class, gender, *and* disability oppression cohere to locate Wilson and the Smiths beyond the pale of appropriate interventions by the very institutions (legal, rehabilitative, and educational) that were designed to nurture and empower them? At which point did disability trump race? When did class become the critical influential factor? At what point did gender become the only perceivable threat? In each of the stories, it is very difficult to unravel and isolate the strands that played an integral part in weaving the violent tapestry of their broken lives.

For Junius Wilson, it was the socio-political context of racial terror and abject poverty in the Jim Crow South that constituted his deafness as "dangerous" difference that could only be contained within the institutional confines of a segregated residential school for the "Colored" deaf. Ironically, this confinement provided Wilson with a cultural community of other deaf students of color while it at the same time alienated him from his community outside the school. Additionally, unlike white deaf students, being black and deaf located him at the lowest rungs of the social hierarchy of the time, providing him with an inferior education that would also play a part in his continued social isolation. On returning home, his disability cast a shadow on his race and gender and contributed to his construction as the dangerously virile young black male—images that led to the false accusation of sexual assault, his incarceration, and ultimately to the final violent act of his castration. During that time, he was put to work in the farm colony as part of the surplus population being utilized to produce profits for the institution. Without financial resources and other social supports, his family could do little to intervene on his behalf, which resulted in him languishing in an institution for 76 years. The institution's refusal to release him even after all charges were dropped against him was justified under a mantle of benevolence. It was this same benevolence that allowed the institution to justify the unequal and oppressive conditions in the institution by arguing that "the lack of facilities are not due to racial biases but the fact [that] Negro patients are willing to accept what is provided to them, 'which is more than they have at home'" (Burch & Joyner, 74).

In an earlier section of this [reading], we wrote that Cassie Smith provided Junius Wilson's story with its unwelcome sequel. At first glance, this assertion may seem far-fetched in the contemporary historical context of the New South where Jim Crow (re)appears as only a distant and shameful memory. Yet, Cassie's story foregrounds an interesting twist to the continuing saga of racial segregation in the New South. In place of Jim Crow, Cassie's ever-changing labels of MR, LD, and ADHD were used as the justification for her continued segregation in an effort to protect the mainstream from a dangerous racialized Other—the economically disadvantaged disabled African American girl. Here, class and race also played a significant role in maintaining this segregation. As educators, we have known privileged white students with similar behavioral problems whose parents were able to corral the school's best resources, were able to access professional help outside the school, and, in the worst case scenario, were able to transfer their child to a private school. Aliya Smith's economic and social disadvantages did not permit her these luxuries. Instead, her disadvantages proved to be a further liability, a signal to the school professionals that there was really no need to "fight" for her daughter Cassie. As a result, even though Cassie had an IEP replete with individualized goals to improve both her behavior and her learning, she never met most of those goals, and nobody cared. This was apparent in her seventh grade report card that listed her as earning As and Bs, even though she was still functionally illiterate and still had little behavior control.

Finally, perhaps most telling is how disability as a "social" not a "clinical" condition was used to establish the benevolence of the special education bureaucracy and in doing so masked the violence that became an inextricable part of Cassie's educational career. Cassie was first MR, then ADHD, and then LD—labels that ebbed and flowed with the passing tides in different contexts. Clearly, given its temporality, "mental retardation" cannot be a robust category. So, could it then be that the educational gatekeepers, when confronted with an allegedly undisciplined, economically disadvantaged, African American girl, fearfully sought the protection of the label "mental retardation"—a label that would justify her incarceration at the tender age of five years old and continue to support her social isolation as it made its punitive march on the successive legs of her young educational career?

We argue here that an intercategorical analysis of intersectionality enables us to foreground the structural context where the social categories of race, class, gender, *and* disability are (re) constituted within the two narratives of Junius Wilson and Cassie Smith. First, we identify disability as the organizing ideological force that is deployed in both narratives as the means to organize the social hierarchies in their respective historical contexts. Here, we describe disability as the very embodiment of the disruption of normativity that is, in turn, symbolic of efficient and profitable individualism and the efficient economic appropriation of those profits produced within capitalist societies. In the early twentieth century, Jim Crow and eugenics served as the two principal mechanisms that patrolled the boundaries of society in order to identify those individuals/communities who were seen as a threat to the normative social order (the status quo) within an incipient capitalist society. The New South replaced those outmoded mechanisms of segregation with more modern systems that were more appropriately in keeping with the times. Thus, for example, in educational contexts the special education bureaucracy with its complex machinery of pseudo-medical evaluations, confusing legal discourses, and overwhelming paperwork administered by a body of intimidating professionals now performs tasks that are not very different from Jim Crow and eugenic ideologies. To put it more simply, special education, instead of being used to individualize education programs to meet the special needs of students, is instead used to segregate students who disrupt the "normal" functioning of schools. Moreover, on the few occasions when Cassie's mother sought to confront them, they invoked their complicated bureaucracy (e.g. using phrases like *manifestation determination*) to further confuse and intimidate her. While we do not deny that Cassie did have significant problems, we argue that the only intervention that was sought by the special education bureaucracy as the most effective was segregation and ultimately incarceration (alternative school and later a very real possibility of prison). Cassie is, no doubt, difficult to manage and perhaps even challenging to care about enough to help her conquer her barriers. But it is her *right* that she *not* be made dispensable.

"Spirit Murder" and the "New" Eugenics: Critical Race Theory meets Disability Studies

The three stories of Eleanor Bumpurs, Junius Wilson, and Cassie and Aliya Smith, however poignant they may appear to be, are not unique. Police brutality, false imprisonment, and educational negligence are commonplace in the lives of people of color—especially those who are located at the margins of multiple identity categories. So common are these practices that CRF scholar Patricia Williams has argued that these kinds of assaults should not be dismissed as the "odd mistake" but rather be given a name that associates them with criminality. Her term for such assaults on an individual's personhood is "spirit murder," which she describes as the equivalent of body murder.

> One of the reasons I fear what I call spirit murder, or disregard for others whose lives qualitatively depend on our regard, is that its product is a system of formalized distortions of thought. It produces social structures centered around fear and hate, it provides a timorous outlet for feelings elsewhere unexpressed ... We need to see it as a cultural cancer; we need to open our eyes to the spiritual genocide it is wreaking on blacks, whites, and the abandoned and abused of all races and ages. We need to eradicate its numbing pathology before it wipes out what precious little humanity we have left. (234)

Clearly, in our educational institutions there are millions of students of color, mostly economically disadvantaged and disabled, for whom spirit murder is the most significant experience in their educational lives. In fact, it is this recognition of spirit murder in the everyday lives of disabled students of color that forges a critical link between disability studies and CRT/F through the intercategorical analysis of intersectionality. In other words, utilizing an intercategorical analysis from the critical standpoint of disability studies will foreground the structural forces in place that constitute certain students as a surplus population that is of little value in both social and economic terms. That most of these students are poor, disabled, and of color is critical to recognize from within a CRT/F perspective. By failing to undertake such an analysis, we could miss several political opportunities for transformative action.

Works Cited

Anzaldúa, Gloria. *Making Face Making Soul: Haciendo Caras: Creative and Critical Perspectives of Women of Color.* San Francisco: Aunt Lute Books, 1990.

Arondekar, Anjali. "Border/Line Sex: Queer Positionalities, or How Race Matters Outside the United States." *Interventions* 7.2 (2005): 236–50.

Artiles, Alfredo J. "The Dilemma of Difference: Enriching the Disproportionality Discourse with Theory and Content." *Journal of Special Education* 32.1 (1998): 32–7.

Artiles, Alfredo J., Beth Harry, Daniel J. Reschly and Philip C. Chinn. "Over-Identification of Students of Color in Special Education: A Critical Overview." *Multicultural Perspectives* 4.1 (2002): 3–10.

Baynton, Douglas. "Disability in History." *Perspectives* 44.9 (2006): 5–7.

Burch, Susan and Hannah Joyner. *Unspeakable: The Life of Junius Wilson.* Chapel Hill: U of North Carolina P, 2007.

Beyond Brown: Pursuing the Promise. Dir. Lulie Haddad, Cyndee Readdean and John J. Valadez. PBS, 2004.

Connor, David J. *Urban Narratives: Portraits in Progress—Life at the Intersections of Learning Disability, Race, and Class.* New York: Peter Lang, 2007.

Connor, David J. and Beth. A. Ferri. "Integration and Inclusion—A Troubling Nexus: Race, Disability, and Special Education." *The Journal of African American History* 90.1/2 (2005): 107–27.

Crenshaw, Kimberlé. "Mapping the Margins: Intersectionality, Identity Politics, and Violence against Women." *Critical Race Theory: The Key Writings that formed the Movement.* Ed. Kimberlé Crenshaw, Neil Gotanda, Gary Pellar, and Kendall Thomas. New York: New Press, 1996. 357–83.

Davis, Angela.Y. *Women, Race, and Class.* New York: Vintage, 1983.

Davis, Lennard J. *Enforcing Normalcy: Disability, Deafness, and the Body.* New York: Verso, 1995.

Erevelles, Nirmala. "(Im) Material Citizens: Cognitive Disability, Race and the Politics of Citizenship." *Disability, Culture, and Education* 1.1 (2002): 5–25.

Erevelles, Nirmala. "Disability and the Dialectics of Difference." *Disability and Society* 11.4 (1996): 519–37.

Espinoza, Leslie and Angela. P. Harris. "Afterword: Embracing the Tar-Baby—LatCrit Theory and the Stick Mess of Race." *California Law Review* 88.5 (1997): 499–559.

Garland-Thomson, Rosemarie. *Extraordinary Bodies: Figuring physical disability in American Culture and Literature.* New York: Columbia UP, 1997.

Gould, Stephen. J. *The Mismeasure of Man.* New York: Norton, 1981.

Haney Lopez, Ian. F. "The Social Construction of Race." *Critical Race Theory: The Cutting Edge*. Ed. Richard Delgado and Jean Stefancic. Philadelphia: Temple UP, 2007. 163–75.
Harris, Angela. "Race and Essentialism in Feminist Legal Theory." *Critical Race Feminism*. Ed. Adrien. K. Wing. New York: New York UP, 1997. 11–26.
Harris, Cheryl I. "Whiteness as Property." *Critical Race Theory: Key Writings that Formed the Movement.* Ed. Kimberlé Crenshaw, Neil Gotanda, Gary Pellar, and Kendall Thomas. New York: New P, 1995. 276–91.
Hill Collins, Patricia. "It's All in the Family: Intersections of Gender, Race, and Nation." *Hypatia* 13.3 (1998): 62–82.
hooks, bell. *Feminist Theory: From Margin to Center.* Cambridge, MA: South End P, 1985.
Hull, Gloria. T., Patricia Bell Scott and Barbara Smith. *All the Women are White, All the Men are Black, But some of Us are Brave.* New York: The Feminist P at CUNY, 1982.
James, Jennifer. C. and Cynthia Wu. "Editors' Introduction: Race, Ethnicity, Disability, and Literature: Intersections and Interventions." *MELUS* 31.3 (2003): 3–13.
Ladson-Billings, Gloria and William F. Tate IV. "Toward a Critical Race Theory of Education." *Teachers College Record* 97.1 (1995): 47–68.
Linton, Simi. *Claiming Disability: Knowledge and Identity.* New York: New York UP, 1998.
Lorde, Audre. *Sister Outside: Essays and Speeches.* Berkeley, CA: The Crossing P Feminist Series, 1984.
McCall, Leslie. "The Complexity of Intersectionality." *Signs: Journal of Women in Culture and Society* 30.3 (2005): 1771–1800.
Parker, Laurence, Donna Deyhle, and Sofia Villenas. *Race is ... Race isn't: Critical Race Theory and Qualitative Studies in Education.* Boulder, CO: Westview P, 1999.
Pastrana, Antonio. "Black Identity Constructions: Inserting Intersectionality, Bisexuality, and (Afro-) Latinidad into Black Studies." *Journal of African American Studies* 8.1–2 (2004): 74–89.
Reid, D. Kim and Michelle G. Knight. "Disability Justifies Exclusion of Minority Students: A Critical History Grounded in Disability Studies." *Educational Researcher* 35.6 (2006): 18–33.
Watts, Ivan and Nirmala Erevelles. "These Deadly Times: Reconceptualizing School Violence by using Critical Race Theory and Disability Studies." *American Educational Research Association* 41.2 (2004): 271–99.
Williams, Patricia. J. "Spirit Murdering the Messenger: The Discourse of Fingerpointing as the Law's Response to Racism." *Critical Race Feminism: A Class Reader.* Ed. Adrien. K. Wing. New York: New York UP, 1997. 229–42.
Wing, Adrien. "Brief Reflections toward a Multiplicative Theory and Praxis of Being." *Critical Race Feminism: A Reader.* Ed. Adrien K. Wing. New York: New York UP, 1997. 27–34.
Yuval-Davis, Nira. "Intersectionality and Feminist Politics." *European Journal of Women's Studies* 13.3 (2006): 193–203.

Questions

1. Erevelles and Minear note that a harmful eugenics ideology is responsible for the historical and continuing association between race and disability and that this association has been used to justify the dehumanizing treatment of people of color and to reconstitute social hierarchies in contemporary contexts. What examples of the way this association between race and disability has been used to give such justifications and reconstitute such hierarchies can you think of?
2. The authors claim that disability is the organizing, grounding principle in the construction of the categories of race, gender, class, and sexuality in capitalist society. What are some ways in which you think disability is at play in the construction of people's identities (e.g., as Black, Asian, female, or working-class)?

End-of-Unit Questions

1. We learned about the specter of ableism and the myriad ways it harms disabled persons, especially multiply marginalized ones. How does this affect the way we should provide healthcare to disabled persons? What are some ways to mitigate the harmful effects of ableism in our institutions of healthcare and medicine to build less ableist and more inclusive and humane institutions?
2. Would it be possible to improve your preferred moral theory by applying this unit's lessons on the problems faced by persons marginalized because of their disability? If yes, how can you refine your preferred moral theory to incorporate these lessons? If no, explain why not. (For example, if you're attracted to care ethics, how can you develop a care ethics approach to tackling bioethical problems that cares for disabled persons more compassionately/considerately?)

Unit III

The Miasma of Cisheteropatriarchy in Healthcare and Medicine

Introduction to the Unit

In this unit, we discuss how bioethical issues are complicated when we center the perspectives/experiences of persons who are marginalized because of their sex, gender, and/or sexuality. It aims to

- educate readers as to the meaning, history, and significance of the concepts of sex, gender, and sexuality;
- give readers a sense of the systemic oppression that women, intersex persons, and LGBTQ+ persons face; and
- acquaint readers with some insightful solutions to the problems of healthcare and medicine that emerge from centering the perspectives/experiences of these marginalized groups.

The Complexity of Biology, Culture, and Development

Sex, gender, and sexuality/sexual orientation are three distinct but interrelated aspects of human experience. We may wonder whether these phenomena of human identity/experience are innate. However, as philosopher of biology Paul

Griffiths (1997, p. 59) has pointed out, innateness is a confused concept that clumps together independent properties that come apart, including these:

- being present at birth
- having an evolutionary explanation
- being insensitive to external variation in development

These properties come apart in part because, as a general matter, the complex evolved traits of adult organisms emerge not just from genes or culture but also from the dynamic, time-sensitive interaction of genes with a richly structured and inherited natural *and* social environment (Griffiths, 1997, p. 61). In short, it's not nature versus nurture but nature *with* nurture. To adequately understand how these aspects of human experience emerge, we need to adopt a nuanced framework that looks at this dynamic, time-sensitive interaction. Indeed, as sexologist Anne Fausto-Sterling (2020) explains, we need to adopt a transdisciplinary framework that brings together[1]

- phenomenology (to study the lived conscious experience of gender/sexuality),
- empirical psychoanalysis (to explore the unconscious psychology of gender/sexuality),
- dynamical systems theory (to understand the development of gender/sexuality within the organism), and
- embodied cognition (to investigate the way gender/sexuality is embodied within the thinking, feeling subject).

This transdisciplinary approach emphasizes the embeddedness of the body (in the womb, in the physical world, in intersubjective interactions) as essential to human development and reveals that personal identity (including gender/sexuality) is inherently relational because of how it develops through embedded processes in a way that allows us to explore it experimentally (Fausto-Sterling, 2020, pp. 297–298). To serve as a tool of liberation, this approach must center not just dominant or normative accounts of the formation of sex/gender/sexuality but also how nonnormative individual differences emerge out of the processes that tend to produce "normal," relatively general characteristics (2020, p. 292). According to this framework, gender and sexuality are emergent properties that are complex, usually stable, and "softly assembled" from bodily, cultural, and intersubjective systems (2020, p. 290). This soft assembly provides stability but also permits change if one or more of the subsystems stabilizing a stable emergent property change. If this happens, currently stable states (one's gender/sexuality) can destabilize, reorganize, and reassemble in new configurations. This makes clear that gender and sexuality are dynamic and potentially fluid phenomena. Fausto-Sterling has fleshed out this framework for the development of sex and gender in humans with empirical work on children, giving a timeline for how, throughout the

1. Such a transdisciplinary framework is also needed for an adequate understanding of complex psychological (e.g., emotional) phenomena.

first three years of development, children come to have "a shaky but still surprisingly sturdy gender/sex identity," with the third year forming an important waypoint in the stabilization of the emerging gender identity, though identity modifications continue "well past this point" (2020, p. 309).

The take-home lesson here is that sex, gender, and sexuality are much more complex and dynamic phenomena than mainstream discussions often lead people to believe.

Binary Biological Models of Sex, Gender, and Sexuality

Mainstream discussions of these phenomena often incorrectly teach that these phenomena are binary and purely biological:

Sex— male/female

- based on bodies and genitalia
- immutable and inherent to identity

Gender— man/woman

- based on binary sex
- immutable and inherent to identity
- (sometimes) social expression of binary sex

Sexuality— straight/gay

- based on genetics
- immutable and inherent to identity

As gender-nonconforming gender scholar Alok Vaid-Menon (2020) explains, these models are based on mistaken assumptions that

- are relatively recent,
- have been told so often that they have become the status quo, and
- are upheld by a system of power designed to create conflict and division, and hence
- have been socially constructed to seem like absolute facts.

Accordingly, we must keep in mind, as McLean (cited in Imani, 2021, p. 132) warns, that discussions about these phenomena are rooted not in science but in power dynamics (which sometimes co-opt pseudo/scientific discourse). These mistaken understandings of these phenomena are ultimately rooted in the Eurocolonial binary.

The Eurocolonial (Sex/Gender/Sexuality) Binary

As McLean and Imani explain, the sex/gender/sexuality binary is a Eurocolonial invention that was socially constructed as a tool of oppression historically used to control the means of production (by controlling human reproduction) (Imani, 2021, p. 134). The work of scholars like Oyèrónkẹ́ Oyěwùmí (1997) shows that before colonization, African societies (and even languages) were not gendered, and the people were organized by age, not by gender; further, the category of "woman" was introduced and implemented through the regimes of European invaders. In many Indigenous cultures in North America and South Asia, even though gender was used as a form of social organization, it was understood not as a mere binary, but as varied.[2] European colonizers socially constructed the sex/gender/sexuality binary, establishing a social gendered hierarchy based on two distinct and opposite sexes, in order to ensure a controlled Indigenous population that could be enslaved and exploited as a labor force (Imani, 2021, p, 134). As part of this imperialist, colonialist construction, the gender expressions of Indigenous peoples came to be regulated through law, policy, and violence.

Despite this history, countless precolonial nonbinary gender identities exist today and are working to rebuild and heal the wounds of Eurocolonialism (Imani, 2021, p. 134). Transgender, nonbinary (e.g., agender or genderfluid), gay, bisexual, and intersex people have always existed and will continue to exist; gender has not always existed, and when it has existed, it has not always been binary. The historical record confirms this time and time again. Moreover, there are thriving communities and peoples that understand themselves outside of gender. In articulating this transdisciplinary framework for understanding these phenomena, Fausto-Sterling (2020, p. 309) notes that we live "in a world in which gender, like nitrogen, oxygen, or carbon dioxide, is one of the predominant atmospheric elements." Gender is a socially produced element, however, not a naturally existing one. And the sex/gender/sexuality binary in our social atmosphere is a toxic element resulting from a history of imperialism and colonialism, one that (as we shall see below) helps constitute a toxic miasma of oppression.

In contrast to the biological models that constitute the Eurocolonial binary, McLean and Imani offer more accurate social constructionist models of these phenomena.

Social Nonbinary Models

Sex

Definition—determination made through application of socially agreed-upon criteria (sex traits) before birth, where sex traits vary widely, offering a "kaleidoscope of possible sex trait combinations" (cited in Imani, 2021, p. 128):

2. Vaid-Menon notes that there is a rich tradition of Indigenous people living outside the gender binary, for example, *two-spirit* among Native Americans, *hijra* in South Asia, *waria* in Indonesia, and *muxe* in Mexico (Vaid-Menon, 2020, p. 39).

- Several chromosome pairings (X, XY, XYY, XXX, XX, XXY)
- Hormones (e.g., testosterone, estrogen) of varying levels
- Internal and external genitalia/sex organs of many shapes that may not align with textbook depictions
- Secondary sex characteristics (e.g., breasts and body hair)

In practice, babies are assigned a sex based primarily (and often exclusively) on what their genitals look like at birth, but this does not change the reality that sex traits vary complexly. Importantly, there is no "normal" or "default" combination of chromosomes, hormones, or look for a vulva, labia, clitoris, scrotum, or penis. There is no such thing as a "normal" or "default" human body. What we claim to be "normal" human bodies says more about our social and cultural context than it says about human biology. **Intersex** persons are those whose bodies do not conform to binary sex combinations.[3] Note that *intersex* is an umbrella term that covers "everything from chromosomal variation to hormone receptors or missing or malfunctioning enzymes involved with hormone synthesis" and that not all intersex persons or families embrace this terminology, with some identifying as male/female instead (Fausto-Sterling, 2020, p. 317).

Gender

Definition—"what we know ourselves to be", consists of "an array of mental and behavioral characteristics that relate to, differ from, and go beyond understandings of masculinity, femininity, and neutrality" (Vaid-Menon, cited in Imani, 2021, p. 133).

On this understanding, gender is "our truth" (Imani, 2021, p. 136). And this understanding is foundational to our margin-centering approach. Whether someone expresses or possesses gender identity is up to that person, and we must respect this fact. Centering marginalized persons requires that we leave it up to individuals to determine their gender identity, regardless of what any external expectations or mandates might claim. Respecting individual autonomy and people's dignity and humanity requires recognizing and respecting people when they autonomously determine and express their gender identity, regardless of whether we understand it or whether it makes us uncomfortable. And despite our recent Eurocolonial history, as Vaid-Menon (2020, p. 55) notes, the self-determination of gender has long been practiced throughout time and space. Possible genders include the following:

- Woman
- Man
- **Nonbinary—**an array of gender identities not conforming to the gender binary
- **Agender—**not having a gender
- **Genderfluid—**having a gender identity that varies over time

3. A bioethical issue of justice in athletics arises for intersex athletes given how gender segregation is practiced. Here there emerges a complex interplay of science, gender, and race, as Fausto-Sterling discusses (2020, pp. 326–334).

- **Bigender—**having two or a combination of gender identities
- **Demigender—**having partial but not full connection to the concept of gender and gender identity(ies)

And there are countless others. There is no fixed number of possible genders and no single way to talk about them.[4] Centering the margins requires creating space for complexity and nuance that has long been silenced and erased. Thus, we should follow Imani in picturing the complexity of gender not as a one-dimensional spectrum (which encourages the thought that nonbinary people have to exist "between" man and woman) but rather as "a fully dimensional universe with constellations, galaxies, and nebulas representing the people who may share communities or similar methods of self-expression and self-understanding" (2021, p. 138). To this we can add that the stars in this universe "do not compete but amplify one another's shine" (Vaid-Menon, 2020, p. 60).

When we are born, we tend to be assigned a sex and a gender. If one's gender identity matches one's assigned gender at birth, then one is **cisgender**. If one's gender identity does not match one's assigned gender at birth, then one is **transgender**. As we shall see, transgender individuals face unique social and healthcare challenges that we must keep in mind as part of our social justice approach to bioethics.

Sexuality

Definition—part of personal identity relating to physical, sexual, romantic, and/or emotional attractions to other people.

As with gender, there is no fixed number of sexualities. Instead, many sexualities (and many ways of talking about them) are possible, including the following:

- **Asexual—**experiences little to no physical, sexual, romantic, or emotional attraction to others
- **Bisexual—**forms physical, sexual, romantic, and/or emotional attraction to two or more genders
- **Gay**[5] **—**forms physical, sexual, romantic, and/or emotional attraction to persons of same gender
- **Heterosexual/straight—**women(men) who form physical, sexual, romantic, and/or emotional attraction to men(women)
- **Omnisexual—**forms physical, sexual, romantic, and/or emotional attraction to all genders
- **Pansexual—**forms physical, sexual, romantic, and/or emotional attraction regardless of gender
- **Polysexual—**forms physical, sexual, romantic, and/or emotional attraction to many genders

As Imani notes, many people grow up thinking that heterosexuality is "the default" and that everyone else needs to figure out and disclose their sexuality, lest they risk "living a lie" (2021, p. 138). This is in

4. For example, Martine Rothblatt (1995) proposes a "chromatic" classification of gender with 343 shades, and Fausto-Sterling (2020, p. 315) notes that, as of 2020, Facebook offers 71 gender self-designation options.
5. Note that the term *homosexual* has a history of being used to pathologize gay people and is scientifically inadequate (cf. Imani, 2021, p. 143; Fausto-Sterling, 2020, p. 11).

part because of the way society centers the experience of heterosexual persons due to **heteronormativity** (unpacked further below). The reality, however, is that there is no default or normal sexuality, and depending on individual contexts, sexuality may or may not be a central part of one's identity at different stages in life. Many discussions (popular and scholarly) about sexuality beyond heteronormativity center around the Kinsey Scale.[6] However, as Imani notes, as groundbreaking as the scale was at the time, the complex nature of human sexuality cannot and should not be understood based entirely on that approach. This approach focuses only on previous sex acts and experiences and is based solely on experiences of and analysis conducted by white men in the US (2021, p. 139).

What the Kinsey Scale seems to get right is that sexuality is not a binary but has a structure closer to a spectrum. What it gets wrong is that this spectrum is not merely one-dimensional and wholly concerned with past sexual experiences. Instead, it is a multidimensional spectrum of physical, romantic, emotional, and sexual attraction to all kinds of different people that may not fall neatly under any label at all. Instead of a spectrum, then, it might be more accurate to speak of a "kaleidoscope of sexuality" (Imani, 2021, p. 130).

Even with these more nuanced understandings of sex, gender, and sexuality, a number of oppressive social constructions (including the Eurocolonial binary) surrounding them create toxic antagonisms that make our social world less valuable than the sum of its parts.

The Toxic Miasma of Cisheteropatriarchy (and Androcentrism/Sexism/Misogyny/Homo/Transphobia)

Building on the idea that gender is a socially produced atmospheric element, we can note that this element nourishes the flourishing of many people who find meaning and joy in these aspects of human experience. Unfortunately, this atmosphere is also marred by many oppressive social constructions that create a toxic atmosphere or miasma[7] around how we embody and experience these phenomena, including the following:

- **Cisnormativity/transphobia**—a socially constructed system that reinforces the idea of the (sex/gender/sexuality) binary, centering cisgender experience as the "default" in human life and discriminating against transgender individuals
- **Heteronormativity/homophobia**—a socially constructed system that reinforces the idea that binary gender individuals must pair themselves with the "opposite" gender in order to form valid relationships; upholds the idea of the binary and delegitimizes/discriminates against LGBTQ+ people and relationships

6. This scale assigns a value from 0 (exclusively heterosexual) to 6 (exclusively gay) based on previous sexual experiences (with intermediate values representing varying degrees of bisexuality). As Fausto-Sterling points out, although multidimensional models of sexuality exist (e.g., Klein, 1990), the linear Kinsey Scale has had long and continuing influence (Fausto-Sterling, 2020, p. 11).
7. This analogy can be found in the work of feminist and queer scholars (e.g., Carney, 2021; Glitzen & Chun, 2021).

- **Patriarchy**—a form of social organization that privileges men and fathers, placing them in positions of power in social structures, including the family, and overvaluing of the masculine
- **Androcentrism**—the view that man is the paradigmatic human being and thus that the male body is the paradigmatic human body (Lindemann, 2012, p. 43).
- **Sexism**—prejudice, stereotyping, or discrimination against people on the basis of sex and/or gender (can be interpersonal, institutional, and/or cultural)
- **Misogyny**—hatred toward and discrimination against women, and undervaluation of the feminine

Together, all these social constructions constitute a toxic miasma of cisheteropatriarchy that affects every aspect of our social world—from our institutions and systems to our interactions and even the way we think, feel, and talk. Its effects can be seen in, for example, political and governmental policies, social norms, media, sexist language, and gendered merchandising. The gender binary is a component of this miasma, for as Vaid-Menon (2020, p. 27) notes, it is concerned with gender norms, not with persons' well-being. Indeed, all these toxic constructions serve to enforce conformity to gender norms that constrain and divide us instead of letting us embody and express who we are.

This toxic miasma systemically harms everyone—but (once again) not equally, with women, intersex, and LGBTQ+ individuals and groups being disproportionately harmed by it. It is an antagonistic organic unity over our social world (including the institutions of healthcare and medicine) that harms everyone but moreover unfairly accommodates and privileges (and thus creates synergies in the lives of) men, straight persons, and cisgender persons and unfairly disadvantages and oppresses (and thus creates antagonisms in the lives of) women, intersex persons, queer persons, and transgender persons.[8] This unjust distribution of synergies and antagonisms itself yields overall antagonisms due to its injustice and inefficiency. Much more can be, should be, and has been said (by feminist and queer scholars) to articulate this miasma and the myriad ways it harms us.[9] Nonetheless, this discussion provides an initial critical lens that we can further articulate.

(Intersectional) Queering of Bioethics

A key part of applying our critical lens to bioethics consists of "queering" (i.e., applying a non-normative lens to what is taken to be standard and ordinary) our approach to bioethics. That is, we need to transform our approach to bioethics from a mainstream one to a "queer" one that centers the needs, perspectives, histories, and concerns of queer persons, adopting an "insider's view" (Wahlert & Fiester, 2014, p. 63).

8. ***Queer*** is an umbrella term for any gender or sexuality that does not correspond to cis/heteronormativity.
9. Complexities arise from the intersection of racialization and gendering. For example, as Patricia Hill Collins (2004) notes, Black people have been and continue to be policed because of how they gender, and Black women are viewed as inherently masculine, aggressive, and less "desirable." Moreover, the toxic miasma of cisheteropatriarchy unjustly extracts emotional labor and energy not only from women but also from **femmes** (persons with queer feminine genders), even within marginalized spaces/communities, and it constructs femininity and femmeness as weaker and lesser (Lakshmi Piepzsna-Samarasinha, 2019, Chapter 8).

The toxic miasma of cisheteropatriarchy is so pervasive that, as Lance Wahlert and Autumn Fiester highlight, cultural norms related to sexuality, gender, and the conventional family can unwittingly reinforce a dominant status quo that marginalizes queer persons despite healthcare providers' good intentions. Wahlert and Fiester note that "even the most sympathetic and well-intentioned cases that include either LGBT persons or queer-related content can play into (rather than redress) long-standing biases about sexuality and gender nonconformity in science and medicine" (2014, p. 62).

Good intentions are not enough to achieve good outcomes for marginalized persons. Wahlert and Fiester (2014) suggest that we "repave the road of good intentions" in bioethics by bringing a queer bioethical lens that centers the perspectives, histories, concerns, and needs of LGBTQ+ persons, lest this road continue proverbially to lead to hell. The same lessons hold concerning the need to bring an intersectional critical lens to bioethical issues, one that is not just queer but also feminist, antiracist, and anti-ableist. Only by bringing this kind of lens to social and bioethical problems, a lens that centers a wide variety of marginalized perspectives, can we repave the road of good intentions for persons marginalized by their race, disability, and/or sex, gender, or sexuality so that it will lead to more inclusive and humane approaches that yield fewer harms and more positive outcomes. The readings further articulate this lens.

Unit Readings

The first reading (Sewell et al., 2018) traces the sexism and androcentrism in the institutions of medicine and healthcare by giving an overview of how and why gender disparities exist in mental health diagnosis, treatment, and access to care.

The second reading (Dargie et al., 2014) enriches our understanding of the kaleidoscope of sexuality and the universe of gender by exploring the diversity in how transgender persons experience their gender and sexuality beyond the binary. It also discusses unique social and health challenges faced by transgender persons

The third reading (Bakhru, 2019) provides a transdisciplinary intersectional approach to reproductive health. It brings together the frameworks of reproductive justice and transnational feminism:

- to connect the toxic miasma of cisheteropatriarchy with neoliberal economic ideology and the forces of globalization, and
- to propose how these frameworks can help us reconceptualize pressing issues and create and sustain movements for social justice and transformation.

The fourth reading (Hutchinson, 2016) further articulates this book's intersectional approach to bioethics by centering Black women's conditions/experiences in its discussion of reproductive health. The reading argues that given the social conditions Black women face (including wealth and healthcare disparities), reproductive justice is a precondition for their mental health, well-being, bodily autonomy, and enfranchisement.

All these readings consider how centering the perspectives/experiences of persons marginalized due to their sex, gender, and/or sexuality can help us better understand the problems faced by marginalized persons, as well as how doing so can provide better solutions to pressing social and bioethical problems.

References

Bakhru, T. S. (2019). Thinking transnationally: Reproductive justice in a globalized era. In T. S. Bakhru (Ed.), *Reproductive justice and sexual rights: Transnational perspectives* (pp. 3–12). Routledge.

Carney, T. (2021). Solving the crimes of patriarchy: Meta-lucidity and middle-aged women in *Happy Valley* and *Broadchurch. Mai: Feminism & Visual Culture.* https://maifeminism.com/solving-the-crimes-of-the-patriarchy-meta-lucidity-and-middle-aged-women-in-happy-valley-broadchurch/

Collins, P. H. (2004). Black sexual politics: African Americans, gender, and the new racism. Routledge.

Dargie, E., Blair, K. L., Pukall, C. F., & Coyle, S. M. (2014). Somewhere under the rainbow: Exploring the identities and experiences of trans persons. The Canadian Journal of Human Sexuality, 23(2), 60–74. https://www.muse.jhu.edu/article/553140.

Fausto-Sterling, A. (2020). Sexing the body: Gender politics and the construction of sexuality. Basic Books.

Glitzen, T., & Chun, W. (2021). *Pandemic surveillance and homophobia in South Korea.* The Social Science Research Council. https://items.ssrc.org/covid-19-and-the-social-sciences/covid-19-fieldnotes/pandemic-surveillance-and-homophobia-in-south-korea

Griffiths, P. E. (2008). What emotions really are. University of Chicago Press.

Hutchinson, S. (2016). Whose bodies? Black Lives Matter and the Reproductive Justice Imperative. *The Humanist, 76*(3), 10.

Imani, B. (2021). Read this to get smarter: About race, class, gender, disability & more. Ten Speed Press.

Klein, F. (1990). The need to view sexual orientation as a multivariable process: A theoretical perspective. In D. P. McWhirter, S.A. Sanders, & J.M. Reinisch (Eds.), *Homosexuality/heterosexuality: Concepts of sexual orientation* (pp. 277-282). Oxford University Press.

Lakshmi Piepzsna-Samarasinha, L. (2019). *Care work: Dreaming disability justice.* Arsenal Pulp Press.

Lindemann, H. (2012). The woman question in medicine: An update. *Hastings Center Report, 42*(3), 38–45.

Oyěwùmí, O. (1997). The invention of women: Making an African sense of Western gender discourses. University of Minnesota Press.

Rothblatt, M. (1995). The apartheid of sex: A manifesto on the freedom of gender. Crown.

Sewell, W. C, Key, W., & Gehlert, S. (2018). Analyzing the problem: Gender disparities in behavioral and mental health care. In C. Moniz & Stephen Gorin (Eds.), *Behavioral and mental health care policy and practice: A biopsychosocial perspective* (pp. 170–182). Routledge.

Vaid-Menon, A. (2020). *Beyond the gender binary.* Penguin.

Wahlert, L., & Fiester, A. (2014). Repaving the road of good intentions: LGBT health care and the queer bioethical lens. *Hastings Center Report, 44*(s4), S56–65. https://doi.org/10.1002/hast.373

Reading 3.1

Analyzing the Problem

Gender Disparities in Behavioral and Mental Health Care

Whitney C. Sewell, Whitney Key, and Sarah Gehlert

Editor's Introduction

In this reading, the authors apply their knowledge of how social determinants of health and well-being affect marginalized populations and offer an overview of how and why gender disparities exist in mental health diagnosis, treatment, and access to care. In their discussion, they

- identify patterns of mental illness and gender-specific mental health outcomes, noting that women face worse mental health outcomes compared to men, despite comparable prevalence rates for some mental illnesses;
- examine how gender disparities in mental health and access to quality mental health services are rooted in social and structural inequity and barriers of a fractured system that leaves many underserved and overlooked;
- show that women's mental health has been stigmatized by historically

misunderstood and improperly diagnosed gender-specific mental health conditions; and

- review mental health policies and programs to promote gender equity in mental health services, noting that the few policies that protect the right of women to access comprehensive healthcare are constantly under scrutiny and at risk of defunding.

Whitney C. Sewell, PhD is a lecturer on population medicine at the Harvard Pilgrim Healthcare Institute. Her work deals with HIV risk perception, discrimination, and patient decision-making. Whitney Key, MPH, MSW is a scholar specializing in health disparities and social determinants of health. Sarah Gehlert, PhD is dean and Ernest P. Larson professor of health, ethnicity, and poverty at the University of Southern California School of Social Work. Her work focuses on social and environmental influences on health, especially the health of vulnerable populations.

Introduction

Gender is a known social determinant of health and well-being, whose interaction with other social determinants, such as race, socioeconomic status, and employment, exacerbates health vulnerabilities. Mounting evidence indicates that gendered inequities in behavioral and mental health are just one consequence of a stratification system that differentially allots opportunities to men and women in a way that affects their quality of life (Denton, Prus, & Walters, 2004; Ross & Bird, 1994). Men and women occupy different social-structural locations that mediate their exposure to risks that are harmful to health, their participation in health-damaging behaviors, and their access to goods and resources that promote well-being (Bird & Rieker, 1999). Many gender-acquired risks arise from women's disproportionate exposure to poverty and socioeconomic disadvantages compared to men. The World Health Organization (WHO) noted that women constitute 70% of the world's poor, and among those employed are significantly underpaid for their work. In addition to the subjugation to disparaged social and economic conditions, gender-based violence and violence exposure disproportionately affects women, increasing their likelihood of experience-adverse mental and physical health outcomes.

Women report worse health than men do and more acute problems, chronic conditions, and disability, yet they tend to live longer than men. Overall, men and women experience comparable rates of mental health problems; however, the type of health problems either experience are distinct. Women experience higher rates of the affective mental health disorders, such as depression and anxiety. In contrast, men are more likely to suffer from antisocial personality disorders and substance abuse.

Empirical evidence has demonstrated that both biological and social processes drive these paradoxical patterns and that gender does matter in understanding and determining disparities in health for men and women.

The goal of this [reading] is to offer an overview of how and why gender disparities exist in mental health diagnosis, treatment, and access to care. In this [reading], we address gender disparities in behavioral and mental health, identify patterns and prevalence of mental illness and gender-specific mental health outcomes, examine gender differences in access to mental health treatment and care, and review mental health policies and programs to promote gender equity in mental health services.

Why Gender Matters

In the examination of various health outcomes, gender disparities are evident, particularly in population health indicators. These indicators provide valuable insight into the incidence, prevalence, and trends of health and help direct preventative measures needed to address disparities. Health risk factors, such as mental illness, obesity, heart disease, smoking, and diabetes, influence two significant population health indicators: life expectancy and mortality.

Policy Analysis

What is the social problem?	There are stark gender disparities in mental health and mental health outcomes, much of which can be mediated by equitable access to resources and services.
Who is affected? What is the extent of the problem?	Women are disproportionately affected by mental illness compared to men; despite instances of comparable prevalence rates, the impact of poor mental health has far worse outcomes for women than men.
What evidence is there that a problem exists?	Multiple national epidemiological studies have provided evidence of the gender disparities in prevalence rates; social scientists have provided further evidence of social determinants such as employment, income, and stable housing as exacerbating existing gender disparities.
How serious is the problem?	Evidence reveals that combined historical and systemic practices have been heavily influenced by bias and stigma in their approach to women's physical and mental health. As such, gender disparities in mental health are a complicated and serious social and structural issue.
What is the perceived cause of the problem?	Lack of access to quality comprehensive health care leaves many individuals untreated and underserved, particularly low-income women. Furthermore, there are dire consequences of policies and programs that treat mental illness and substance use separately.
What explanations exist for the problem?	Women face multiple gender-specific social determinants of health, including health insurance, income, employment, housing, bias, and stigma that moderate their likelihood to be exposed to acute and chronic stressors and/or trauma that leads to mental illness. These determinants also influence their access to resources and services that can improve their mental health outcomes.

Life expectancy at birth measures the number of years a cohort of infants would live if the group experiences the present age-specific mortality rate. According to recent data from the Centers for Disease Control and Prevention (CDC), as of 2015, the total population life expectancy at birth in the United States was 78.8 years. The life expectancy was 76.3 years for males and 81.2 years for females. Since 2004, the life expectancy at birth has increased 1.4 years for males and 1.1 years for females; however, there remains a substantial 4.9-year disparity between males and females.

Despite reporting worse health outcomes than men, women tend to live longer—this is referred to as the "morbidity paradox" (Gorman & Read, 2006). How do we explain these gender differences in health and health outcomes? Evidence suggests it is the combined impact of social and behavioral factors that contribute to gender health disparities. Behaviorally, men are more likely to engage in health-damaging behaviors. As men age, they smoke more than women do (Bar-beau, Krieger, & Soobader, 2004), and they consume more alcohol and more often than do women (Chan, Neighbors, Gilson, Larimer, & Alan Marlatt, 2007; Johnson, Gruenewald, Treno, & Taff, 1998). However, men also exercise, including walking and high-impact exercise, more frequently than do women (Ross & Bird, 1994; Trost, Owen, Bauman, Sallis, & Brown, 2002). Socially, men and women navigate distinct types of social embeddedness and locations that mediate their exposure to health risks, health-damaging behaviors, and access to health-promoting resources, goods, and services (Bird & Rieker, 1999). [...] Here it is worth noting that while men engage in more health-damaging behaviors, there are social-structural systems of power and access that protect them and reduce their risk of detrimental outcomes.

Consistent with the exposures to socioeconomic and social-structural inequities, women are exposed to greater stressful life events and chronic stressors in their daily life (Matheson et al., 2006). These exposures are linked to depression, which subsequently impacts blood pressure, immune functioning, and damaging health behaviors such as excessive smoking and drinking (Ross & Bird, 1994). Recent evidence suggests that the differences in health behaviors and outcomes are temporal, as men and women age this gender gap begins to close, particularly in middle and late life (Gorman & Read, 2006). This is directly linked to the higher rates of depression among women, compared to men, as well as many other gender differences in patterns of mental illness.

Gender Differences in Patterns of Mental Illness

Epidemiological studies have shown that there are no gender-significant differences in lifetime prevalence rates of severe mental disorders such as schizophrenia and bipolar disorder; however, there are stark gender differences in less-severe yet high-prevalence affective disorders such as depression and anxiety. Psychiatric epidemiology reveals that the prevalence of major depressive disorder among women is nearly double than that of men (Kessler, 2003). Furthermore, the disparity and increased risk of depression for women persists across the life span from youth to older adulthood (Kessler, Chiu, Demler, & Walters, 2005).

The following patterns in prevalence of mental illness, according to findings from the National Comorbidity Survey Replication study (Kessler, 2003), demonstrate that women are disproportionately affected by mental health issues. In affective disorders, 46 million women (29%) suffer from depression compared to 28 million (18%) of men over their lifetimes. Additionally, 54 million women (34%) experience anxiety during their lifetimes, compared to 36 million men (23%). In contrast to these rates, men have higher rates of externalized mental health problems in their lifetimes than women have. According to the study, 8 million men (5%) are affected by antisocial personality disorder, compared to 1.5 million women (1%). In addition, 54 million men (35%) experience substance abuse disorders versus 29 million women

(18%). Decreasing the gender disparities would improve mental and physical health outcomes for millions of men and women nationwide. Evidence shows that these patterns in gender disparities exist on a global level, further necessitating the commitment to improving mental health globally (WHO, 2001).

Gendered Mental Health Conditions

Throughout recorded history, certain mental disorders have been attributed to women by virtue of their association with the female reproductive system and sexuality. This attribution began with hysteria (Tasca, Rapetti, Carta, & Fadda, 2012), which is no longer recognized as a mental condition, and continues with premenstrual dysphoric disorder, a current diagnosis in the *Diagnostic and Statistical Manual of Mental Disorders* (*DSM–5*; American Psychiatric Association, 2013).

Hysteria

Hysteria is difficult to define because descriptions of its nature and origins have varied markedly over time. In her 1965 text on the history of hysteria, Veith wrote that "much of what has been called hysteria at various periods would no longer be so described, and much of what is now recognized as symptomatic of hysteria was earlier attributed to other diseases" (Veith, 1965, p. vii). The first written description was by the ancient Egyptians, who identified the source of hysterical disorders as the uterus, with symptoms arising when it moved from its natural position (Cosmacini, 1997). The Greeks later attributed it to the lack of a normal sexual life (Cosmacini, 1997). Over time, the locus of hysteria shifted from the uterus to the brain and nervous system. Another major shift occurred in 1697, when Thomas Syndham first characterized hysteria as an emotional disorder that could simulate almost any disease rather than as a physical condition or disease in and of itself (North, 2015).

The term "hysteria" appeared in various forms in psychiatric nosology until the middle of the 20th century. It was replaced by "conversion symptoms" in the American Psychiatric Association's first publication of the *Diagnostic and Statistical Manual of Mental Disorders* (American Psychiatric Association, 1952). "Hysterical neurosis" remained in *DSM* until the publication of *DSM-III* (American Psychiatric Association, 1980).

The shift from the uterus to the brain and nervous system as the origin of hysteria and the change in terminology from "hysteria" to "conversion symptoms" seem to represent a shift from an exclusive attribution to women to a broader attribution by gender. Rather than focusing on reproductive functioning or sexuality, conversion symptoms suggest neurological disease, and occur in situations in which neither physical examination nor diagnostic testing can provide an explanation for their occurrence. Conversion symptoms are generally acute in onset and may follow unresolved psychological conflict. They are see in a variety of *DSM* diagnoses, such as conversion disorder, somatization disorder, and other conditions not exclusive to women. Yet, the fact that conversion disorder, which first appeared in *DSM-IV* (American Psychiatric Association, 2000), is described in *DSM-5* as being two to six times more likely in woman suggests that some attribution to women's reproductive system and sexuality persists (American Psychiatric Association, 2013).

Premenstrual Dysphoric Disorder

Premenstrual dysphoric disorder (PMDD) was included as a provisional diagnostic category in the appendix of *DSM-III-R* (American Psychiatric Association, 1987; then called late luteal phase dysphoric disorder), remained as an appendix item in *DSM-IV* (American Psychiatric Association, 1994), and became a formal diagnosis in *DSM-5* (American Psychiatric Association, 2013).

Although the idea of premenstrual symptoms affecting mood has existed since the time of Hippocrates (Gehlert, Song, Chang, & Hartlage, 2009), efforts to capture exactly how it occurs have largely been unsuccessful. Premenstrual syndrome (PMS) was described in the 1950s (Greene & Dalton, 1953) as a condition in which symptoms appear ten to seven days before menstruation and remit upon its onset. Since that time, over 150 symptoms have been attributed to the condition (Gehlert, Song, Chang, & Hartlage, 2009).

A subtype of PMS with the primary feature of debilitating mood symptoms was proposed in the 1970s. It was first named "late luteal phase dysphoric disorder" in *DSM-III-R* (American Psychiatric Association, 1987) and then renamed "premenstrual dysphoric disorder" in *DSM-IV* (American Psychiatric Association, 1994). It remained in appendices of *DSM* as part of "Criterion Sets and Axes provided for further study" until 2012, when it was included in *DSM-5* as a diagnostic category (Premenstrual Dysphoric Disorder DSM-5 625.4 [N94.3]). According to *DSM-5*, it occurs in 3% to 8% of women, but varies greatly by geography (American Psychiatric Association, 2013).

PMDD is defined in *DSM-5* (American Psychiatric Association, 2013) by a set of four research criteria that are required for diagnosis. The first of these is that at least five from among a list of eleven symptoms, one of which must be affective, are present for most of the last week of the luteal phases and absent in the week post-menses. The second criterion is that PMDD must interfere markedly with work, school, or interpersonal relationships. The third criterion is that the first three criteria are confirmed by prospective daily ratings for two consecutive menstrual cycles.

The PMDD diagnosis remains controversial because of lingering ambiguity about its origins and nature (Gehlert, Song, Chang, & Hartlage, 2009; Gehlert, Chang, & Song, 2010). Some authors have questioned the implications of PMDD as the only *DSM-5* disorder attributable exclusively to women. Chrisler and Caplan (2002) have argued that PMDD is a culture-bound syndrome and therefore not appropriate as a diagnostic category, a notion that seems to be supported by *DSM-5* language about PMDD's wide geographic variation. In a 2013 interview on National Public Radio, Gehlert also expressed concern that PMDD's status as a psychiatric diagnosis could be used to gain power over socioeconomically vulnerable women in situations such as custody hearings or in disputes over employment or housing (Standen, 2013).

Gender Bias and Stigma

Employment plays an important role in determining women's and men's relative wealth, power, and prestige. This generates gender inequalities in the distribution of resources, benefits, and responsibilities. The workplace can be a setting where gender inequalities are both manifested and sustained, with consequent impacts on health. The number of women engaged in the workforce has increased dramatically in both developing and developed countries over the past few decades. According to World Bank estimates, from 1960 to 1997, women have increased their numbers in the global labor force by 126% (World Bank, 2001). Today, women make up about 42% of the estimated global working population, making them essential commodities to the global economy (Messing & Ostlin, 2006).

Employment can differ depending on gender. In the developing countries, women and men work at different tasks in agriculture (London et al., 2002; Kisting in WHO, 2005), mining, manufacturing, and services (Acevedo, 2002; Parra Garrido, 2002). Women are more likely to work in the informal economy sector and they do specific types of informal work, such as domestic work, street vending, and sex work. In the industrialized countries, women and men also commonly perform different tasks and work in different sectors, although some job titles in white-collar work are occupied by both women and men, such as medicine, law, and business. However, women are more likely than men to spend more time in the house and are primarily responsible for the family well-being (Messing & Ostlin, 2006).

In industrialized countries, there has been a rise in nonstandard forms of employment, such as short-term contracts and subcontracting (Quinlan et al., 2001). Women hold specific types of nonstandard work, such as part-time work and one-person independent contracting (Cranford et al., 2003). Available evidence suggests that as a group, women suffer more from growing competitive pressures and cost-saving strategies, which can be associated with lack of security, limited possibilities for training and career advancement, and inadequate social security coverage in terms of old-age pensions, health insurance, and maternity protection (Messing & Ostlin, 2006).

Women are increasingly choosing to enter traditionally male jobs, such as engineering and technical jobs, and this trend has been increasing over the past decade (Asselin, 2003). By entering a male-dominated workforce, such women are exposed to discrimination, which may put their health at risk. For example, women's mental health may be directly affected because they may feel forced to take risks to prove that they are able to do the job (Messing & Elabidi, 2003).

Women are more reluctant to argue for full protection for their health, especially where the health problems concerned imply gender differences. A study in Canada demonstrated that women in food processing plants were subjected to severe cold temperatures and irregular work schedules. These conditions were associated with problems with their menstrual cycles, which lead to an absence of work (Mergler & Vézina, 1985; Messing et al., 1992, 1993). This could be appropriately treated through the occupational health and safety system, yet women have never argued for this. In fact, trade unionists approached about this issue felt that it would not be a good strategy to argue for inclusion of work-related menstrual problems in the occupational health and safety system, due to fears of a negative effect on employment possibilities for women (Messing et al., 1992).

Women do, however, feel more empowered to advocate for protection for possible damage to their fetus from dangerous working conditions (Turcotte, 1992). This could be because protecting children is seen as an appropriate maternal role. Because women house the fetus and nurse the child, the child is exposed to chemicals, toxins, and other workplace exposures that women are exposed to in the workplace.

Men and women behave and react differently to various situations. Men are more likely to have higher self-esteem and confidence, while women are more emotionally expressive (Lindelöw & Bildt-Thorbjornsson, 1998). Male–female differences in education, socialization, and upbringing may lead to differences in the behavior and expression of individuals. This has been studied in many facets regarding the way workers manage their illnesses (Alexanderson, 1998), their perception of risk (Gustafson, 1998), and the propensity to take sick leave or to seek treatment (Alexanderson et al., 1994, 1996). These differences may be attributed to why women's work-related sick leave lasts longer on the average than does men's (Islam et al., 2001).

In general, women are exposed to some psychosocial risk factors at work more often than men are, such as negative stress, psychological and sexual harassment, and monotonous work (Arcand et al., 2000). Because of the traditional male-dominated hierarchy in the workplace, women have less control over their work environment, which is associated with cardiovascular, mental, and musculoskeletal ill health (Hall, 1989). The combination of paid and unpaid work affects women's health (Brisson et al., 1999). Consequently, work-related fatigue, repetitive strain injury, infections, and mental health problems are more common among women than among men (Östlin, 2002).

There is an underestimation of women's work-related injuries and diseases because women's occupational injuries and illnesses are underdiagnosed (Kraus, Peek, Silberman, & Anderson, 1995) and women's claims for compensation for some health problems are preferentially refused (Lippel, 1999, 2003). When it comes to mental and behavioral health disorders, only 12% of the women's claims were accepted against 35% of the men's (Lippel, 2003). This systematic discrimination based on gender is incredibly harmful for women in the workplace.

Policy and Mental Health Promotion

Economic Policy and Women's Health

With the implementation of the Affordable Care Act (ACA), health insurance coverage was expanded by the requirement of individuals and employers to purchase insurance and by the expansion of Medicaid. By expanding the opportunities for coverage, the ACA names coverage an essential benefit. The ACA created essential health benefits defined by 10 components: ambulatory services, emergency services, hospitalization, maternity/newborn care, pediatric care, prescription drugs, laboratory services, preventive/wellness services, rehabilitative/habilitative services, and mental health and substance abuse care (Frank, Beronio, & Glied, 2014). By naming behavioral health (with substance abuse as a provision) as an essential benefit, insurance providers cannot deny services for this care.

However, in 2017, there has been a large effort to repeal and replace the ACA with a more conservative plan. In May 2017, the House of Representatives passed the American Health Care Act (AHCA) which, among other things, would eliminate the essential benefit clause and has the ability to deny coverage for pre-existing conditions (Kaiser Family Foundation, 2017). The essential benefits clause is incredibly important for women because it includes maternity and newborn care, services that are very expensive and can be a determining factor when individuals/families start planning. According to an article in the *New York Times*, women with insurance pay out of pocket an average of $3,400 compared to two decades ago; women typically paid nothing other than a small fee if they opted for a private hospital room or television (Rosenthal, 2013). From 2004 to 2010, the prices that insurers paid for childbirth—one of the most universal medical encounters—rose 49% for vaginal births and 41% for caesarean sections in the United States, with average out-of-pocket costs rising fourfold (Rosenthal, 2013). The average total price charged for pregnancy and newborn care was about $30,000 for a vaginal delivery and $50,000 for a caesarian section, with commercial insurers paying out an average of $18,329 and $27,866 (Rosenthal, 2013). In 2011, 62% of women in the United States covered by private plans that were not obtained through an employer lacked maternity coverage. However, even for women who do have coverage, insurers demanded higher copayments and deductibles and excluded many pregnancy-related services (Rosenthal, 2013).

Although these costs are directly related to the act of the childbirth process, they do not reflect the costs incurred for any post-partum counseling. Post-partum depression is a common illness that one in ten new mothers face each year (CDC, 2017). The costs of depression in the U.S. totaled $83.1 billion dollars in 2000, including $26.1 billion for direct medical costs, $5.4 billion for suicide-related mortality costs, and $51.5 billion for workplace costs (absenteeism, presenteeism, and disability) (Santoro, Peabody, & Schoenman, 2010). The specific costs of maternal depression are unknown; however, women with depression generally have more expensive medical claims than do men with depression, and pregnant women with untreated depression are at risk for costly complications, such as preterm birth. Children of depressed mothers may also have higher lifetime medical spending due to the adverse effects of postpartum depression on the child's own health. In fact, children with depressed mothers have been found to use health care services, including office and emergency room visits, more frequently than do children of healthy women (Santoro, Peabody, & Schoenman, 2010).

When undiagnosed and untreated, depression during pregnancy may lead to premature births, and this has substantial costs as well. In 2005, costs for all preterm births totaled at least $26.2 billion, or $51,600 for every infant born prematurely (Santoro & Peabody, 2010). Medical care for premature infants comprised 65% or $16.9 billion of the total costs, maternal delivery costs were $1.9 billion (7%), early intervention and special education services were $1.7 billion (6%), and lost household and labor market productivity totaled $5.7 billion (22%) (Santoro et al., 2010). The first-year medical costs are 10 times higher for preterm infants than full-term infants, including costs for both inpatient and outpatient care. In 2007, average medical costs for preterm infants were $49,033 compared to $4,551 for full-term infants (Santoro, Peabody et al., 2010).

The essential benefit clause is also important for women who may be victims of sexual assault. Standard public health practices after the trauma of sexual assault, such as testing and treatment of sexually transmitted infections, may not be covered with the repeal of this clause, and the subsequent counseling for the individual may be viewed as a pre-existing condition by the insurance company, possibly resulting in an increased premium or counseling services not being available in the plan again.

In July 2017, the Senate proposed two bills: The Health Care Freedom Act and the Better Care Reconciliation Act. These bills aimed to include services that are included under the ACA that the AHCA proposed to eliminate. Both included the prohibition of the pre-exiting conditions exclusion; however, the essential benefits clause was only included in the Health Care Freedom Act (Kaiser Family Foundation, 2017).

Both bills, however, prohibited federal funding of Planned Parenthood for one year. Although the Senate did propose legislation that would be more equitable for women by including essential benefits and the prohibition of excluding pre-existing conditions, the cut to the funding of Planned Parenthood is detrimental, as Planned Parenthood is an affordable option for the community when it comes to reproductive health, counseling, and other services.

Economic Policy and Equity

Health insurance is the strongest predictor of access and outcomes to health care, not just because it reduces the cost of care to the recipient. Payers design the behavioral health care delivery system through their network development and benefit design activities. Those with health insurance have greater access and better process and outcomes (Han, Gfroerer, & Colliver, 2010). However, obtaining health insurance has been difficult for the non-group market (e.g., those without group (employer)-based health insurance). Obtaining health insurance on the individual market was difficult because it is difficult to spread risk, a key to any insurance, within an individual or among an unknown group. To manage this possibility, health insurers did not enter the non-group market. If they did, the plans excluded those with pre-existing conditions and had limited benefits, narrow networks of providers, and lifetime limits. This led to health plans that were very expensive and did not provide many benefits, when they were available.

This is particularly true of behavioral health. Prior to the ACA, only one-third of health plans on the individual market offered any type of substance use disorder benefit, and those that did had strict controls with regard to cost sharing, lifetime limits, provider networks, etc. (Montz et al., 2016). However, these coverages did not include mental and behavioral health packages, therefore treatment and subsequent coverage was not active during this time. Mental health and substance abuse were treated as two separate diseases, while today we know that the two are intrinsically related.

Highlights

- Despite comparable prevalence rates for some mental illnesses, women face far worse mental health outcomes compared to men
- Gender disparities in mental health are rooted in social and structural inequity
- Gender-specific mental health conditions that affected women were historically misunderstood and improperly diagnosed, therefore stigmatizing women's mental health
- Women face social and structural barriers to access to quality mental health services
- The few policies protecting the rights of women to have access to comprehensive health care are constantly under scrutiny and at risk of defunding
- Access to quality affordable comprehensive health care is a significant contributor to gender disparities in mental health, and the current fractured system leaves many underserved and overlooked

Additional Websites

Allies for Reaching Community Health Equity—Women's Wealth & Health Equity Summit: https://healthequity.globalpolicysolutions.org/resources/training-and-events/womens-wealth-health-equity-summit/
Kaiser Family Foundation–Women's Health: www.kff.org/state-category/womens-health/
World Health Organization—Women and Gender Equity: www.who.int/social_determinants/themes/womenandgender/en/

References

Acevedo, D. (2002). *El trabajo y la salud laboral de las mujeres en Venezuela: Una vision de Genero*. Universidad de Carabobo, Dirección de Medios y Comunicaciones.

Alexanderson, K., Leijon, M., Akerlind, I., Rydh, H., & Bjurulf, P. (1994). Epidemiology of sickness absence in a Swedish county in 1985, 1986 and 1987: A three year longitudinal study with focus on gender, age and occupation. *Scand J Soc Med*. 22:27–34.

Alexanderson, K., Sydsjö, A., Hensing, G., Sydsjö, G., & Carstensen, J. (1996). Impact of pregnancy on gender differences in sickness absence. *Scand J Soc Med*. 24:169–76.

Alexanderson, K. (1998). Measuring health. Indicators for working women. In Å. Kilbom, K. Messing, & C. Bildt-Thorbjörnsson (Eds.), *Women's health at work* (pp. 121–161). Stockholm: National Institute of Working Life.

American Psychiatric Association. (1952). *Diagnostic and statistical manual of mental disorders* (1st ed.). Washington, DC: American Psychiatric Association.

American Psychiatric Association. (1980). *Diagnostic and statistical manual*, (3rd ed., *DSM-III*). Washington, DC: American Psychiatric Association.

American Psychiatric Association. (1987). *Diagnostic and statistical manual of mental disorders* (*DSM-IV-R*). Washington, DC: American Psychiatric Association.

American Psychiatric Association. (1994). *Diagnostic and statistical manual of mental disorders* (*DSM-IV*). Washington, DC: American Psychiatric Association.

American Psychiatric Association. (2000). *Diagnostic and statistical manual of mental disorders* (*DSM-IV-TR*). Washington, DC: American Psychiatric Association.

American Psychiatric Association. (2013). American Psychiatric Association, 2013: Diagnostic and statistical manual of mental disorders (5th ed.). *American Journal of Psychiatry*. Retrieved from http://doi.org/10.1176/appi.books.9780890425596.744053

Arcand, R., Labrèche, F., Messing, K., Stock, S., & Tissot, F. (2000). Environnement de travail et santé. In *Enquête sociale et de santé 1998* (pp. 525–570). Québec: Institut de la statistique du Québec.

Asselin, S. (2003). Professions: convergence entre les sexes? *Données sociodémographiques en bref*, *7*(3), 6–8.

Barbeau, E. M., Krieger, N., & Soobader, M. J. (2004). Working class matters: Socioeconomic disadvantage, race/ethnicity, gender, and smoking in NHIS 2000. *American Journal of Public Health*, *94*(2), 269–278. Retrieved from http://doi.org/10.2105/AJPH.94.2.269

Bird, C. E., & Rieker, P. P. (1999). Gender matters: an integrated model for understanding men's and women's health. *Social Science & Medicine*, *48*(6), 745–755. Retrieved from http://doi.org/10.1016/S0277-9536(98)00402-X

Brisson, C., Laflamme, N., Moisan, J., Milot, A., Masse, B., & Vezina, M. (1999). Effect of family responsibilities and job strain on ambulatory blood pressure among white-collar women. *Psychosomatic Medicine*, *61*, 205–213.

Chan, K. K., Neighbors, C., Gilson, M., Larimer, M. E., & Alan Marlatt, G. (2007). Epidemiological trends in drinking by age and gender: Providing normative feedback to adults. *Addictive Behaviors*, *32*(5), 967–976. Retrieved from http://doi.org/10.1016/j.addbeh.2006.07.003

Chrisler, J. C., & Caplan, P. (2002). The strange case of Dr. Jekyll and Ms. Hyde: How PMS became a cultural phenomenon and a psychiatric disorder. Annual Review of Sex Research, *13*(1), 274–306.

Cosmacini, G. (1997). *The long art: The history of medicine from antiquity to the present*. Rome: Oxford University Press.

Cranford, C. J., Vosko, L. F., & Zukewich, N. (2003). The gender of precarious employment in Canada. *Relations industrielles/Industrial Relations*, *58*(3): 454–479.

Denton, M., Prus, S., & Walters, V. (2004). Gender differences in health: A Canadian study of the psychosocial, structural and behavioural determinants of health. *Social Science and Medicine*, *58*(12), 2585–2600. Retrieved from http://doi.org/10.1016/j.socscimed.2003.09.008

Frank, R. G., Beronio, K., & Glied, S. A. (2014). Behavioral health parity and the Affordable Care Act. *Journal of Social Work in Disability & Rehabilitation*, *13*(1–2), 31–43.

Gehlert, S., Song, I. H., Chang, C-H., & Hartlage, S. A. (2009). The prevalence of premenstrual dysphoric disorder in a randomly selected group of urban and rural women. *Psychological Medicine*, *39*(1), 129–136.

Gorman, B. K., & Read, J. G. (2006). Gender disparities in adult health: An examination of three measures of morbidity. *Journal of Health and Social Behavior*, *47*, 95–110. Retrieved from http://doi.org/10.1177/002214650604700201

Greene, R., & Dalton, K. (1953). The premenstrual syndrome. *British Medical Journal*, *1*(4818), 1007.

Gustafson, P. E. (1998). Gender differences in risk perception: theoretical and methodological perspectives. *Risk Analysis*, *18*(6), 805–811.

Hall, E. (1989). Gender, work control and stress: A theoretical discussion and an empirical test. *International Journal of Health Services*, *19*, 725–745.

Han, B., Gfroerer, J. C., & Colliver, J. D. (2010). Associations between duration of illicit drug use and health conditions: Results from the 2005–2007 national surveys on drug use and health. *Annals of Epidemiology*, *20*(4), 289–297.

The Henry J. Kaiser Family Foundation. (2017). *Health reform implementation timeline*. Retrieved from http://kff.org/interactive/implementation-timeline/

Islam, S., Velilla, A. M., Doyle, E. J., & Ducatman, A. M. (2001). Gender differences in workrelated injury/illness: Analysis of workers compensation claims. *American Journal of Industrial Medicine*, *39*, 84–91.

Johnson, F. W., Gruenewald, P. J., Treno, A. J., & Taff, G. A. (1998). Drinking over the life course within gender and ethnic groups: A hyperparametric analysis. *Journal of Studies on Alcohol*, *v59*(n5), *568*(13). Retrieved from http://doi.org/10.15288/jsa.1998.59.568

Kessler, R. C. (2003). Epidemiology of women and depression. *Journal of Affective Disorders*, *74*(1), 5–13. Retrieved from http://doi.org/10.1016/S0165-0327(02)00426-3

Kessler, R. C., Chiu, W. T., Demler, O., & Walters, E. E. (2005). Prevalence, severity, and comorbidity of 12-month DSM-IV disorders in the national comorbidity survey replication. *Archives of General Psychiatry*, *62*(6), 617. Retrieved from http://doi.org/10.1001/archpsyc.62.6.617

Kraus, J., Peek, C., Silberman, T., & Anderson, C. (1995). The accuracy of death certificates in identifying work-related fatal injuries. *American Journal of Epidemiology*, *141*, 973–979.

Lindelöw, M., & Bildt-Thorbjornsson, C. (1998). Psychological differences between men and women. In Å. Kilbom, K. Messing, & C. Bildt-Thorbjörnsson (Eds.), *Women's health at work*. Solna: National Institute of Working Life.

Lippel, K. (1999). Workers' compensation and stress: Gender and access to compensation. *International Journal of Law and Psychiatry*, *22*(1), 79–89.

Lippel, K. (2003). Compensation for musculo-skeletal disorders in Quebec: Systemic discrimination against women workers? *International Journal of Health Services*, *33*(2), 253–282.

London, L., De Grosbois, S., Wesseling, C., Kisting, S., Rother, H. A., & Mergler, D. (2002). Pesticide usage and health consequences for women in developing countries: Out of sight out of mind? *International Journal of Occupational and Environmental Health*, *8*(1), 46–59.

Matheson, F. I., Moineddin, R., Dunn, J. R., Creatore, M. I., Gozdyra, P., & Glazier, R. H. (2006). Urban neighborhoods, chronic stress, gender and depression. *Social Science & Medicine*, *63*(10), 2604–2616. Retrieved from http://doi.org/10.1016/j.socscimed.2006.07.001

Mergler, D., & Vézina, N. (1985). Dysmenorrhea and cold exposure. *Journal of Reproductive Medicine*, *30*(2), 106–11.

Messing, K., & Elabidi, D. (2003). Desegregation and occupational health: How male and female hospital attendants collaborate on work tasks requiring physical effort. *Policy and Practice in Health and Safety*, *1*(1), 83–103.

Messing, K. & Ostlin, P. (2006). *Gender, equality, work and health: A review of the evidence*. World Health Organization. Retrieved from www.who.int/gender/documents/Genderworkhealth.pdf

Messing, K., Saurel-Cubizolles, M. J., Bourgine, M., & Kaminski, M. (1992). Menstrual cycle characteristics and work conditions of workers in poultry slaughterhouses and canneries. *Scandinavian Journal of Work, Environment & Health*. *18*(5), 302–309.

Messing, K., Saurel-Cubizolles, M. J., Bourgine, M., & Kaminski, M. (1993). Factors associated with dysmenorrhea among workers in French poultry slaughterhouses and canneries. *Journal of Occupational Medicine*, *35*(5), 493–500.

Montz, E., Layton, T., Busch, A. B., Ellis, R. P., Rose, S., & McGuire, T. G. (2016). Risk-adjustment simulation: Plans may have incentives to distort mental health and substance use coverage. *Health Affairs*, *35*(6), 1022–1028.

North, C. S. (2015). The classification of hysteria and related disorders: historical and phenomenological considerations. *Behavioral Sciences*, *5*(4), 496–517.

Östlin, P. (2002). Gender inequalities in health: the significance of work. In S. Wamala & J. Lynch (Eds.), *Gender and socioeconomic inequalities in health*. Lund: Studentlitteratur.

Parra Garrido, M. (2002). La salud de las mujeres trabajadoras en América Latina. In K. Messing (Ed.), *El trabajo de las mujeres: Comprender para transformar*. Madrid: Catarata.

Quinlan, M. C., Mayhew, C., & Bohle, P. (2001). The global expansion of precarious employment, work disorganization, and consequences for occupational health: A review of recent research. *International Journal of Health Services*, *31*, 335–414.

Rosenthal, E. (2013, June 30). American way of birth, costliest in the world. *New York Times*, pp. 1A.

Ross, C. E., & Bird, C. E. (1994). Sex stratification and health lifestyle: Consequences for men's and women's perceived health. *Journal of Health and Social Behavior*, *35*(2), 161. Retrieved from http://doi.org/10.2307/2137363

Santoro, K., Peabody, H., & Schoenman, J. (2010). *Identifying and treating maternal depression: Strategies and considerations for health plans*. National Institute for Health Care Management. Retrieved from www.nihcm.org/pdf/FINAL_MaternalDepression6-7.pdf

Standen, A. (2013). *Should severe premenstral symptoms be a mental disorder?* National Public Radio. Retrieved from https://owl.english.purdue.edu/owl/resource/560/10/

Tasca, C., Rapetti, M., Carta, M. G., & Fadda, B. (2012). Women and hysteria in the history of mental health. *Clinical Practice and Epidemiology in Mental Health: CP & EMH*, *8*, 110–119. Retrieved from http://doi.org/10.2174/1745017901208010110

Trost, S. G., Owen, N., Bauman, A. E., Sallis, J. F., & Brown, W. (2002). Correlates of adults' participation in physical activity: Review and update. *Medicine and Science in Sports and Exercise*, *34*(12), 1996–2001. Retrieved from http://doi.org/10.1249/01.MSS.0000038974.76900.92

Turcotte, G. (1992). How pregnant workers see their work, its risks and the right to precautionary leave in Quebec. *Women Health, 18*(3), 79–95.
Veith, I. (1965). *Hysteria: The history of a disease.* Chicago: University of Chicago Press. Retrieved from https://books.google.com/books?id=YLzKMgEACAAJ
WHO. (2001). Department of mental health and substance dependence gender disparities in mental health world. *Mental Health a Call for Action by World Health Ministers, 48*(5), 1–25.

Questions

1. What are some historically misunderstood and improperly diagnosed gender-specific mental health conditions that have stigmatized women's mental healthcare? Can you think of examples of ways in which this stigma continues today?
2. The authors note that the few policies that protect the right of women to access to comprehensive healthcare are constantly under scrutiny and at risk of defunding. What are some ways to ensure that these policies are adequately implemented, funded, and defended from such threats?

Reading 3.2

Somewhere Under the Rainbow

Exploring the Identities and Experiences of Trans Persons

Emma Dargie, Karen Blair, Caroline Pukall, Shannon Coyle

Emma Dargie, Karen L. Blair, Caroline F. Pukall, and Shannon M. Coyle, "Somewhere Under the Rainbow: Exploring the Identities and Experiences of Trans Persons," *The Canadian Journal of Human Sexuality*, vol. 23, no. 2, pp. 60–74.

Editor's Introduction

This reading discusses a study the authors conducted aimed at improving upon the psychological literature on transgender persons. This literature tends to assume that transgender persons are best understood within rigid and binary definitions of gender and sexuality and focuses on diagnostics, medical management, and risk factors. The authors' study instead explores the gender and sexual identities of transgender persons, investigating whether there are group differences and examining factors that predict better psychological and physical well-being in LGBT persons. The results of this study depict diverse gender identities and sexual orientations among trans persons that do not adhere to the gender binary. Using data from this study, the authors build on their research investigating the human sexuality of LGBTQ persons to argue for the importance of

- acknowledging the complexity and diversity of the gender and sexual identities of trans persons in research and practice, which motivates frameworks beyond the binary; and
- the role of social and personal support as potential sources of protection for trans persons, which helps foster cultural acceptance and celebration of transgender identities.

Emma Dargie, PhD is a psychotherapist with a client-centered, evidence-based, sex-positive, LGBTQ-positive approach to therapy. Karen L. Blair, PhD is assistant professor of psychology and director of the Social Relations, Attitudes, and Diversity Lab at Trent University. Her research interests include the social determinants of health and the interactions between developmental, social, health, and LGBTQ psychology. Caroline F. Pukall, PhD is a professor of psychology at Queen's University who focuses on human sexuality, especially sexual function, dysfunction, and health. Shannon M. Coyle, MA is a research associate in the Sexual Health Research Lab at Queen's University and a part-time professor at St. Lawrence College. Her work on human sexuality and health investigates the needs, experiences, and fulfillments of transgender persons.

The literature on transgender/transsexual-spectrum persons is limited. Most studies are based on the assumption that trans persons are best understood within rigid and binary definitions of gender and sexuality and they tend to focus on diagnostics, medical management and risk factors. Researchers and clinicians may also assume that people who challenge cultural norms of gender and sexuality can be grouped together. Such assumptions about the specific experiences of trans person can be harmfully incorrect. The goals of the present study were to explore the gender and sexual identities of trans persons, to investigate group differences, and to examine factors that predict better psychological and physical well-being. Participants took part in an online study and provided information about their gender and sexual identity, social support, relationship quality, and mental/physical health. Results depicted diverse gender identities and sexual orientations among trans persons and emphasized that while many challenges faced by sexual and gender minorities are similar, trans persons report unique mental and physical health outcomes. Also, greater social support and relationship quality predicted mental, but not physical, health among trans persons. These results highlight the importance of acknowledging the complexity of trans identities and the key role of social and personal support.

Introduction

If all of us, including transgender people, are to be able to express our authentic selves, as well as to increase our capacity for intimacy and sexual autonomy, a new sexual revolution is necessary. This revolution would entail the collapse of limited, hierarchical models and a move away from reductionist binary constructs of gender and toward the creation of pleasure-based models of sexuality encompassing the wealth and breadth of human desire and experiences. Bockting & Iantaffi, 2008, p. 368

In Western societies, the concept of gender nonconformity is becoming widely recognized in both theoretical and practical research disciplines. Individuals who reject the rigid two-sex binary system often fall under the umbrella term 'trans,' indicating that they do not identify with their birth-assigned gender and may self-identify or be defined by a variety of terms reflecting diverse and complex identities. (see Tables 3.2.1 and 3.2.2 for detailed definitions and examples). For trans persons, living authentically may or may not involve physical changes to their body. Indeed, if it was widely understood that there is no "right" way to perform maleness and femaleness, this attitude would create more space for individuals who reject traditional gender norms so that they can live authentically, without fear of judgment and persecution. Exploring gender non-conformity may help facilitate ethical and responsible discussions about trans persons' gender identities as well as their mental and physical health.

Table 3.2.1 Definitions of Common Terms Pertinent to the Discussion of Sex and Gender

Term	**WPATH Definition**
Gender Dysphoria	Distress that is caused by a discrepancy between a person's gender identity and that person's sex assigned at birth
Gender Identity	A person's intrinsic sense of being male (a boy or a man), female (a girl or a woman), or an alternative gender
Gender Identity Disorder	Strong and persistent cross-gender identification and a persistent discomfort with one's sex or sense of inappropriateness in the gender role of that sex, causing clinically significant distress or impairment in social, occupational, or other important areas of functioning.
Sex	Assigned at birth as male or female, usually based on the appearance of the external genitalia.
Transgender	Adjective to describe a diverse group of individuals who cross or transcend culturally defined categories of gender. The gender identity of transgender people differs to varying degrees from the sex they were assigned at birth
Transsexual	Individuals who seek to change or who have changed their primary and/or secondary sex characteristics through feminizing or masculinizing medical interventions (hormones and/or surgery), typically accompanied by a permanent change in gender role.

Note: All definitions are quotes from the WPATH SOC, pp. 221–222

Table 3.2.2 Binary Categorizations Expanded to Capture Complex Identities

Gender Identity	Male	Cisgender male Transman; Trans; Transgender; Transsexual FtM Drag King

Binary Categorizations Expanded to Capture Complex Identities

	Female	Cisgender female Transwoman; Trans; Transgender; Transsexual MtF Drag Queen
	Other	Genderqueer; Pan-gender; Bi-gender; No gender Intersex Boygirl; Girlboy Two-spirited
Sexual Orientation	Heterosexual	Heterosexual Straight
	Non-heterosexual	Gay Lesbian Bisexual Pansexual; Polysexual Queer Asexual
Relationship Composition	Same-sex	Both partners cisgender One partner trans Both partners trans
	Mixed-sex	Both partners cisgender One partner trans Both partners trans

Note: These examples are not inclusive of all identities and relationship experiences.

Although research on trans persons is growing, it is limited in content and methodology, e.g., many studies are based on small subsets of specific trans identities, they rely heavily on clinical samples, and/or the focus is on diagnostics and pathology (e.g., Asscheman et al., 2011; Dhejne et al., 2011; Docter & Fleming, 2001). Some research studies claim to have comprehensive population samples, including individuals who self-identify as Lesbian, Gay, Bisexual, or Transgender/Transsexual (LGBT), but sampling may yield few trans persons, if any, who are actually included in the final sample (Blumer, Green, Knowles, & Williams, 2012). For example, one study on the impact of discrimination on access to health care for older gay men, lesbians, bisexuals and transgender individuals, had a sample composed of only 1.5% trans persons; 2 out of a 132 participants (Jackson, Johnson, & Roberts, 2008). The assumption that people who self-identify within the LGBT acronym should be considered one sub-population in research is misleading and contributes to the conflation of sex and gender. Lumping the "T" with the "LGB" in research further erases trans persons' experiences since results may not generalize to trans persons.

For example, LGB and trans persons face different and unique barriers when accessing health care due to the varied (in)visibility of their identities. While a lesbian may be repeatedly questioned about the possibility of unplanned pregnancy, a trans man may never be asked about the same possibility or may face significant barriers when attempting to access gynecological services, such as a routine pap smear. Many of these challenges are reinforced through systemic erasure (Bauer et al., 2009), such as the continued use of computer systems that do not acknowledge the possibility of women with testicular cancer or men undergoing hysterectomies (Coyle, 2011). To combat the continued erasure, systemic ignorance, and misrepresentation of trans persons' realities, researchers and clinicians must move away from a rigid two-sex binary system and the practice of lumping sexual and gender minorities together as one distinct group. Given the close relationship between clinical practice, policy and research, it is imperative that researchers begin to understand and reflect upon the complex identities of trans persons to provide the basis of a more ethical, informed, and evidence-based knowledge set from which future research, clinical practice and policy can draw.

The Complexity of Trans Identities

The classification of "trans" does not begin to describe the multi-faceted and often fluid nature of trans identities, both in terms of gender and sexual orientation (Carrera, DePalma, & Lameiras, 2012). Even in studies that offered comparatively comprehensive array of gender and identity options to choose from, Iantaffi and Bockting (2011) found that 29.5% of 1229 participants in an online survey chose an "other" option when reporting their gender. Similarly, in a college sample of trans-gender persons, 37% of participants did not identify as Female-to-Male (FtM; i.e., trans man) or Male-to-Female (MtF; i.e., trans woman) (Dugan, Kusel, & Simounet, 2012). While a long list of categories and labels might seem superfluous, qualitative research has illustrated the importance trans persons place on their fluid, non-binary identities. Nagoshi, Brzuzy, and Terrell (2012) interviewed 11 transgender individuals about their experience of gender roles, gender identity, and sexual orientation. Participants differentiated between the gender expressed by their physical characteristics, and the gender represented by their choices and actions (i.e., gender roles). Furthermore, all participants reported experiencing both masculine and feminine characteristics and tended to identify gender as fluctuating.

The complexity of trans identities was apparent in an online survey of 292 trans persons (Kuper, Nussbaum, & Mustanski, 2012), in which the majority of participants did not adhere to typical binary definitions of gender, with 55.1% identifying as genderqueer. Further, most endorsed multiple identity descriptors, and reported that their identities shifted over time. Similar patterns emerged when expressing sexual orientation. Over one third (37.7%) selected pansexual or queer as their sexual orientation, which may indicate that participants sought a definition that did not require them to identify themselves as strictly male or female. As such, clinicians and researchers may need to take a detour from the two-sexed gender binary system to better understand gender identity. Poorly considered research designs and clinical practices that do not take into account the diversity among trans persons could convey stigma and be seen as lack of compassion for an already-marginalized group of people.

Another important factor to take into consideration is the sexual orientation of trans persons. Researchers must take care to avoid assumptions about trans persons' sexual orientations before and after transitioning, if they indeed choose to transition. In one European study of 170 individuals identifying as MtF or FtM (Nieder et al., 2011), researchers found great variability in sexual orientations, especially among trans women. Other researchers have also reported diversity in sexual orientation (Weyers et al., 2009), in addition to variability in sexual orientation before and after gender reassignment surgery (GRS, sometimes referred to as sex reassignment surgery), with one in four trans women reporting a change in sexual orientation following surgery. Nagoshi and colleagues (2012) found that the concepts of sexual and gender identity were not straightforward for their trans participants, with some viewing the constructs as inherently separate and others articulating that their orientation and gender identity mutually influenced one another. Indeed, many participants expressed difficulty in disentangling their gender identity from their sexual identity. Thus, if research is to accurately reflect the experiences of trans persons and draw conclusions regarding how to best provide care and education, it should include a detailed assessment of both gender identity and sexual orientation throughout and following any processes of transition.

Mental and Physical Health

A primary goal of clinical literature is often to determine if certain markers are predictive of better mental and physical functioning. Many studies have examined the mental and physical health of trans persons, yet the results have been inconclusive. Some studies have reported that trans individuals fare poorer than their cisgender counterparts (i.e., people whose gender identity matches their assignation at birth), in that they have higher mortality rates, more suicide attempts and greater incidences of psychopathology and substance abuse when compared with their cisgender counterparts (e.g., Asscheman et al., 2011; Dhejne et al., 2011). Other studies have suggested that trans persons, as a group, fare no better or worse than cisgender persons with respect to mental and physical functioning. For example, Fisher et al. (2013) indicated that patients attending their Gender Identity Disorder clinic reported a prevalence of psychiatric disorders that was only slightly higher than the general population of Europe. Other researchers established that health-related quality of life is similar for trans persons and cisgender persons (Motmans, Meier, Ponnet, & T'Sjoen, 2012; Weyers et al., 2009; Wierckx et al., 2011). These studies indicate that the emotional, psychological, and physical functioning of trans persons is not straightforward, providing justification for a more concrete approach to understanding the predictors of mental and physical health outcomes for trans persons.

Some authors have begun to investigate whether variation in sexual orientation, social support, and relationship status predict positive functioning. Bockting, Benner, and Coleman (2009) found no major differences in psychological adjustment, sexual satisfaction, and gender identity/social sex role between FtMs identifying as gay or bisexual when compared to cisgender gay and bisexual men. Weyers and colleagues (2009) noted that trans persons who are in a romantic relationship have better mental health, vitality, and social functioning. Other research has also indicated that a positive association exists with social support and romantic relationship well-being and mental and physical health among sexual minority populations (Blair & Holmberg, 2008), suggesting that having a healthy and socially supported relationship may serve a protective purpose for some trans people.

The Current Study

To provide comprehensive care, researchers and clinicians should work toward designing studies capable of reflecting the complex identities of trans persons, while describing, without pathologizing, common patterns observed in trans spectrum persons. Since trans persons are often considered as a homogeneous group, the current study sought to explore differences among trans persons in addition to comparing trans persons to a broader group of cisgender LGB persons. Consequently, the current study examines the similarities and differences in experiences of social support, relationship satisfaction and health between trans persons and cisgender LGB individuals in an attempt to determine the appropriateness of combining sexual and gender minorities as a singular group for the purposes of social and psychological research. To do so, five research questions were examined:

1. How do trans persons describe their sexual orientation and gender identity?

Based on similar past findings, it was hypothesized that trans persons would report diversity in sexual and gender identity(ies) (Carrera et al., 2012; Iantaffi & Bockting, 2011; Kuper et al., 2012; Nagoshi et al., 2012).

2. Are there differences between trans women and trans men on measures of social support, relationship quality, physical and mental health?

It was hypothesized that these groups would differ, though no directionality was specified since such differences are not often explored, and preliminary findings in the literature have been inconclusive (e.g., Motmans et al., 2012).

3. Are there differences between trans persons in same-sex relationships and those in mixed-sex relationships?

Based on similar findings in the relationship literature, it was hypothesized that trans persons in mixed-sex relationships would fare similarly as those in same-sex relationships (e.g., Kurdek, 2004).

4. Do measures of relationship quality, social support, and physical/mental health differ from cisgender LGB persons?

It was hypothesized that LGB persons would fare better than trans persons since trans persons have many additional challenges to face (e.g., Hendricks & Testa, 2012; Iantaffi & Bockting, 2011).

5. Do social support and relationship quality predict physical and mental health?

Based on findings in the LGB literature, it was hypothesized that both variables would uniquely predict both physical and mental health outcomes (e.g., Blair & Holmberg, 2008).

Method

Participants

Participants were recruited as a part of a larger study on romantic relationships through listservs, websites, print advertisements, re-contacting past participants, and snowball methods. Participants were invited to take part if they were over the age of 18 and fluent in English.

Initially, 3597 people visited the survey website. Of those, 1559 were eligible and provided answers to at least the sociodemographic questions. Twenty-seven individuals identified as trans women, 32 as trans men, 4 as "other" (genderqueer or cross-dresser), while one person declined to indicate their gender. Examination of this participant's answers to questions addressing gender indicated that they experienced low identification with male and female genders. A smaller group of individuals completed all of the questionnaires relevant to this study: 15 trans women and 21 trans men. The initial descriptive analyses were conducted on the larger group (n = 64), while the subsequent inferential analyses were performed on the smaller group that completed all questionnaires (n = 36).

For inferential analyses that involved comparisons with cisgender persons, the sample consisted of 689 LGB-identified participants who had also completed all questionnaires. Relevant sociodemographic characteristics for each of group can be found in Tables 3.2.3 and 3.2.4. To summarize, an equal number of males and females participated, though more trans men participated than trans women. Participants were in their early thirties, and the majority reported being in a same-sex relationship. Most were seriously dating their partner(s), while only a few were casually dating. The rest were married or in a domestic partnership. Most had at least some college or university education, though income levels varied.

Sociodemographic and Relationship Characteristics of the Full and Smaller Trans Samples

		Full Sample ***M (SD)***	**Sub-Sample** ***M (SD)***
Age		32.77 (10.96)	30.22 (10.25)
		n (%)	*n* (%)
Gender	MtF	27 (42.2%)	15 (41.7%)
	FtM	32 (50.0%)	21 (58.3%)
	Other	4 (6.3%)	
	Not specified	1 (1.6%)	

Sociodemographic and Relationship Characteristics of the Full and Smaller Trans Samples

Relationship Type	Mixed Sex	24 (37.5%)	13 (36.1%)
	Same Sex	38 (59.4%)	23 (63.9%)
	Decline Response	2 (3.1%)	
Education	High School or Less	9 (14.1%)	5 (13.9%)
	Some College/University	26 (40.6%)	15 (41.7%)
	College Degree	11 (17.2%)	7 (19.4%)
	Undergraduate Degree	10 (15.6%)	5 (13.9%)
	Graduate Degree	8 (12.5%)	4 (11.1%)
Income	< $20,000	36 (56.3%)	22 (61.1%)
	$20,000–75,999	18 (28.1%)	9 (24.9%)
	$76,000þ	4 (6.3%)	1 (2.8%)
	Decline Response	6 (9.4%)	
Relationship Stage	Casually Dating	3 (4.7%)	1 (2.8%)
	Seriously Dating	31 (48.5%)	22 (61.2%)
	Married/Domestic Partnership	30 (46.8%)	13 (36.1%)

Sociodemographic and Relationship Characteristics of the Cisgender LGB Sample (N = 689)

		M (SD)
Age		32.92 (11.69)
		n (%)
Gender	Male	332 (48.2%)
	Female	357 (51.8%)
Relationship Type	Mixed Sex	59 (8.7%)
	Same Sex	621 (90.1%)
	Decline Response	9 (1.3%)
Sexual Orientation	Homosexual	547 (79.4%)

Table 8.2.4 Sociodemographic and Relationship Characteristics of the Cisgender LGB Sample (N = 689)

	Bisexual	90 (13.1%)
	Queer	38 (5.5%)
	Pansexual	14 (2.0%)
Education	High School or Less	109 (15.8%)
	Some College/University	240 (34.8%)
	College Degree	100 (14.5%)
	Undergraduate Degree	125 (18.1%)
	Graduate Degree	115 (16.3%)
	Decline Response	0
Income	< $20,000	217 (31.5%)
	$20,000–75,999	336 (48.8%)
	$76,000+	71 (10.3%)
	Decline Response	65 (9.4%)
Relationship Stage	Casually Dating	21 (3.0%)
	Seriously Dating	419 (60.8%)
	Married/Domestic Partnership	233 (33.8%)
	Decline Response	4 (.6%)

Measures

Kinsey Scale (Kinsey, Pomeroy, & Martin, 1948; Kinsey, Pomeroy, Martin, & Gebhard, 1953). This measure consists of a single question that assesses the sexual attraction and behaviour of individuals toward members of the same and opposite sex. Participants select a response on a 7-point scale (0 = *exclusively heterosexual*, 6 = *exclusively homosexual*).

Sexuality Questionnaire (SQ; Alderson, 2012). This questionnaire was designed to capture various components of sexual and gender identity. Participants rated the extent to which they identified as male and female, as well as 'traditional' masculine and feminine gender roles. Finally, participants were asked to rate the extent to which they identified with a range of identities (i.e., heterosexual, bisexual, gay or lesbian, queer, transsexual, no label, or other) and their comfort with their label(s) at present and during adolescence.

Social Network Support (SNS; Sprecher & Felmlee, 1992). This measure was designed to capture perceived social support for one's romantic relationship(s). Higher scores on this measure are indicative of greater perceived social support. The alpha for the overall measure of perceived social support for the relationship in the current study was .82.

Multidimensional Scale of Perceived Social Support (MSPSS; Zimet, Dahlem, Zimet, & Farley, 1988). This 12-item scale measures perceptions of perceived social support from one's family, friends, and significant other. Higher scores represent greater amounts of social support. The authors reported good reliability ($a = .88$), similar to the current study, $a = .90$.

Hendrick's Relationship Assessment Scale (RAS; Hendrick, 1988). This seven-item scale measures general relationship satisfaction. Higher scores on this scale are related to greater levels of satisfaction. The authors of this scale reported high reliability (Cronbach's alpha = .86), similar to the current study, $a = .88$.

Rubin Love Scale (RLS; Rubin, 1970). This 13-item measure is used to assess the extent to which participants love their partners. Higher scores on this scale are indicative of greater love for one's partner. The author reported high internal consistency, ($a = .84$). In the current study, participants responded to the statements using a 7-point scale rather than a 9-point scale, due to a programming error at the time of survey creation. Given that a mean score is used for this measure, the scale was not discarded. The internal consistency within this sample remained high, $a = .87$.

Trust (Rempel, Holmes, & Zanna, 1985). This 17-item scale addresses the level of trust present in one's romantic relationship. Higher scores on this measure indicated greater levels of trust for one's partner. The authors reported good reliability, $a = .81$, similar to the current study ($a = .91$).

Commitment (IMSCS; Rusbult, Martz, & Agnew, 1998). This scale measures commitment to one's partner and relationship. Higher scores are indicative of greater commitment to one's partner. The authors report excellent reliability ($a > .92$). The Cronbach's alpha for the present study was $a = .88$.

Center for Epidemiologic Studies Depression Scale (CES-D; Radloff, 1977). This 20-item scale measures the frequency of depressive symptoms over the past week. Higher scores represent more symptoms. Radloff demonstrated that this measure has high reliability (as > 0.84). For this sample, high reliability was achieved, $a = .93$.

State Trait Anxiety Inventory Trait Version (STAI-T; Spielberger et al., 1983). This 20-item questionnaire measures anxiety. Spielberger reported that the STAI-T has high test-retest reliability (rs > 0.73), internal consistency (αs > 0.89), and construct validity (high correlations between the STAI-T and other trait anxiety measures, rs > 0.73). For this sample, high reliability was achieved, $a = .94$.

Perceived Stress Scale (PSS; Cohen, Kamarck, & Mermelstein, 1983). This 10-item measure determines how much stress an individual experiences in general. Cohen and colleagues reported that the PSS has adequate reliability (αs > 0.84) and validity (e.g., adequately predicts health outcomes, rs > 0.52). For this sample, high reliability was achieved, $a = .90$.

Cohen-Hoberman Inventory of Physical Symptoms (CHIPS; Cohen & Hoberman, 1983). This 33-item scale measures the occurrence of various relatively minor physical symptoms over the past month. Higher scores reflect more minor health problems. Past research indicates that this scale is reliable, $a = .89$ (Aspinwall & Taylor, 1992), similarly to the current study, $a = .93$.

Procedure

Interested participants were invited to visit the study's website. After reading a description of the study, participants answered a series of screening questions used to determine eligibility and to personalize the questionnaires. Participants progressed through the survey at their own pace with the ability to save their work and return at a later time. Participants were compensated with participation points that they could use to enter into various prize draws. Our institutional ethics review board approved this study.

Results

Data Considerations

Prior to conducting any analyses, the data were cleaned and evaluated for violation of assumptions. A Missing Values Analysis was conducted to determine the extent of missing data. For all questionnaires but Social Network Support (SNS), less than 1% of the data were categorized as missing. For all other measures, missing values were imputed using the item mean. No imputation was performed on demographics or sexual/gender identity questionnaires. Scores for each scale were then calculated, but only if the participant had originally completed at least 85% of the items for each individual scale. For all pairwise comparisons, Bonferroni-corrected significance levels were used. Otherwise, the significance level was set at $p < .05$.

Because the sample size was small, it was not prudent to conduct most multivariate analyses, thus we opted instead for multiple *t*-test analyses. There was, however, enough power (.80) to detect a large effect for multiple regressions with two predictors at the $p < .05$ level (Cohen, 1992).

Gender and Gender Roles

Histograms were generated from responses to the SQ to explore the extent to which trans persons identify with aspects of gender (*male, female*), gender role (*masculine, feminine*), and with the label "transsexual" (Figure 3.2.1). An examination of these data indicated that the experience of each of these traits is not uniform for trans persons when grouped on gender identity.

When considering gender, the majority of trans men strongly identified as experiencing male gender, and the majority of trans women strongly identified as experiencing female gender. Some trans women also indicated some identification with male gender (55.5%), and some trans men indicated identification with female gender (50.0%), though typically at fairly low levels (i.e., they selected "unsure" or "low" when asked the extent to which they actually viewed themselves as male or female). Though there were few genderqueer/other responses, the experience of gender in these individuals tended to fall somewhat in the middle, not identifying strongly as male or female.

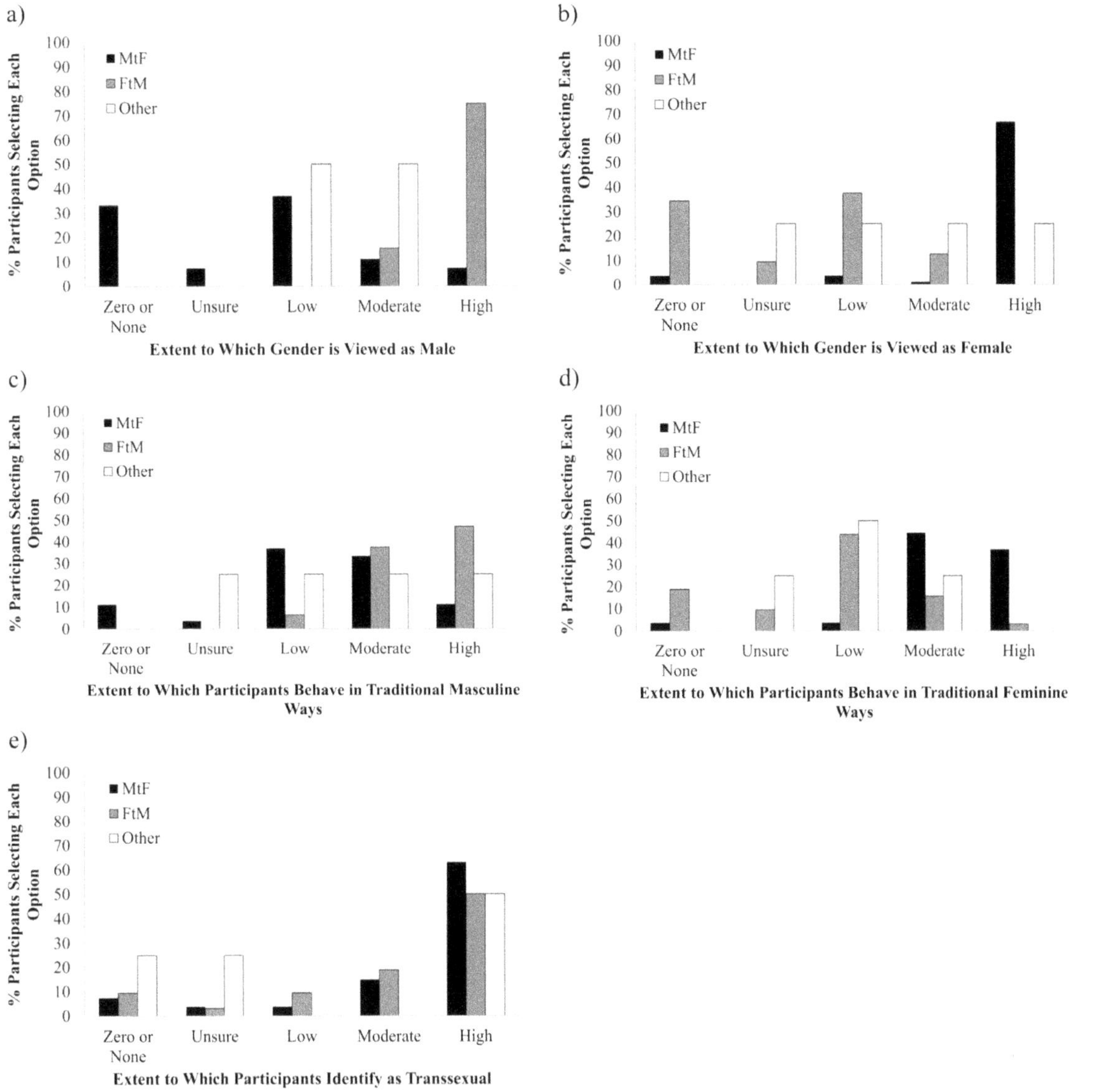

Figure 3.21 Histograms depicting the percentage of participants who endorsed various identification with male and female gender, masculine and feminine gender roles, and the term transsexual. Note. A minority of participants did not provide responses for each of the items: a. 1 MtF, 3 FtMs; b. 4 MtFs, 2 FtMs; c. 1 MtF, 3 FtMs; d. 3 MtFs, 3 FtMs; e. 2 MtFs, 3FtMs

When considering 'traditional' gender roles, a more diverse pattern emerged. The majority of trans women expressed moderate or high identification with traditional feminine gender roles (as defined by the SQ), and trans men did so with traditional masculine gender roles. However, the majority of both groups expressed low or moderate identification with the gender role associated with their birth-assigned gender. The genderqueer/other persons reported gender role identifications that tended toward the middle of the gender identity spectrum.

When considering identification with the term "transsexual," the patterns for trans men and trans women were fairly consistent. The majority expressed a high or moderate identification with the term, though some (11.9%) did not identify with the term transsexual at all or were unsure. Finally, half of the "other" category (n = 2) identified with transsexual, and half did not or were unsure.

Sexual Identity and Orientation

Histograms were generated to explore participants' various sexual orientation identity categories. The degree to which participants identified as heterosexual or homosexual was first explored (Figure 3.2.2). The majority of trans men indicated that they did not identify as strictly heterosexual or homosexual. One third of trans women identified as exclusively homosexual, whereas participants in the "other" category were more likely to identify in a similar pattern to the trans men, neither strictly heterosexual nor homosexual.

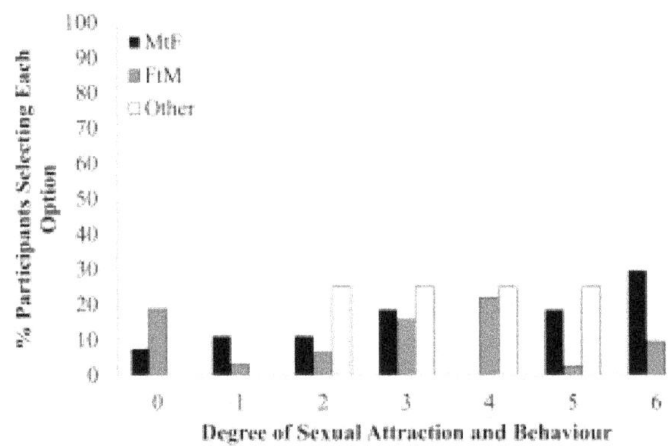

Figure 3.2.2 Histogram predominantly predominantly equally predominantly predominantly exclusively endorsed various degrees of sexual attraction and behaviour. Note. heterosexual; heterosexual, only incidentally homosexual; heterosexual, but more than incidentally homosexual; heterosexual and homosexual (bisexual); homosexual, but more than incidentally heterosexual; homosexual, only incidentally heterosexual; homosexual. One MtF person and 4 FtM persons declined to answer this question.

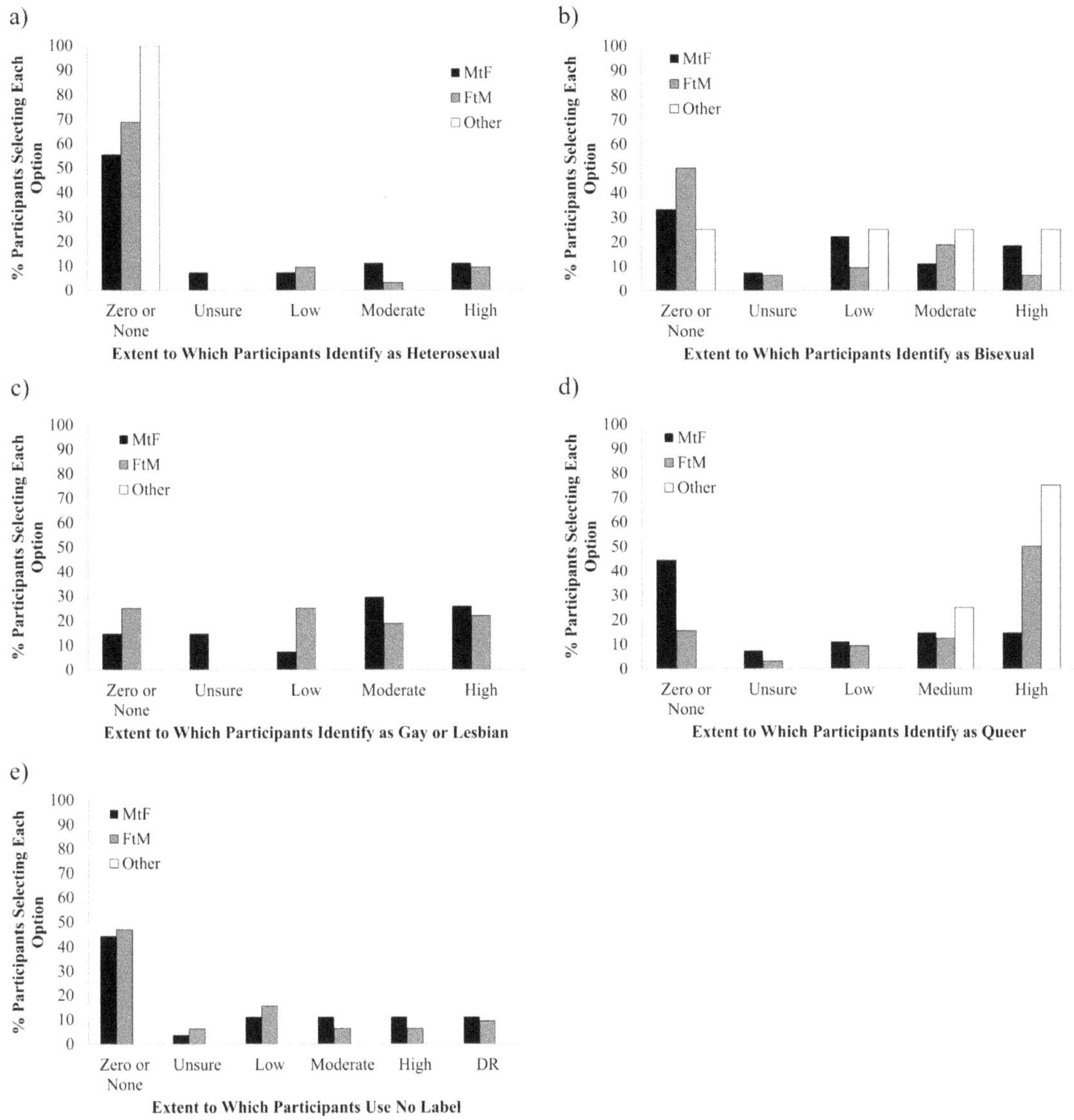

Figure 3.2.3 Histograms depicting the percentage of participants who endorsed various identification with the terms heterosexual, bisexual, gay or lesbian, queer, or no label. Note. Two MtF persons and three FtM persons did not answer these questions.

Participants also rated the extent to which they identified with several sexual orientation labels (Figure 3.2.3). The majority of trans men and trans women indicated no identification with the label "heterosexual," though 25% indicated that they at least 'somewhat' identified as heterosexual. None of those in the "other" category identified as heterosexual (Figure 3.2.3a). When asked about the label "bisexual," the majority of trans men did not identify with this term, though almost a third reported moderate or high identification. The majority of trans women, on the other hand, reported at least some identification with this label. Those in the "other" category reported a range of identification (Figure 3.2.3b).

When considering the label "gay or lesbian" patterns were fairly consistent between trans men, trans women, and those in the "other" category. Each of the groups was relatively evenly distributed between zero and none/unsure, low, moderate, and high (Figure 3.2.3c). For the label "queer," the majority of trans women did not endorse this descriptor or were unsure how it applied to them. The majority of trans men and those in the "other" category expressed moderate to high identification with the term (Figure 3.2.3d). Finally, there were some people who chose to not identify themselves with a label (Figure 3.2.3e).

Comparisons Based on Gender Identity and Relationship Composition. Independent-samples *t*-tests were computed to determine whether trans women (n = 15) differed significantly from trans men (n = 21) when it came to symptoms of depression, stress, anxiety, physical symptoms, global social support, support for the relationship, commitment, love, relationship satisfaction, and trust. After implementing Bonferroni corrections for multiple comparisons (.05/10 = .005), there were no significant differences between the groups, *ps* > .04.

The same procedure was applied to comparing those in same- (n = 23) and mixed-sexed (n = 13) relationships. After using the same Bonferroni-corrected significance levels ($p < .005$), none of the tests were significant, *ps* > .04.

Comparisons with Cisgender LGB Persons. Independent-samples *t*-tests were conducted to determine if trans persons (n = 36) reported different outcomes than cisgender persons (n = .689) on measures of relationship quality, social support, mental, and physical health. No differences were observed for the relationship quality variables (commitment, love, relationship satisfaction, trust), or social support for one's relationship *ps* > .13.

When it came to global social support, cisgender LGB persons (M = 4.08, SD = .70) reported experiencing significantly more social support than trans persons (M = 3.70, SD = .64), $t(715) = 3.03$, p = .003, *Cohen's d* = .57. Similar patterns emerged for mental and physical health. Cisgender LGB persons (M = 14.80, SD = 11.99) reported significantly fewer symptoms of depression than trans persons (M = 26.00, SD = 13.16), $t(720) = 5.29$, $p < .001$, *Cohen's d* = .60. Cisgender LGB persons (M = 16.77, SD = 7.63) also reported fewer symptoms of stress than trans persons (M = 22.06, SD = 6.81), $t(719) = 3.96$, $p < .001$, *Cohen's d* = .73. Fewer symptoms of anxiety were reported by cisgender LGB persons (M = 38.17, SD = 11.76) than trans persons (M = 50.62, SD = 11.17), $t(720) = 6.04$, *Cohen's d* = .72. Finally, cisgender LGB persons (M = 20.77, SD = 18.26) experienced significantly fewer physical health problems than trans persons (M = 38.59, SD = 23.07), $t(720) = 5.48$, $p < .001$, *Cohen's d* = .86.

Predicting Mental and Physical Health Outcomes for Trans Persons. Before conducting multiple regression analyses to predict physical and mental health, a series of Pearson correlations were conducted to investigate the relationships between two clusters of variables. The first cluster consisted of the mental and physical health variables. As expected, a moderate-strong positive relationship was found between each pair of variables (*rs* > .56). Next, the correlations between the relationship quality variables were assessed. As expected, a moderate-strong relationship was found between each pair of variables (*rs* > .43). Since the RAS had the strongest pattern of relationships with the other variables (*rs* > .61), it was selected to include in the multiple regression to account for relationship quality.

For each multiple regression (MR), global social support and relationship satisfaction were the predictors. For symptoms of depression, the MR was significant, $R^2 = .22$, adjusted $R^2 = .18$, $F(2, 33)$ =

4.71, $p = .02$. When examined individually, however, neither predictor reached significance (social support: *beta* = –.27, $p = .12$; relationship satisfaction: *beta* = –.28, $p = .11$). For symptoms of stress, the MR was significant, $R^2 = .39$, adjusted $R^2 = .35$, $F(2, 33) = 10.55$, $p < .001$. When examined individually, however, only relationship satisfaction reached significance (social support: *beta* = –.28, $p = .07$; relationship satisfaction: *beta* = –.45, $p = .01$). For experiences of anxiety, the MR was significant, $R^2 = .24$, adjusted $R^2 = .20$, $F(2, 33) = 5.32$, $p = 01$. When examined individually, however, only social support reached significance (social support: *beta* = –.39, $p = 03$; relationship satisfaction: *beta* $R^2 = -.18$, $p = .29$). For physical complaints, the MR was not significant, $R^2 = .02$, adjusted $R^2 = -.04$, $F(2, 33) = .27$, $p = .77$.

Discussion

The purpose of this study was to explore nuances of trans persons' gender identity(ies), sexual orientation(s), social support, and their physical and mental health.

Gender and Gender Roles

When asked to describe their gender and adherence to 'traditional' masculine and feminine behaviours, trans persons reported a wide range of experiences. The majority identified quite strongly with the gender to which they transitioned, though many also expressed some identification with the gender they were assigned at birth. The complexity of gender identities expressed by participants underscores the importance of clinicians and researchers using multidimensional assessments of gender identity and ceasing their over-reliance on a binary understanding of gender. The gender expressions of participants in the current study echo those discussed in past research (Kuper et al., 2012; Nagoshi et al., 2012), particularly those that emphasize the importance of fluid, non-binary understandings of gender (Diamond & Butterworth, 2008). These patterns also call into question any therapeutic practices with trans persons that utilize goals of strict adherence and identification with either male or female gender identities and, alternatively, suggest that a focus should be placed on self-exploration and acceptance.

An even more interesting pattern emerged when considering 'traditional' gender roles. As expected, trans men identified more with traditional masculine roles and trans women identified more with traditional feminine gender roles. A substantial percentage of participants reported experiencing low or moderate identification with traditional roles for the gender they were assigned at birth. Rather than interpreting such patterns as an indication that some trans persons have not 'fully transitioned,' this pattern of dually identifying with multiple 'traditional' gender roles underscores the multiplicities of gender and the often arbitrary nature of assigning specific tasks, hobbies, or personal qualities to a particular gender. Since trans persons must engage in a great deal of self-discovery and personal reflection, they may embody the traits that best reflect their own experiences, rather than restricting themselves to qualities common to only one gender.

Finally, participants' responses to the label "transsexual" illustrate the importance of inclusive and diverse language in research and clinical practice. While the majority of trans persons identified with this term to a high or moderate degree, it was by no means universal. As indicated by the Standards of Care (SOC) published by the World Professional Association for Transgender Health (WPATH; Coleman et al., 2012), there are several terms that can, and should, be used to capture the identities and experiences of trans persons (Table 3.2.2).

Though few genderqueer persons responded to this survey, their responses indicate that much diversity exists within categories of gender identity. Many clinicians and researchers currently understand trans persons in terms of their abilities to approximate the gender and gender roles associated with their gender identity, to the exclusion of those associated with their gender assigned at birth. It may be more authentic and realistic to accept that many trans persons (and for the sake of argument, many cisgender persons), simultaneously, and comfortably, occupy both male and female identities and their supposed corresponding gender roles, or expressions of femininity and masculinity.

Though clinicians and researchers might endeavour to understand trans person in terms of unilateral understandings of gender and gender roles, a more inclusive and authentic approach would be ideal. For example, in addition to questions addressing one's identification with masculinity and femininity, a comprehensive set of questions might include personality traits and experiences that could be experienced regardless of one's gender expression (e.g., emotional intelligence, aggression). Overall, the results of this study underscore that trans-spectrum identities are capable of moving beyond rigid gender binaries, with many participants reporting on their gender and gendered experiences in fluid and individual manners.

Sexual Identity and Orientation

While the concepts of gender identity and gender expression are both central to discourses on trans persons, this study also aimed to simultaneously explore the importance of including sexual identity and orientation as part of these discourses. Trans persons reported a wide range of attractions and sexual behaviours, with only a minority reporting exclusive identification as heterosexual or homosexual. Similar results were observed when participants were asked to rate the strength of their identification with various orientation descriptors (e.g., gay/lesbian, bisexual, queer, heterosexual). Indeed, a minority of participants identified as heterosexual (Figure 3.2.3). It is also possible that trans persons would hesitate to identify with the term heterosexual for reasons other than the type of person to which they are attracted (i.e., due to the continuous perpetuation of systemic heterosexism). The category of 'heterosexual' is often associated with 'straight' culture rather than 'queer' culture; therefore potentially making trans persons feel the need to reject the term to maintain a link to the queer community and/or queer identity. Clinicians and researchers should be aware of the negative connotations that may underlie the use of heterosexist and presumptuous terminology. Awareness should also be cultivated about the assumptions that are made when asking this type of question. Identifying with such orientation labels requires referencing one's own gender identity as well as the gender identity of one's partner, which can prove problematic for those who are gender nonconforming.

These results also suggest that clinicians and researchers should not assume that trans persons identify as either heterosexual or gay/lesbian. Perhaps an approach that fosters self-exploration and acceptance for sexual orientation as well as gender identify would be of greatest benefit to those engaging in some form of gender transition.

Comparing 'Types' of Trans Persons

Findings in the literature have suggested that there are some differences between trans men and trans women, particularly when it comes to physical and mental health (e.g., Asscheman et al., 2011; Dhejne et al., 2011; Motmans, Meier, Ponnet, & T'Sjoen, 2012). Similar differences were hypothesized in the current study, though none emerged. While it is possible that the sample size was too small to detect systematic differences, the type of samples each past study used might also explain this discrepancy. The previously mentioned studies used clinical samples of trans persons (e.g., those seeking GRS at a gender clinic), while the current study used a community sample. Perhaps those seeking 'treatment' are at greater risk for negative outcomes, which manifest differently in trans men and trans women. Alternatively, trans persons seeking treatment may be more inclined to provide the responses to researchers/clinicians that they think will most efficiently and effectively lead to the provision of services they desire (i.e., hormone therapy or surgery). Consequently, the power imbalances that exist when researchers are also the gatekeepers to treatment call into question the validity of such research findings. The current findings may also suggest that trans persons are more similar than they are different with respect to mental health and physical health. Each embody an identity that transcends Western cultural norms, which may be linked to the experience of minority stress (Hendricks & Testa, 2012). Perhaps such challenges have similar impacts on physical and mental health regardless of the directionality of one's transition. This conjecture must be considered with caution, however, given the small sample size.

It is also possible that there is something unique about this sample. For example, the participants in this study required access to a private computer and needed to be in a romantic relationship. These requirements imply a measure of economic stability, social support, and social skill. Perhaps these resources were protective against greater impairment that would have differentiated these groups. It is also possible that cohort effects may be a more powerful predictor for variations in psychological and physical health outcomes. A qualitative study comparing trans men who transitioned in the 1980s to those who transitioned in the 2000s revealed a more open conceptualization of gender and sexual identity among the younger sample, as well as a far less strict adherence to the gender binary and less inclination to seek GRS (Yerke & Mitchell, 2011). Similarly, Dhejne and colleagues (2011) reported that individuals who began transitioning before 1989 drove the reported mortality effect up, leading them to highlight that during that time the availability of quality GRS, hormonal treatment, and psychosocial care was limited. Such circumstances may have contributed significantly to poorer psychological and mental health rather than the patients' status as a trans person. The results of the current study would have been more comprehensive if knowledge regarding when (if at all) participants began their transition and, more specifically, what social circumstances were prevalent at that time.

Comparing Trans and Cisgender LGB Persons

This study also compared trans persons to cisgender LGB identified persons on outcomes of relationship quality, social support, and mental/physical health. The lack of differences between the two groups in relationship quality indicators implies that the trans participants had similar experiences with their romantic relationships as cisgender participants, which is congruent with literature on same- and mixed-sex couples. For example, Kurdek (2004) reported that relationship quality was relatively similar for both heterosexual couples and gay/lesbian couples, and that these relationships function in much the same way. Peplau and Fingerhut (2007) reached similar conclusions to Kurdek (2004), and Patterson (2000) also reported that relationship quality might not differ as a function of sexual orientation. Consequently, while a great deal of the relationships literature has begun to conclude that sexual identity does not play a crucial role in determining relationship outcomes (Blair, 2012), the results of this study provide cursory evidence that differences based on gender identity may be equally negligible, with trans and cisgender individuals reporting similar levels of relationship functioning. Further research should examine the romantic relationships of non-clinical samples of trans persons and their partners to further understand the role that gender identity, specifically transgender identities, may or may not play in predicting relationship well-being.

In addition, trans and cisgender persons in the current sample did not differ in their perceptions of social support for their relationships, although it is possible that there may have been differences if the comparison group also included those in non-stigmatized, mixed-sex relationships (Blair & Holmberg, 2008). Given the similarities in relationship quality and perceived levels of support for one's relationship, it appears that the participants in the current study did not experience great challenges with respect to their romantic relationships. These findings are particularly positive given the well-established link between healthy romantic relationships and positive mental and physical health outcomes (e.g., Weyers et al., 2009). Future research should examine how relationship well-being and perceived support for one's relationship might vary as a function of relationship composition (e.g., same- or mixed-sex, one or more partners identifying as transgender; see Table 3.2.2) as well as the extent to which trans identified individuals within the relationship are able to "pass" as cisgender. It is possible that the challenges and benefits associated with one's ability/desire to "pass" may play an important role in predicting relationship well-being and functioning.

Several differences emerged, however, when considering mental and physical health, with trans persons faring poorer than cisgender persons. Trans persons reported more symptoms of depression, anxiety, stress, and physical complaints. Of note, trans persons scored above a commonly-used clinical cutoff for significant symptoms of depression, while cisgender persons did not (16.00; Boyd, Weissman, Thompson, & Myers, 1982). These findings suggest that, at least for this sample, being a gender minority is associated with greater psychological and physical strain beyond that which might be associated with identifying as a sexual minority. The results from this study support the need for making informative resources available to trans persons to assist them in coping with the physical and psychological obstacles they may face while transitioning and living in cissexist Western society.

Trans persons in this study also reported significantly less general social support than cisgender LGB persons. This finding may reflect the fact that while there has been a gradual societal acceptance of sexual minorities in Western countries, understanding of non-binary and diverse gender expressions is lacking. Trans persons still face a great deal of discrimination and stigma in their personal and professional lives (Bauer et al., 2009; Coyle, 2011). The full impact of the varying types of stress experienced by trans persons is still unknown, though the results from this study suggest that trans persons do indeed experience discrepancies in their mental and physical well-being when compared to other populations.

The differences observed in this study provide evidence that individuals falling under the LGBT acronym should not always be considered a homogeneous group for the purposes of research. Assuming that all LGBT individuals share similar experiences can be particularly problematic given the fact that the literature on trans persons is relatively sparse, which may create a greater reliance on the larger LGB literature in attempts to gain insight about trans persons and their experiences. Such a process could easily result in misinformation and misunderstandings, given that the results of studies with LGB populations, or ones with predominantly LGB participants and only a few trans participants, may not accurately represent the experiences of trans identified persons. The results of the current study indicate that findings in the LGB literature might not apply to trans persons the same way as they would apply to LGB persons, particularly when addressing mental and physical health. Thus while we encourage inclusive research methods, we remind researchers that gender and sexual identity are separate constructs, and it may be inappropriate to consider trans participants as necessarily belonging to the "LGBT" portion of the sample. Furthermore, it is important to note that trans persons can simultaneously represent both the "T" and the "L," "G," or "B" (e.g., a trans man who identifies as gay), and it may therefore be necessary to examine how various combinations of identities might predict better or worse mental and physical health outcomes.

Predicting Physical and Mental Health

The combination of greater general social support and higher relationship satisfaction predicted fewer symptoms of depression, stress and anxiety for trans participants in the current study. This finding aligns with previous literature highlighting the importance of having healthy romantic relationships and positive social support for trans and LGB persons (Blair & Holmberg, 2008; Kurdek, 2003, 2004; Weyers et al., 2009). Neither social support nor relationship satisfaction emerged as unique and significant predictors of depression, indicating that it was the specific interaction between these two concepts—having both a greater sense of social support *and* high relationship satisfaction—that played an important role in predicting positive mental health outcomes.

Greater relationship satisfaction was associated with lower levels of stress for trans persons in the current study. This pattern may indicate that healthy relationships are a particularly important element in reducing stress for trans persons or that experiencing problems in one's relationship may be an important aspect to consider when addressing concerns of stress among trans identified individuals. Conversely, it may also be that those experience higher levels of stress in other aspects of their life may then have difficulty maintaining a healthy and satisfying relationship.

Increased perceptions of general social support were associated with lower levels of anxiety. It is reasonable to assume that feeling socially accepted and experiencing fewer instances of rejection would make it easier for an individual to function in the world with fewer symptoms of anxiety. Social support may be particularly salient for trans persons, given the potential magnitude of consequences associated with a lack of support, including familial and societal rejection, as well as threats of violence or even death. Consequently, social support may play a crucial role in creating a sense of acceptance and safety for trans persons, which then translate into lower levels of anxiety. Further research should examine the specific ways in which trans persons perceive support and how they make attributions for the support that they do or do not receive from their social network members.

General social support and relationship satisfaction did not emerge as significant predictors of physical health symptoms. This finding contradicts much of what is reported with cisgender samples (both LGB and heterosexual), where relationship satisfaction and social support play important roles in predicting physical health outcomes (e.g. Blair & Holmberg, 2008; Blair, 2012; Kiecolt-Glaser & Newton, 2001). Consequently, the discrepancies in physical health reported between the trans and cisgender samples within the current study do not appear to be associated with levels of support or relationship satisfaction, indicating that researchers and clinicians may need to look to other factors to better understand the predictors of health outcomes for trans persons. Of note, it is quite likely that the current study did not measure some potentially salient predictors of physical health outcomes for trans persons, such as their stage of transitioning, their satisfaction with transitioning, complications associated with GRS, or social support specifically for their gender identity and the associated health-related issues. Other relationship factors may have also played a role, such as their sexual satisfaction (Holmberg, Blair, & Phillips, 2010).

Overall, these results indicate that both relationship satisfaction and general social support are important predictors of mental health status among trans persons. Further research should examine potential causal directions between these variables as well as investigate further into understanding what the most important predictors of physical health are among trans identified individuals.

Limitations

The inclusive nature of this study represents a step toward a comprehensive and accepting clinical literature dedicated to the well being of trans persons. There are, however, some limitations that merit acknowledgement. Although participants were invited to articulate their identities in multiple ways, it is difficult for survey research to accurately capture each individual's nuanced identity, such that we have limited information about how each participant conceptualizes their own gender and sexual identity. In addition, the experiences of the trans persons within the current sample may not generalize to trans persons who are single, given that previous research has indicated that trans persons in relationships report better quality of life than single trans persons (e.g., Motmans, Meier, Ponnet, & T'Sjoen, 2012).

The small sample size of this study made most multivariate statistical procedures unadvisable due to a lack of power. The use of multivariate analyses could have drastically reduced the type I error rate, and increased the ability to detect more nuanced effects. The small sample size is also problematic since it may reduce the generalizability of these results. Future research should endeavour to expand these results by obtaining larger sample sizes and applying more sophisticated statistical analyses.

Future Directions

While the findings of this study contribute to a more comprehensive understanding of trans persons' identities, social support, and mental/physical health, the canon of literature is still quite sparse. Future research would benefit from a more inclusive and wide-reaching examination of various subgroups of trans persons, such as genderqueer persons and individuals with varying desires with respect to their process of transitioning. Methodological approaches should be ethically sound and combine qualitative and quantitative research that captures individual experiences as well as more global trends. Future research should also address experiences of transphobia and cissexim as predictors of mental and physical health, in addition to investigating the role of romantic relationships and social support. It may also be interesting to have a better understanding of what forms of gender presentation and identity are most likely to elicit negative societal responses, with the aim of developing educational interventions designed to promote a non-binary understanding of gender and reduce gender-identity-based discrimination. Future research should be informed not only by current findings in the literature, but also through dialogues with the trans community at every stage of the research process. Such research should also be done at various time points in a person's transition, if undertaken, and also take the sociopolitical climate into account (e.g., capture participants' experiences with transphobic public and health policies, discriminatory practices, etc.).

Conclusions

The implications of this study are threefold: 1) Gender and sexual orientation/identity experiences are very diverse among trans persons, and should be acknowledged and addressed as such in research and clinical practice; 2) Though many of the challenges faced by LGB persons are similar to those faced by trans persons, their physical and psychological functioning may differ systematically, particularly when it comes to social support as well as physical and mental health; 3) Social support and relationship quality may prove to be powerful sources of protection for trans persons, providing impetus for fostering cultural acceptance and celebration of trans identities.

References

Alderson, K. (2012). Sexuality Questionnaire. Retrieved from http://www.kevinalderson.ca/resources/SQ.pdf

Aspinwall, L.G., & Taylor, S.E. (1992). Modeling cognitive adaptation: a longitudinal investigation of the impact of individual differences and coping on college adjustment and performance. *Journal of Personality and Social Psychology*, *63*(6), 989–1003. Retrieved from http://www.ncbi.nlm.nih.gov/pubmed/1460565. http://dx.doi.org/10.1037/0022-3514.63.6.989 Medline:1460565

Asscheman, H., Giltay, EJ., Megens, J.AJ., de Ronde, W.P., van Trotsenburg, M.A.A., & Gooren, LJ.G. (2011). A long-term follow-up study of mortality in transsexuals receiving treatment with cross-sex hormones. *European Journal of Endocrinology*, *164*(4), 635–642. http://dx.doi.org/10.1530/EJE-10-1038 Medline:21266549

Bauer, G.R., Hammond, R., Travers, R., Kaay, M., Hohenadel, K.M., & Boyce, M. (2009). "I don't think this is theoretical; this is our lives": how erasure impacts health care for transgender people. *The Journal of the Association of Nurses in AIDS Care*, *20*(5), 348–361. http://dx.doi.org/10.1016/j.jana.2009.07.004 Medline:19732694

Blair, K.L. (2012). *Perceived social support for relationships as a predictor of relationship well-being and mental and physical health in*

same-sex and mixed-sex relationships: A longitudinal investigation. (Doctoral Dissertation, Queen's University). Retrieved from http://qspace.library.queensu.ca/
Blair, K.L., & Holmberg, D. (2008). Perceived social network support and well-being in same-sex versus mixed-sex romantic relationships. *Journal of Social and Personal Relationships*, *25*(5), 769–791. http://dx.doi.org/10.1177/0265407508096695
Blumer, M.L.C., Green, M.S., Knowles, SJ., & Williams, A. (2012). Shedding light on thirteen years of darkness: content analysis of articles pertaining to transgender issues in marriage/couple and family therapy journals. *Journal of Marital and Family Therapy*, *38*(Suppl 1), 244–256. http://dx.doi.org/10.1111/j.1752-0606.2012.00317.x Medline:22765337
Bockting, W., Benner, A., & Coleman, E. (2009). Gay and bisexual identity development among female-to-male transsexuals in North America: emergence of a transgender sexuality. *Archives of Sexual Behavior*, *38*(5), 688–701. http://dx.doi.org/10.1007/s10508-009-9489-3 Medline:19330439
Boyd, J.H., Weissman, M.M., Thompson, W.D., & Myers, J.K. (1982). Screening for depression in a community sample. Understanding the discrepancies between depression symptom and diagnostic scales. *Archives of General Psychiatry*, *39*(10), 1195–1200. Retrieved from http://archpsyc.jamanetwork.com/. http://dx.doi.org/10.1001/archpsyc.1982.04290100059010 Medline:7125849
Carrera, V., DePalma, R., & Lameiras, M. (2012). Sex/gender identity: Moving beyond fixed and "natural" categories. *Sexualities*, *15*(8), 995–1016. http://dx.doi.org/10.1177/1363460712459158
Cohen, J. (1992). A power primer. *Psychological Bulletin*, *112*(1), 155–159. http://dx.doi.org/10.1037/0033-2909.112.1.155 Medline:19565683
Cohen, S., & Hoberman, H.M. (1983). Positive events and social supports as buffers of life change stress. *Journal of Applied Social Psychology*, *13*(2), 99–125. http://dx.doi.org/10.1111/j.1559-1816.1983.tb02325.x
Cohen, S., Kamarck, T., & Mermelstein, R. (1983). A global measure of perceived stress. *Journal of Health and Social Behavior*, *24*(4), 385–396. http://dx.doi.org/10.2307/2136404 Medline:6668417
Coleman, E., Bockting, W., Botzer, M., Cohen-Kettenis, P., DeCuypere, G., Feldman, J., …, & Zucker, K. (2012). Standards of care for the health of transsexual, transgender, and gender-nonconforming people, version 7. *International Journal of Transgenderism*, *13*(4), 165–232. http://dx.doi.org/10.1080/15532739.2011.700873
Coyle, S.M. (2011). *A mixed methods investigation of the needs, experiences, and fulfillments of trans persons accessing Ontario health care services.* (Master's Thesis, Queen's University). Retrieved from http://qspace.library.queensu.ca/
Dhejne, C., Lichtenstein, P., Boman, M., Johansson, A.L.V., Långström, N., & Landén, M. (2011). Long-term follow-up of transsexual persons undergoing sex reassignment surgery: cohort study in Sweden. *PLoS ONE*, *6*(2), e16885. http://dx.doi.org/10.1371/journal.pone.0016885 Medline:21364939
Diamond, L.M., & Butterworth, M.R. (2008). Questioning gender and sexual identity: Dynamic links over time. *Sex Roles*, *59*(5-6), 365–376. http://dx.doi.org/10.1007/s11199-008-9425-3
Docter, R.F., & Fleming, J.S. (2001). Measures of transgender behavior. *Archives of Sexual Behavior*, *30*(3), 255–271. http://dx.doi.org/10.1023/A:1002795929547 Medline:11330116
Dugan, J.P., Kusel, M.L., & Simounet, D.M. (2012). Transgender college students: An exploratory study of perceptions, engagement, and educational outcomes. *Journal of College Student Development*, *53*(5), 719–736. http://dx.doi.org/10.1353/csd.2012.0067
Fisher, A.D., Bandini, E., Casale, H., Ferruccio, N., Meriggiola, M.C., Gualerzi, A., …, & Maggi, M. (2013). Sociodemographic and clinical features of gender identity disorder: an Italian multicentric evaluation. *Journal of Sexual Medicine*, *10*(2), 408–419. http://dx.doi.org/10.1111/j.1743-6109.2012.03006.x Medline:23171237
Hendrick, S.S. (1988). A generic measure of relationship satisfaction. *Journal of Marriage and the Family*, *50*(1), 93–98. http://dx.doi.org/10.2307/352430
Hendricks, M.L., & Testa, R.J. (2012). A conceptual framework for clinical work with transgender and gender nonconforming clients: An adaptation of the minority stress model. *Professional Psychology, Research and Practice*, *43*(5), 460–467. http://dx.doi.org/10.1037/a0029597
Holmberg, D., Blair, K.L., & Phillips, M. (2010). Women's sexual satisfaction as a predictor of well-being in same-sex versus mixed-sex relationships. *Journal of Sex Research*, *47*(1), 1–11. http://dx.doi.org/10.1080/00224490902898710 Medline:19381998
Iantaffi, A., & Bockting, W.O. (2011). Views from both sides of the bridge? Gender, sexual legitimacy and transgender people's experiences of relationships. *Culture, Health & Sexuality*, *13*(3), 355–370. http://dx.doi.org/10.1080/13691058.2010.537770 Medline:21229422
Jackson, N.C., Johnson, M.J., & Roberts, R. (2008). The potential impact of discrimination fears of older gays, lesbians, bisexuals and transgender individuals living in small- to moderate-sized cities on long-term health care. *Journal of Homosexuality*, *54*(3), 325–339. http://dx.doi.org/10.1080/00918360801982298 Medline:18825868
Kiecolt-Glaser, J.K., & Newton, T.L. (2001). Marriage and health: his and hers. *Psychological Bulletin*, *127*(4), 472–503. http://dx.doi.org/10.1037/0033-2909.127.4.472 Medline:11439708
Kinsey, A., Pomeroy, W., & Martin, C. (1948). *Sexual Behaviour in the Human Male.* Philadelphia: W.B. Saunders.
Kinsey, A., Pomeroy, W., Martin, C., & Gebhard, P. (1953). *Sexual Behaviour in the Human Female.* Philadelphia: W.B. Saunders.
Kuper, L.E., Nussbaum, R., & Mustanski, B. (2012). Exploring the diversity of gender and sexual orientation identities in an online sample of transgender individuals. *Journal of Sex Research*, *49*(2-3), 244–254. http://dx.doi.org/10.1080/00224499.2011.596954 Medline:21797716
Kurdek, L. (2003). Differences between Gay and Lesbian cohabiting couples. *Journal of Social and Personal Relationships*, *20*(4), 411–436. http://dx.doi.org/10.1177/02654075030204001

Kurdek, L. (2004). Are Gay and Lesbian cohabiting couples really different from heterosexual married couples? *Journal of Marriage and the Family, 66*(4), 880–900. http://dx.doi.org/10.1111/j.0022-2445.2004.00060.x
Motmans, J., Meier, P., Ponnet, K., & T'Sjoen, G. (2012). Female and male transgender quality of life: socioeconomic and medical differences. *Journal of Sexual Medicine, 9*(3), 743–750. http://dx.doi.org/10.1111/j.1743-6109.2011.02569.x Medline:22188877
Nagoshi, J.L., Brzuzy, S., & Terrell, H.K. (2012). Deconstructing the complex perceptions of gender roles, gender identity, and sexual orientation among transgender individuals. *Feminism & Psychology, 22*(4), 405–422. http://dx.doi.org/10.1177/0959353512461929
Nieder, T.O., Herff, M., Cerwenka, S., Preuss, W.F., Cohen-Kettenis, P.T., De Cuypere, G., ..., & Richter-Appelt, H. (2011). Age of onset and sexual orientation in transsexual males and females. *Journal of Sexual Medicine, 8*(3), 783–791. http://dx.doi.org/10.1111/j.1743-6109.2010.02142.x Medline:21143416
Patterson, C. (2000). Family relationships of Lesbians and Gay men. *Journal of Marriage and the Family, 62*(4), 1052–1069. http://dx.doi.org/10.1111/j.1741-3737.2000.01052.x
Peplau, L.A., & Fingerhut, A.W. (2007). The close relationships of Lesbians and gay men. *Annual Review of Psychology, 58*(1), 405–424. http://dx.doi.org/10.1146/annurev.psych.58.110405.085701 Medline:16903800
Radloff, L.S. (1977). The CES-D Scale: A self-report depression scale for research in the general population. *Applied Psychological Measurement, 1*(3), 385–401. http://dx.doi.org/10.1177/014662167700100306
Rempel, J.K., Holmes, J.G., & Zanna, M.P. (1985). Trust in close relationships. *Journal of Personality and Social Psychology, 49*(1), 95–112. http://dx.doi.org/10.1037/0022-3514.49.1.95http://www.ncbi.nlm.nih.gov/entrez/query.fcgi?cmd=Retrieve&db=PubMed&list_uids=11474726&dopt=Abstract
Rubin, Z. (1970). Measurement of romantic love. *Journal of Personality and Social Psychology, 16*(2), 265–273. Retrieved from http://www.ncbi.nlm.nih.gov/pubmed/5479131. http://dx.doi.org/10.1037/h0029841 Medline:5479131
Rusbult, C.E., Martz, J.M., & Agnew, C.R. (1998). The Investment Model Scale: Measuring commitment level, satisfaction level, quality of alternatives, and investment size. *Personal Relationships, 5*(4), 357–387. http://dx.doi.org/10.1111/j.1475-6811.1998.tb00177.x
Spielberger, C.D., Gorsuch, R.L., Lushene, R., Vagg, P.R., & Jacobs, G.A. (1983). *Manual for the State-Trait Anxiety Inventory.* Palo Alto, CA: Consulting Psychologists Press.
Sprecher, S., & Felmlee, D. (1992). The influence of parents and friends on the quality and stability of romantic relationships: A three-wave longitudinal investigation. *Journal of Marriage and the Family, 54*(4), 888–900. http://dx.doi.org/10.2307/353170
Weyers, S., Elaut, E., De Sutter, P., Gerris, J., T'Sjoen, G., Heylens, G., ..., & Verstraelen, H. (2009). Long-term assessment of the physical, mental, and sexual health among transsexual women. *Journal of Sexual Medicine, 6*(3), 752–760. http://dx.doi.org/10.1111/j.1743-6109.2008.01082.x Medline:19040622
Wierckx, K., Van Caenegem, E., Elaut, E., Dedecker, D., Van de Peer, F., Toye, K., ..., & T'Sjoen, G. (2011). Quality of life and sexual health after sex reassignment surgery in transsexual men. *Journal of Sexual Medicine, 8*(12), 3379–3388. http://dx.doi.org/10.1111/j.1743-6109.2011.02348.x Medline:21699661
Yerke, A.F., & Mitchell, V. (2011). Am I man enough yet? A comparison of the body transition, self-labeling, and sexual orientation of two cohorts of female-to-male transsexuals. *International Journal of Transgenderism, 13*(2), 64–76. http://dx.doi.org/10.1080/15532739.2011.622125
Zimet, G.D., Dahlem, N.W., Zimet, S.G., & Farley, G.K. (1988). The Multidimensional Scale of Perceived Social Support. *Journal of Personality Assessment, 52*(1), 30–41. http://dx.doi.org/10.1207/s15327752jpa5201_2

Questions

1. The authors' study explores the gender identities and sexual orientations of transgender persons. What are some ways in which transgender persons' experiences of gender and sexuality do not adequately fit within the (sex/gender/sexuality) binary?

Thinking Transnationally

Reproductive Justice in a Globalized Era

Tanya Saroj Bakhru

Editor's Introduction

In this reading, Tanya Saroj Bakhru uses her background in feminist critiques of globalization and reproductive health to outline an interdisciplinary, intersectional, transnational approach to the issue of sexual and reproductive health. Her discussion brings together the frameworks of reproductive justice and transnational feminism to provide a nuanced understanding of the role the forces of globalization have played in the sexual and reproductive lives of gendered bodies in the 21st century. In articulating this perspective, Bakhru centers the interrogation of present-day globalization and neoliberal economic ideology to these topics and discusses how transnational feminism and reproductive justice can provide conceptual reconfigurations of pressing issues and create and sustain movements for justice and social transformation. Tanya Saroj Bakhru, PhD is a professor of women, gender, and sexuality studies at San Jose State University. Her areas of interest include feminist critiques of globalization, reproductive health and justice, and transnational women's health.

My reasons for thinking transnationally about women's lives are both deeply personal and political. My paternal grandmother, who I called Amma, was born in 1916 in the city of Rohri located in the Indian state of Sindh. Rohri is now in present-day Pakistan but had been a part of the British imperial project for 200 years. Amma was named Nirmala Ahuja by her parents. However, when she was married at the age of 14, she became Heer Bakhru. Pursuant to custom, my grandfather's family changed both her first and last name, signaling a key shift: separate from her birth family, her obligation now belonged to her husband's family. A year later, Amma's first child was born but died in infancy. My father, Keshoolal, was born shortly thereafter, when she was 17.

At the time of the Partition of India in 1947, my grandparents and their four children lived in the city of Quetta. As my dad tells it, one night there was a riot in their town. Unrest between Muslim and Hindu groups had escalated as the end of British occupation drew near. My grandparents, my dad, his brothers, and sister hid anxiously in the bathroom while fighting and rioting continued outside their home. The next morning, the British Army occupied the city, promising residents they would provide safe passage out of town so long as they left all their belongings behind. That night was the beginning of my family's yearlong journey as refugees—moving from Mumbai (Bombay) to Nagpur and eventually settling in Varanasi (Banaras). Once settled, Amma had two more children. Eventually in 1960 my father immigrated to the United States and sponsored, one by one, each of his family members to join him.

I often reflect on my grandmother's experiences, her role in our family, and the gendered limitations to which she was subjected: To what extent did she have a choice in the number and spacing of her children? What, if any, was her escape from intimate partner violence? How did she manage the constraints she faced while raising children within a deeply patriarchal society—especially against the backdrop of British colonization? What would reproductive justice have looked like for her? I had so many unanswered questions, since she passed away when I was a teenager. I have spent years trying to excavate her story through interviews with my dad, aunt, and uncles.

Amma's lived experience and mine, a queer woman and new parent, born and living in the United States, are temporally and spatially discrete. However, we are connected through bloodlines and legacies of not only violence but also resilience and resistance. Furthermore, we are linked by common themes of the struggle for bodily autonomy, the residual impacts of colonization and intergenerational trauma, family violence, and a desire for reproductive freedom. Recognizing these connections, across time and space, national boundaries, and various identity categories are vital to building the solidarities necessary to create a more equitable world. How can we understand the lived reproductive and sexual experiences of marginalized peoples, especially women, in seemingly contrasting social and geographic places and build alliances between individuals and communities? This question drives the formation of this book.

Why is a book of this kind needed? In the present moment, the need for justice, and reproductive justice in particular, feels critically urgent. We have reached an apex of neoliberalism "marked by market-based governance practices on the one hand (the privatization, commodification, and proliferation of difference) and authoritarian, national-security driven penal state practices on the other" (Mohanty, 2013, p. 970). While these trends have emerged around the world, no other event embodies the full realization of such ideologies than the election of Donald Trump in 2016 to President of the United States.

The election of Donald Trump is but one specific event and there has been much rumination about the causes of his ascension to political power. One idea put forth argues that Trump is a symbol of hyper-capitalism and its reliance on racist and sexist ideology to enact and prop up oppressive structures around the world. As Naomi Klein (2017) articulates in her book, *No Is Not Enough: Resisting Trump's Shock Politics and Winning the World We Need*, for Trump "the presidency is in fact the crowning extension of the Trump brand" (p. 5) and the completion of decades-long effort by proponents of neoliberalism to destroy the public sphere and create a fully corporate state. She further explains that among the main pillars of Trump's political and economic project are

> the deconstruction of the regulatory state; a full-bore attack on the welfare state and social services (rationalized in part through bellicose racial fear mongering and attacks on women for exercising their rights); the unleashing of a domestic fossil fuel frenzy (which requires the sweeping aside of climate science and the gagging of large parts of the government bureaucracy); and a civilizational war against immigrants and "radical Islamic terrorism" (with ever-expanding domestic and foreign theatres).
>
> (p. 5)

Klein's book was published in mid-2017, in the early days of the Trump presidency. As time progresses and Trump remains in office, however, we can see these concepts further materialize through the implementation of a stream of severe policies and practices. There are many examples, but in the context of the work presented in this [reading], three stand out in particular. This first includes the reinstatement and expansion of the Global Gag Rule/Mexico City Policy, entitled the Policy Protecting Life in Global Health Assistance. This policy restricts "using US foreign aid for abortion-related activities, [and] requires foreign nongovernmental organizations receiving US global health assistance to certify that they do not use their own non-US funds to provide abortion services" (Human Rights Watch, February 14, 2018). The Policy Protecting Life in Global Health Assistance extends the Global Gag Rule/Mexico City Policy restrictions to billions of dollars in U.S. global health assistance, such as maternal and child health programs, prevention and treatment of tuberculosis, malaria, infectious diseases, neglected tropical diseases, and water, sanitation, and hygiene programs.

Second, sweeping tax cuts made to corporations have resulted in increases in taxes for low- and moderate-income families and increases in the national deficit by over a trillion dollars. This increase in national debt is then used to justify cuts to social welfare services as a 'remedy' to the aforementioned budget deficit. Proposed cuts include, for example, funding for the Supplemental Nutrition Assistance Program (SNAP) upon which many low-income women and children rely (National Women's Law Center, 2018).

President Trump's third draconian policy and practice includes the forced separation of children from their parents who have entered the United States without documentation, frequently seeking asylum, and having been detained as a result. What makes this act particularly harsh is that it was conceived as a means to deter 'illegal immigration' across the U.S. border. As Attorney General Jeff Sessions stated in May 2018, "If you don't want your child to be separated, then don't bring them across the border illegally. It's not our fault that somebody does that." Children who are removed from their parents are placed in the custody of the Office of Refugee Resettlement in shelters and facilities around the country (Burnett, 2018). It has been documented that, "Detention and family separation, even for short periods of time, have serious adverse consequences for mental well-being, particularly for those who have already suffered trauma" (Human Rights Watch, February 28, 2018). Many women who migrate, and especially those who are seeking asylum, are fleeing violence, economic crises, and conflict that are often by-products of the economic restructuring that is a hallmark of globalization (Baran & Hafiz, 2017).

The Policy Protecting Life in Global Health Assistance, Trump tax cuts, and increased immigrant detention and family separation are only a few examples (the list goes on) of the many practices with racist, xenophobic, and misogynistic ramifications taking place under the Trump Administration. Under such conditions of social and economic crisis, it is women, particularly those who are most marginalized due to their citizenship status, socioeconomic class, or race, that become the 'shock absorbers' of such policies and practices and shoulder the heaviest burdens. Although, the Trump Administration is not the only example of trends towards authoritarianism and of patriarchal rule in the current era (as Madeleine Albright (2018) points out, authoritarianism is on the rise in Eastern Europe, North Korea, the Philippines, Turkey, and Russia), the size and scope of the United States in terms of its economic and political influence make its global influence far and wide reaching.

Against the background just described, this [reading] takes an intersectional, interdisciplinary, and transnational approach, to present work that will provide the reader with a nuanced and in depth understanding of the role that forces of globalization have played in sexual and reproductive lives of gendered bodies in the 21st century. [This reading] draws on two primary conceptual frameworks to explore and make sense of the reproductive and sexual experiences of various groups of women and marginalized people around the world: reproductive justice and transnational feminism.

Reproductive justice is an intersectional, human rights based framework that

> makes the link between the individual and community, addresses government and corporate responsibility, fights all forms of population control (eugenics), commits to individual/community leadership development that results in power shifts, and puts marginalized communities at the center of the analysis.
>
> (Ross, Roberts, Derkas, Peoples, & Toure, 2018, p. 19)

While the reproductive justice movement is rooted in the work and lived experiences of African American women, it involves theory, strategy, and practice that applies to everyone and has brought American reproductive politics into rhythm with work already being done by feminist groups around the world.

Reproductive justice offers a holistic model of theory and activism focused on three principles: (1) the right not to have children; (2) the right to have children; and (3) the right to parent children one already has. It points to the sense that "our collective sexual consciousness has been warped by misogyny, slavery, and colonialism" (Ross et al., 2018, p. 175). While reproductive justice centers the experiences of Black women in America, it also brings to light the ways that systems of oppression like white supremacy, sexism, and capitalism work together in determining the worth, utility, and value of certain bodies over others—a framework that is wide reaching and illuminating when understood in a global context.

The epistemological trajectory of reproductive justice intersects with transnational feminism as both paradigms locate an interrogation of current day globalization and neoliberal economic ideology at the center of analysis. Because globalization and neoliberal economic ideology aim to undermine the public sphere, social welfare networks "naturalize capitalist values as if they are inevitable" (Ross et al., 2018, p. 21). Thus, it is critical that any exploration of the reproductive experiences of marginalized individuals interrogate and complicate notions of "choice" to advocate for justice.

As Andrea Smith (2005) has so succinctly articulated, when we rely on choice as our main framework for understanding women's reproductive and sexual experiences, reproductive health matters become configured from a commodity perspective. Consequently, the processes and circumstances that inform how individuals and communities perceive and negotiate their sexual and reproductive freedoms are obscured. When reproductive rights are embedded in notions of 'free' choice, all the social, political, and economic factors that surround how choices are made become hidden. In addition, when approaching reproductive health from a commodity perspective, the notion that women and marginalized groups have inherent rights is lost. What remains is the idea that choices should only be made if one can afford them or if one is deemed a legitimate choice-maker (Smith, 2005). Examples of this ideology play out time and again in varying historical and geographic contexts [...]. Against a global backdrop of legacies of colonialism, exploitation, and economic, social, and political disenfranchisement that carry on through generations, we need more than choices. We need justice.

This quest for justice compels many feminist scholars and activists to frame their work within a transnational context. Transnational feminist frameworks include a commitment to addressing the asymmetries of globalization/capitalist re-colonization as well as the implementation of an intersectional set of understandings, tools, and practices such as paying attention to the raced, classed, and gendered ways that globalization and capitalist patriarchies (re)structure colonial and neo-colonial relations of domination and subordination. As I have discussed in previous work (Bakhru, 2008) transnational feminist scholarship acknowledges the simultaneously constituting relationships between the local and global, employs tools of constant contextualization and historicization, and challenges hegemonic views of global capitalism (Mies, 2007; Bhavnani, 2007; Kim, 2007). Transnational feminism also grapples with the complex and contradictory ways that individual and collective agencies are shaped by and in turn shape processes of globalization. It juxtaposes women and marginalized people in similar contexts, in different geographical spaces, rather than as a homogeneous category across the world (Nagar & Swarr, 2010, p. 5). In a transnational feminist framework, contexts, links, and relationships that are material and temporal between the local and global take our focus. "What is emphasized are relations of mutuality, coresponsibility, and common interests, anchoring the idea of feminist solidarity" (Mohanty, 2003, p. 242). It is through such conceptual reconfigurations of pressing issues that we can create and sustain movements for justice and social transformation.

Over the past several decades, a visible transnational women's health movement has emerged and gathered momentum. Responding to the negative impacts of globalization, the rise of antifeminist and fundamentalist political and religious forces, and the HIV/AIDS pandemic, transnational coalitions formed and leadership emerged from the Global South (Petchesky, 2003, p. 1). United Nations (UN) conferences such as the International Conference on Population and Development (ICPD) in 1994 and the World Conference on Women in 1995 along with the non-governmental organizations associated with those conferences recognized sexual and reproductive health as crucial and complex concepts, including control and decision-making over one's body, and the full realization of gender equality. These conferences strengthened connections between gender equality, justice, education for women, and girls' empowerment and reproductive health. The ICPD in particular "emphasized the ineluctable relationship between poverty, underdevelopment, and women's reproduction" (Ross et al., 2018, p. 43). In fact, some of the founders of the reproductive justice movement in the United States participated in the 1994 ICPD Conference and found solidarity with women from the Global South who were already implementing a human rights framework to push back against the forces of globalization and the use of women's fertility as a means to neoliberal economic ends (Ross et al., 2018, p. 44).

In the finding of feminist solidarity, transnational women's health movements have, in recent years, moved in the direction of being able to see the interconnections between communities of women and look at the "broader pattern and structures of domination and exploitation" (Mohanty, 2013, p. 967) that circumscribe the experiences outlined in this [reading]. If scholars, activists, or policymakers fail to see the points of connection between various groups of people, we run the risk of interpreting sexual and reproductive health decisions and actions as only occurring at the individual level or as private matters. In the work presented here, by using reproductive justice and transnational feminism as theoretical lenses, my hope is to show a history of reproductive and sexual lived experiences that connect across time and place.

[...] This [reading] is intended to provide academics and students with a challenging and thought provoking look into sexual and reproductive health matters from a transnational perspective. Like my own search to understand myself in my grandmother's story, my hope is that the work presented in this [reading] will help the reader understand their own reproductive and sexual experiences in a more nuanced and contextualized way that links us to each other in a quest for justice and liberation.

Bibliography

Adoptive Couple v. Baby Girl, 133 S. Ct. 2552 (2013).

Albright, M. (2018). *Fascism: A Warning.* New York: Harper Press.

Bakhru, T. (2008). Negotiating and Navigating the Rough Terrain of Transnational Feminist Research. *Journal of International Women's Studies, 10*(2), 198–216.

Baran, A., & Hafiz, S. (2017). Trump's First 100 Days: Immigrant Women and Families on the Frontlines. Retrieved from https://webelongtogether.org/sites/default/files/WBT100days_report.pdf.

Bhavnani, K. (2007). Interconnections and Configurations: Toward a Global Feminist Ethnography. In Hese-Biber, S. (Ed.). *Handbook of Feminist Research.* London: Sage.

Burnett, J. (2018, May 30). What Happens When Parents and Children are Separated at the U.S.–Mexico Border. *Npr.org.* Retrieved from www.npr.org/2018/05/30/615585043/what-happens-when-parents-and-children-are-separated-at-the-u-s-mexico-border.

Heltberg, R., Hossain, N., Reva, A., & Turk, C. (2013). Coping and Resilience During the Food and Financial Crises. *Journal of Development Studies, 49*(5), 705–718.

Human Rights Watch. (2018, February 14). Trump's "Mexico City Policy" or "Global Gag Rule": Questions and Answers. *Hrw.org*. Retrieved from www.hrw.org/news/2018/02/14/trumps-mexico-city-policy-or-global-gag-rule.
Human Rights Watch. (2018, February 28). In the Freezer: Abusive Conditions for Women and Children in US Immigration Holding Cells. *Hrw.org*. Retrieved from www.hrw.org/report/2018/02/28/freezer/abusive-conditions-women-and-children-us-immigration-holding-cells.
Kim, H.S. (2007). The Politics of Border Crossings: Black, Postcolonial, and Transnational Feminist Perspectives. In Hese-Biber, S. (Ed.). *Handbook of Feminist Research*. London: Sage.
Klein, N. (2007). *The Shock Doctrine: The Rise of Disaster Capitalism*. New York: Picador.
Klein, N. (2017). *No Is Not Enough: Resisting Trump's Shock Politics and Winning the World We Need*. Chicago: Haymarket Books.
Luibhéid, E. (2004). Childbearing Against the State? Asylum Seeker Women in the Irish Republic. *Women's Studies International Forum, 27*, 335–349.
Mendoza, R. (2009). Aggregate Shocks, Poor Households, and Children: Transmission Channels and Policy Responses. *Global Social Policy, 9*, 55–78.
Mies, M. (2007). A Global Feminist Perspective on Research. In Hese-Biber, S. (Ed.). *Handbook of Feminist Research*. London: Sage.
Mohanty, C.T. (2003). *Feminism Without Borders: Decolonizing Theory, Practicing Solidarity*. Durham, NC: Duke University Press.
Mohanty, C.T. (2013). Transnational Feminist Crossings: On Neoliberalism and Radical Critique. *Signs: Journal of Women in Culture and Society, 36*(4), 967–991.
Nagar, R., & Swarr, A. (2010). *Critical Transnational Feminist Praxis*. New York: Suny Press.
National Women's Law Center. (2018, April). What's in the Tax Cuts and Jobs Act of 2017: Provisions that Impact Women and Families. Retrieved from https://nwlc-ciw49tixgw5lbab.stackpathdns.com/wp-content/uploads/2018/04/Tax-Cuts-and-Job-Act-2017.pdf.
Petchesky, R. (2003). *Global Prescriptions: Gendering Health and Human Rights*. New York: Zed Books.
Ross, L.J., Roberts, L., Derkas, E., Peoples, W., & Toure, P.B. (Eds.). (2018). *Radical Reproductive Justice: Foundations, Theory, Practice, Critique*. New York: Feminist Press.
Smith, A. (2005). Beyond Pro-Choice Versus Pro-Life: Women of Color and Reproductive Justice. *NWSA Journal, 17*(1), 119–140.

Question

1. Bakhru argues that our collective sexual consciousness has been warped by misogyny, slavery, and colonialism. Can you think of particular examples of this warping?

Reading 3.4

Whose Bodies? Black Lives Matter and the Reproductive Justice Imperative

Sikivu Hutchinson

Sikivu Hutchinson, "Whose Bodies? Black Lives Matter and the Reproductive Justice Imperative," *The Humanist*, vol. 76, no. 3, pp. 10–11.

Editor's Introduction

This reading uses an intersectional perspective on reproductive health to highlight Black women's health conditions and experiences. In it, Sikivu Hutchinson explains that reproductive justice has always been about more than unrestricted access to abortion and birth control and that because of wealth and healthcare disparities, Black women's reproductive justice is a precondition for mental health, wellness, bodily autonomy, and community enfranchisement. Hutchinson thus brings her unique Black, feminist, humanist perspective to bear on this topic in a way that helpfully

- situates reproductive justice within the Black Lives Matter movement, broadening this movement's scope by making explicit connections between

anti-abortion legislation, reactionary misogyny, anti-Black propaganda, and economic justice activism; and
- calls for bringing together humanist, feminist, and progressive voices in the struggle for racial and reproductive justice.

Sikivu Hutchinson is a US feminist, author, novelist, playwright, and director. In 2020, she was the recipient of the Harvard Humanist of the Year award. In her work, she highlights the cultural influences of African American humanist and atheist social thought and explores the emergence of Black atheist and freethought activism, amplifying the voices of African American nonbelievers.

Over the past several years toxic canards like "abortion is black genocide" and "the most dangerous place for a black child is the womb," which are often cloaked in civil rights rhetoric, have been used to smear abortion and demonize black women's bodies. In 2009, when conservative organizations began targeting communities of color with anti-abortion billboard propaganda, black and Latina women's organizations fought back with their own billboards and media campaigns. These unrelenting assaults on the reproductive rights and self-determination of black women are epitomized by the wave of anti-abortion and anti-contraception state laws that have rocked the nation. One of the most egregious recent examples is a Missouri bill dubbed the "All Lives Matter Act," which would define a fertilized egg as a person with rights. This blatant appropriation of the Black Lives Matter mantle is just another example of the right wing's efforts to undermine black liberation struggle by distorting the language of human rights.

To bolster its claims that abortion is genocide, images of Planned Parenthood founder Margaret Sanger are stamped with Nazi swastikas. Historically revisionist assessments of Planned Parenthood conveniently omit the connection many early-twentieth-century progressive black activists made between family planning, birth control, abortion, and black liberation. Tellingly, Ida B. Wells, Martin Luther King, Malcolm X, and Mary McLeod Bethune supported Sanger's controversial work with the Birth Control Federation of America.

This past February, in an effort to address this tactic, Black Lives Matter (BLM) activists publicly aligned with reproductive justice activists. Historically, reproductive justice has always been about more than just unrestricted access to abortion and birth control. Under slavery and Jim Crow, black women had little to no control over their reproductive destinies. In addition to having the least wealth of any group in the United States, black women, according to the Center for Disease Control and Prevention statistics, are also more likely to get abortions—precisely because of wealth and health care disparities. Thus, for black women, reproductive justice is a precondition for mental health, wellness, bodily autonomy, and community enfranchisement. Spearheaded nationally by the Atlanta-based African-American women's organization Sister Song, the concept of reproductive justice draws upon the notion of intersectionality, which situates women's right to self-determination within a broader economic justice and human rights framework. As Sister Song notes:

> Reproductive justice is a positive approach that links sexuality, health, and human

> rights to social justice movements by placing abortion and reproductive health issues in the larger context of the well-being and health of women, families, and communities because reproductive justice seamlessly integrates those individual and group human rights particularly important to marginalized communities. We believe that the ability of any woman to determine her own reproductive destiny is directly linked to the conditions in her community and these conditions are not just a matter of individual choice and access.

Discussing the relationship between Black Lives Matter activism and reproductive justice in a February 9 statement published at the daily news site *Color Lines*, BLM co-founder Alicia Garza maintained:

> I think from our perspective, reproductive justice is very much situated within the Black Lives Matter movement. And the way we that talk about that is that essentially, it's not just about the right for women to be able to determine when and how and where they want to start families, but it is also very much about our right to be able to raise families, to be able to raise children to become adults.... And that is being hindered by state violence in many different forms. One form being violence by law enforcement or other state forces, and the other form of crisis through poverty and lack of access to resources and lack of access to health communities that are safe and sustainable. So we certainly understand that BLM and reproductive justice go hand in hand.

This is an important juncture in the BLM movement because it further broadens its scope, making an explicit connection between anti-abortion legislation, reactionary misogynist, anti-black "messaging," and economic justice activism. BLM's embrace also comes at critical moment in the national mobilization over women's rights. As the Supreme Court weighs HB2, a Texas law requiring that doctors who perform abortions at local health clinics have hospital admitting privileges, the threat to health care for poor and working class women has deepened. If the court upholds this dangerous law, Texas would be left with as few as nine abortion clinics, and other states would have the right to enforce similar laws. The insidious implications of this shift should be a catalyst for further intersectional organizing—bringing together humanist, feminist, and progressive voices against the forces of religious and political fascism.

Questions

1. What are the key ways in which a reproductive justice approach to women's reproductive health goes beyond approaches that emphasize the right to choose and access to birth control?
2. From an intersectional perspective, what are the advantages of taking a reproductive

justice approach to this bioethical issue?

3. What is lost in emphasizing only reproductive rights?

End-of-Unit Questions

1. We learned about the miasma of cisheteropatriarchy and the many ways it harms everyone, especially multiply marginalized persons. How does this affect how we should provide healthcare to women and to intersex, queer, and transgender persons? What are some ways to mitigate the harmful effects of this miasma (with its many facets) in our institutions of healthcare and medicine to build less oppressive and more inclusive and humane institutions?
2. Would it be possible to improve your preferred moral theory by applying the lessons from this unit concerning the problems faced by persons marginalized because of their sex, gender, and/or sexuality? If yes, how can you refine your preferred moral theory to incorporate these lessons? If no, explain why not. (For example, if you're attracted to Kantian ethics, how can you develop a Kantian approach to solving bioethical problems in a way that adequately respects the autonomy of women and intersex, queer and transgender persons?)

Unit IV

Morality and Mortality

Introduction to the Unit

In this unit, we discuss moral/bioethical issues related to mortality. It aims to

- educate readers as to different views of the nature of death, and
- show how the bioethical issues of abortion and physician-assisted suicide are complicated when we center the perspectives/experiences of marginalized persons of different kinds.

Concepts/Definitions of Death

Death is an inevitable part of life, one that raises many ethical questions, especially in biomedical contexts, where sometimes the only way for healthcare providers to relieve suffering may be to end a patient's life, or where a patient in agony may request help in ending their life.[1] In contending with these difficult questions, we must recognize that the concept of death is disputed and not easily definable. Indeed, there are at least three different views available:

1. **Cardio-respiratory view—**A person is dead when they do not breathe and have no heartbeat.

1. This section is partially inspired by Vaughn (2022, p. 652).

This was traditionally the biomedical definition of *death*, but many people have criticized it given that modern medicine can maintain people's breathing and heartbeat indefinitely, despite the loss of brain function.

2. **Whole brain view—**A person is dead when all their brain functions permanently cease.

Some hold that this view of death avoids some of the problems of the cardio-respiratory one. However, some argue against this view, holding that an individual should be considered dead when their consciousness is permanently lost and thus advocate for:

3. **Higher brain view—**A person is dead when their higher brain functions (responsible for consciousness) permanently cease.

A person in a persistent vegetative state (who is wakeful but without consciousness or intentional behavior and with little chance of significant improvement) counts as dead according to the higher brain view but not the whole brain view.

Not only is there no consensus on the official concept/definition of *death*, but philosophers have plausibly argued that defining *human death* is not solely up to medicine but requires looking to philosophical, cultural, and religious factors.[2] Given this, Alireza Bagheri (2007) argues that it is more ethical to allow people to choose their preferred definition of *death*. Our margin-centering approach fits nicely with this proposal, making room for the self-determination of marginalized persons in accordance with their preferred cultural and religious values (which may lead them to different commitments regarding the connection of life/death to the functioning of the body/brain).

With these basic considerations in hand regarding how to understand death, we turn to two concrete bioethical issues related to death/mortality: abortion and euthanasia/physician-assisted suicide.

The Ethics of Abortion

Our intersectional margin-centering approach, together with the overturning of *Roe v. Wade* (and the dismantling of federal protections of abortion rights this constitutes), requires that we address this issue from the perspective of gendered bodies who face multiple forms of marginalization. Feminists such as Professor of American Culture and Women's Studies Andrea Smith forcefully argue that adequately doing so requires moving beyond the "pro-choice versus pro-life" paradigm that has shaped much discussion.

2. For example, see Olick (1991) and Veatch (1993).

Reproductive Justice: Beyond Pro-Choice Versus Pro-Life

Smith (2005) argues that this standard paradigm for understanding reproductive rights further marginalizes women from marginalized communities, including economically disadvantaged women, women of color, and women with disabilities. Neither of these standard positions "endows women with inherent rights to their body—the pro-life position pits fetal rights against women's rights whereas the pro-choice position argues that women should have freedom to make choices rather than possess inherent rights to their bodies regardless of their class standing" (Smith, 2005, p. 134). Smith argues that when reproductive rights are thought of in terms of "free" choice, the social, political, and economic factors that shape such choices are obscured in a way that both masks and reifies how systems of oppression like cisheteropatriarchy and white supremacy underpin the reproductive choices women make (Smith, 2005). This approach thus leads to the idea that choices should be made only if one can afford them and if one is deemed a legitimate choice-maker—conditions that many marginalized pregnant persons do not meet, precisely because they are oppressed/marginalized.

As Bakhru eloquently puts it in the reading from the previous unit, "Against a global backdrop of legacies of colonialism, exploitation, and economic, social, and political disenfranchisement that carry on through generations, we need more than choices. We need justice" (2019, p. 7). Centering the perspectives of multiply marginalized women thus leads to the reproductive justice conceptual framework as a holistic model for theory and activism advocated for in the last unit's readings. This focuses on three principles (Ross et al., 2018):

1. the right not to have children
2. the right to have children
3. the right to parent the children one already has

In adopting this framework, our approach highlights bodily autonomy as an inherent right of persons and thus is staunchly and adamantly in favor of the legality of and safe access to abortion, seeing legality and access as necessary conditions for the physical, social, and mental health and well-being; bodily autonomy; and community enfranchisement of women. A reproductive justice framework makes clear that, as Smith (2005) rightly argues, even if a fetus is a person, it does not follow that abortion should be criminalized.[3] According to this framework, it is possible to hold that the fetus is a person whose life has value and still hold that (in certain circumstances) this life must be ended.

3. Indeed, even if the fetus is a person (with a right to life), it does not follow that terminating this life constitutes murder, as Judith Jarvis Thomson (2004) has famously argued using an analogy between pregnancy and providing life-sustaining connection to a famous violinist. In short, a right to life does not entitle a person to whatever is required for them to stay alive.

Calling Out Insidious Rhetoric

From our margin-centering perspective, talk of an "abortion debate" is to be called out as a deliberate rhetorical trick being played by anti-abortion advocates. The reality is that, as the World Health Organization points out, abortion is a simple, common, and (when performed by a skilled healthcare provider in sanitary conditions) safe procedure, and lack of access to safe, timely, affordable, and respectful abortion care poses a risk to the physical, mental, and social well-being of women and girls (World Health Organization, 2023). Criminalizing abortion dangerously neglects these realities and violates a human right recognized by the United Nations Human Rights Committee (UN CCPR 2019).[4] To this we can add that the criminalization of abortion creates significant antagonisms in the lives of pregnant persons, making their lives less valuable than the sum of their parts by jeopardizing their health and well-being. The reality is that abortion is a key part of healthcare for all persons who are or could become pregnant, including willingly pregnant persons who must terminate their pregnancy for their own health.

Given the current criminalization of abortion in many parts of the US, it is important for proponents of abortion to go on the offensive in advocating for safe, legal, timely, and affordable access to abortion. This requires calling out the deceptive rhetoric of the anti-abortion position. As Smith has argued, this view gains plausibility by positioning itself as "ethically pure" in allying with the "sanctity of life" (2005, p. 121). However, this is a rhetorical trick. As Methodist pastor Dave Barnhart (2018) articulated in a viral post, "the unborn" are an insidiously convenient group to advocate for. They (unlike "the incarcerated, addicted, or chronically poor") are uncomplicated moral subjects who make no political demands, and once they are born, you can neglect them, as they "cease to be unborn. . . . You can love the unborn and advocate for them without substantially challenging your own wealth, power, or privilege, without reimagining social structures, apologizing, or making reparations to anyone" (Barnhart, 2018). In other words, the anti-abortion position gains false appeal by advocating for the value of the sanctity of life in the abstract. When we scrutinize what protecting this value by itself concretely entails, however, we realize that it consists of something vacuous and harmful: allowing the unborn to be born at all costs, even if it (predictably) harms many who are already vulnerable, including economically disadvantaged women, Indigenous women, women of color, and even the very innocent lives of the unborn that this position purports to protect once they come into this world.

Our discussion thus argues that there are many good reasons not to criminalize abortion and, upon scrutiny, no good reason to do so.[5] When we lose sight of these realities and debate human rights (e.g., bodily autonomy) as negotiable (on a par with, e.g., the implications of minority religious views), we fall prey to insidious rhetoric that is used to justify the stripping away of these rights. Much more can be, should

4. This committee (re)affirmed (1) that safe, legal, and effective access to abortion is a human right protected under the right to life; (2) that preventable maternal mortality and morbidity violate the right to life; and (3) that the right to life begins at birth.
5. The only way for an anti-abortion position to have any degree of plausibility is if it is coupled with strong feminist, social justice commitments to protect and care for pregnant persons and children after they are born (e.g., Schouten, 2017). The right-wing, anti-abortion position and current circumstances in the US fail to meet this crucial condition.

be, and has been said about this topic.[6] But the discussion so far provides a critical, margin-centering lens through which to look at the ethics of abortion. We now discuss another bioethical issue related to mortality: physician-assisted suicide.

Euthanasia/Physician-Assisted Suicide

There are a couple of related phenomena here worth distinguishing:[7]

- **Euthanasia—**"good death" (from *eu*, the Greek word for "good/well," and *thanatos*, the Greek word for "death"), meaning "to bring about the death of a person/patient for their own sake"
- **Passive euthanasia—**"letting die" by withdrawing life support or by not doing something that would prolong life (e.g., removing a feeding tube, failing to perform necessary surgery)
- **Active euthanasia—**"mercy-killing" by actively taking an action to hasten the death of a patient
- **Voluntary euthanasia—**A competent patient voluntarily requests or agrees to euthanasia (communicating their wishes while competent or through instructions to be followed if they lose competence).
- **Nonvoluntary euthanasia—**performed on a patient whose consent cannot be obtained (because the patient lacks competence or has not previously disclosed their preferences)
- **Physician-assisted suicide—**bringing about one's own death with the help of a physician (through the physician prescribing, providing, or explaining the medical means for the patient to commit suicide)

These all concern the killing or letting die of a person for their own good. The question of whether to end one's life is especially pressing given that, arguably, for most people death comes either too soon or too late. A group of moral philosophers who "differ on many issues of public morality and public policy" came together to argue in an *amicus curiae* brief that respect for fundamental principles of liberty and justice justifies the establishment of a constitutionally protected right to exercise the time and manner of one's death (Dworkin et al., 1997).[8] There are thus not inconsiderable reasons in favor of the value and legality of physician-assisted suicide in at least certain cases. This bioethical issue is, however, further complicated when we take an intersectional margin-centering approach.

6. For example, as Daniel Williams (2015) has noted, between the late 1960s and the 1980s the anti-abortion movement transformed from a liberal movement linked to human rights generally to a politically conservative campaign linked to moral order and "family values." This history is further complicated by conservative use of "pro-life" rhetoric and other culture war–fueling rhetorical strategies to galvanize their base, using "dog whistle politics" (i.e., racially coded appeals) after the civil rights movement made it no longer fashionable to be explicitly racist (Haney-López, 2014).
7. This section is partially inspired by Vaughn (2022, pp. 649–650).
8. An *amicus curiae* or "friend of the court" brief is written by a nonparty to a case and is intended to inform/guide the court. This brief was submitted for the U.S. Supreme Court case of *Washington v. Glucksberg*, in which the crucial question was whether the relevant right to commit suicide includes a right to assistance in doing so.

Multiple Marginalization and Abuse

Our intersectional margin-centering approach requires us to highlight the possibility of abuse of legal euthanasia and physician-assisted suicide to end life. Given the ableism and social and economic marginalization they face, disabled persons are especially vulnerable to such abuse. Some disability advocates and physicians argue that, for example, Canada's euthanasia law, which allows people with disabilities to choose to be killed in the absence of any other medical issue, discriminates against disabled persons by allowing disability-related suffering (largely caused by ableist lack of support and marginalization) to justify the termination of a person's life (cited in Herx et al., 2020). It is therefore critical to be aware of the possibility of this kind of abuse when advocating for the goodness/rightness/legality of euthanasia/physician-assisted suicide and to implement adequate safeguards against it, especially if we are in favor of these.

Our discussion so far makes clear that this is a complex bioethical issue, one that requires nuanced engagement. This unit's readings provide some more of this nuance.

Unit Readings

The previous unit included readings on reproductive justice, so this unit's readings focus on the bioethical issue of physician-assisted suicide.

The first reading (Fleischer & Zames, 2011) details some of the history of the disability rights movement as it relates to physician-assisted suicide. In doing so, it discusses this bioethical issue from a perspective that centers persons with disabilities, raising worries about the dangers of legalizing physician-assisted suicide leading to legalizing disability discrimination and arguing that most of the time adequate support and pain management leads to people asking for suicide to change their mind.

The second reading (Davis, 1998) discusses this same bioethical issue from a feminist perspective, drawing and qualifying an analogy between the rationality of suicide and that of contraception.

Both readings provide nuance to this key biomedical issue by centering the perspective of persons marginalized because of their disability or gender.

References

Bagheri, A. (2007). Individual choice in the definition of death. *Journal of Medical Ethics*, *33*(3), 146–149.

Bakhru, T. S. (2019). Thinking transnationally: Reproductive justice in a globalized era. In T. S. Bakhru (Ed.), *Reproductive justice and sexual rights: Transnational perspectives* (pp. 3–12). Routledge.

Barnhart, D. (2018, June 25). *"The unborn" are a convenient group to advocate for. They never make demands of you; they are morally uncomplicated*. . . Facebook. https://www.facebook.com/dave.barnhart/posts/10156549406811031

Davis, D. S. (1998). Why suicide is like contraception: A woman-centered view. In M. P. Battin, R. Rhodes, & A. Silvers (Eds.), *Physician assisted suicide: Expanding the debate*. Routledge.

Dworkin, R., Nagel, T., Nozick, R., Rawls, J., Scanlon, T., & Thomson, J. J. (1997, March 27). Assisted suicide: The philosophers' brief. *The New York Review of Books*, 41–47.

Fleischer, D. Z., & Zames, F. (2011). "Not dead yet" and physician-assisted suicide. In *The disability rights movement: From charity to confrontation* (pp. 132–148). Temple University Press.

Haney-López, I. (2014). Dog whistle politics: How coded racial appeals have reinvented racism and wrecked the middle class. Oxford University Press.

Herx, L., Cottle, M., & Scott, J. (2020). The "normalization" of euthanasia in Canada: The cautionary tale continues. *World Medical Journal*, *66*(2), 28–37. https://www.wma.net/wmj_2_2020_web/

Olick, R. S. (1991). Brain death, religious freedom, and public policy: New Jersey's landmark legislative initiative. *Kennedy Institute of Ethics Journal*, *1*(4), 275–292.

Ross, L. J., Roberts, L., Derkas, E., Peoples, W., & Toure, P. B. (Eds.). (2018). *Radical reproductive justice: Foundations, theory, practice, critique*. Feminist Press.

Schouten, G. (2017). Fetuses, orphans, and a famous violinist: On the ethics and politics of abortion. *Social Theory and Practice*, *43*(3), 637–665.

Smith, A. (2005). Beyond pro-choice versus pro-life: Women of color and reproductive justice. *NWSA Journal*, *17*(1), 119–140.

Thomson, J. J. (2004). A defense of abortion. In H. J. Gensler, E. W. Spurgin, & J. C. Swindal (Eds.), *Ethics: Contemporary Readings* (pp. 267–274). Routledge.

UN CCPR. (2019, September 3). *General comment No. 36 on Article 6: Right to life* [UN Report CCPR/C/GC/36/Art.6]. https://www.ohchr.org/en/calls-for-input/general-comment-no-36-article-6-right-life

Vaughn, L. (2022). *Bioethics: Principles, issues, and cases*. Oxford University Press.

Veatch, R. M. (1993). The impending collapse of the whole-brain definition of death. *Hastings Center Report*, *23*(4), 18–24

Williams, D. K. (2015). The partisan trajectory of the American pro-life movement: How a liberal Catholic campaign became a conservative evangelical cause. *Religions*, *6*(2), 451–475.

World Health Organization. (2023). *Abortion*. https://www.who.int/health-topics/abortion

Reading 4.1

"Not Dead Yet" and Physician-Assisted Suicide

Doris Fleischer and Frieda Zames

Editor's Introduction

This reading is a chapter from *The Disability Rights Movement: From Charity to Confrontation*, a comprehensive history of this ongoing movement. In the reading, the authors employ their encyclopedic knowledge of the disability rights movement and its history to discuss the issue of physician-assisted suicide from a perspective that centers persons with disability. In their discussion, they give nuanced treatments of

- the experiences of disabled persons who oppose ableist assumptions about needing to be pitied or to have their suffering ended by physician-assisted suicide;
- key legal decisions regarding physician-assisted suicide and their consequences given the social context of ableist societies both in the

Netherlands and United States, articulating the dangers of inflexible laws and the potential for legalizing disability discrimination;

- the relevance of pain management given that most people asking for suicide almost always change their minds once their pain is under control;
- how focusing on curing disabilities inadvertently sends the pernicious message that disabled people are not whole unless cured and directs resources toward costly research with uncertain future applications instead of toward accommodating living disabled persons;
- the importance of providing people who become disabled with knowledge of the possibilities of community living arrangements and opportunities for putting their knowledge and skills to use professionally with the help of assisted technologies; and
- the key distinction between terminal illness and disability and the fact that often policy decisions reflect a confusion between these as well as ableist complacency or even arrogance in judging the value of a life.

Doris Fleischer, PhD, is senior university lecturer in humanities and social sciences at the New Jersey Institute of Technology. Her research and teaching range widely on issues related to disability rights. The late Frieda Zames was a professor emeritus of mathematics at the New Jersey Institute of Technology. She was disabled by a childhood bout of polio and her pioneering activism starting in the 1970s helped secure rights for people with disabilities and led to the Empire State Building and all Metropolitan Transportation Authority buses in New York City being made wheelchair accessible.

With increasingly sophisticated technology for life-sustaining treatment, doctors frequently are given the awesome responsibility of determining when a life should end. Anthropologist Margaret Mead observed that "society is always attempting to make the physician into a killer—for instance, to kill the defective child at birth.... It is the duty of society to protect the physician from such requests."[1] People with disabilities are particularly vulnerable to judgments that their lives are not worth living.[2]

Opposition to "the Death Train"

On January 8, 1997, while the U.S. Supreme Court was hearing *Vacco v. Quill*—a case involving the

1. Nat Hentoff quoted Margaret Mead in "We Hear the Death Train Coming," *Village Voice*, February 4, 1997, 12. See also Michael Specter, "The Dangerous Philosopher," *The New Yorker*, September 6, 1999, 46–55. For a comprehensive analysis of some of the cases and issues discussed in this [reading], see Gregory E. Pence, *Classic Cases in Medical Ethics* (New York: McGraw Hill, 2000).
2. "People with physical and mental disabilities ... still continue to be segregated, institutionalized, tortured in the name of behavior management, abused, raped, euthanized and murdered" (Norman Kune and Emma Van Der Klift, "A Credo For Support," *Moebius Syndrome News*, 1995).

constitutionality of state laws prohibiting physician-assisted suicide-people from many parts of the nation demonstrated in front of the Court. Many of the demonstrators, people with severe disabilities—blind people, deaf people, people in motorized wheelchairs—displayed signs proclaiming the sardonic name of their organization, Not Dead Yet, in "spooky-shaped" letters evoking the spirit of Halloween.

The organization was founded in Spring 1996 in reaction to public support for legalization of assisted death that had been promoted by the well-publicized suicides aided by Jack Kevorkian.[3] Mark O'Brien—journalist, poet, and member of Not Dead Yet, as well as the subject of the 1997 Academy Award-winning documentary "Breathing Lessons"—responds to the Kevorkian ethic:

> It is tempting to pity a man in an iron lung. But pity has become a lethal weapon. On January 8 [1997], the Supreme Court heard arguments in favor of killing people like me—out of pity—to end our suffering. An iron lung has been my second skin since the 1955 polio epidemic. For forty years, people have said, "That poor thing—how he must suffer! He's terminally ill, you know." I'm not "suffering," "terminal," or even "ill." Don't waste your pity on me. I want to live. Every year, the practitioners of mercy death kill thousands of people against our will—out of pity. If the Supreme Court declares mercy death legal, that's like declaring open season on people with disabilities. We are not contagious or dangerous. And we aren't affiliated with any political party. We are people who hear the death train. We will not board that train willingly.[4]

In the amicus curiae briefs submitted by Not Dead Yet and American Disabled for Attendant Programs Today (ADAPT), attorneys Diane Coleman and Stephen Gold-supporting former New York State attorney general Dennis Vacco's effort to uphold the constitutionality of the state's ban on physician-assisted suicide—contended that "the creation of a right to assisted suicide for a class of individuals based on health status or disability is a lethal form of discrimination that violates the ADA."[5] The disability community was concerned about the potentially ominous consequences of physician-assisted suicide for those people whose quality of life may be considered unacceptable by members of the medical profession.

Responding to the much publicized November 22, 1998, "60 Minutes" spectacle of Kevorkian injecting Thomas Youk—a man with amyotrophic lateral sclerosis (ALS)—with lethal chemicals,[6] Coleman, founder and president of Not Dead Yet, asserted: "Reporters ignore the fact that most of Kevorkian's victims have been disabled, not terminal, ignore the discrimination and oppression that drove each of them to despair—ignore the injustice in a society that helps people die, *but refuses to help us* [people with

3. Although he is frequently referred to as Dr. Jack Kevorkian, not only was his Michigan medical license revoked in 1991, but also "the only remedies he 'prescribes' are poisons" (Michael Betzold, "The Selling of Dr. Death," *The New Republic,* May 26, 1997, 22–23).
4. Mark O'Brien, "Maybe You'd Rather Die Than Be Me," *DIA Activist,* January 1997, 3.
5. Nadina LaSpina quoted Diane Coleman and Stephen Gold in "We Want To Live," *New York Able,* January 1997, 7.
6. The CBS program "60 Minutes" presented Jack Kevorkian's videotape of his euthanasia of Thomas Youk. Although in their response to this "60 Minutes" broadcast producers of the November 23, 1998, ABC program "Nightline" decided against disability representation, on February 28, 1999, "60 Minutes" presented people living meaningful lives with ALS.

disabilities] *live with the basic respect and the simple supports we deserve*."[7] Kevorkian, who claims he has helped more than 130 people commit suicide, was found guilty of second-degree murder in the Youk case, after prosecutors had unsuccessfully attempted to convict him in five former cases.[8]

Michael Betzold explains in his 1997 exposé of journalist Jack Lessenberry, "The Selling of Dr. Death," how Kevorkian became a national hero.[9] A personal friend of Kevorkian and his attorney Geoffrey Fieger, Lessenberry reported on Kevorkian for the *New York Times* from 1993 until publication of the Betzold exposé, thus playing a major role in shaping that newspaper's approach to assisted suicide.[10] Betzold reveals that "in his writings and statements, Kevorkian advocates a society that allows euthanasia for the dying, the disabled, the mentally ill, infants with birth defects, and comatose adults; and he sanctions experiments prior to their death and organ harvesting. He envisions a global system of death on demand run by doctors who operate without oversight from government or ethicists."[11]

Critic of physician-assisted suicide Nat Hentoff of New York City's *Village Voice* notes:

> It's a bitter irony [that a] quintessentially liberal judge [Ninth Circuit Court Judge Stephen Reinhardt] has opened the door wide not only to assisted suicide but also to euthanasia, because the majority of the resultant dead will be the poor, the disabled, and other vulnerable people. Many of them will persuade themselves to die because they feel nobody thinks their lives are worth preserving. Or that keeping themselves alive will cost too much, thereby burdening their families and companions.[12]

The Supreme Court

Reversing the 1996 rulings in the Second Circuit Court of Appeals in *Vacco v. Quill* and in the Ninth Circuit Court of Appeals in *Washington v. Glucksberg* the U.S. Supreme Court on June 26, 1997, unanimously upheld state criminal laws against physician-assisted suicide.[13] Prior to *Quill,* competent adults in New York State had the right to refuse medical treatment, and physicians were allowed to honor the requests of such patients to withhold or terminate life support. At the same time, intentionally assisting another person to commit or attempt suicide was a felony according to New York State law.

The Second Circuit Court of Appeals recognized that the right to refuse life-sustaining treatment

7. Diane Coleman, letter to Not Dead Yet Members and Supporters, January 25, 1999.
8. Pam Belluck, "Dr. Kevorkian Is a Murderer, the Jury Finds," *New York Times,* March 27, 1999, A1, A9. Jack Kevorkian was found guilty of murder in Pontiac, Michigan, on March 26, 1999.
9. Michael Betzold, *Appointment with Dr. Death* (Troy, Mich.: Momentum Books, 1993). References to Jack Lessenberry from Michael Betzold, "The Selling of Dr. Death," *New Republic,* May 26, 1997, 22–28.
10. "Lessenberry has also published pieces flattering toward Kevorkian and Fieger in *Esquire, George, Vanity Fair* and other publications" (Betzold, "The Selling of Dr. Death," 25).
11. Betzold, "The Selling of Dr. Death," 22.
12. Nat Hentoff, "Class Warfare to the Death," *Village Voice,* May 21, 1996, 12.
13. John Gresham of New York Lawyers for the Public Interest provided information about *Vacco v. Quill,* 117 S.Ct. 2293 (1997). See *Washington v. Glucksberg* 117 S.Ct. 2258 (1997).

gives those patients who become dependent on life support the opportunity to have some control over the timing of their death. Finding no rational basis for the state allowing patients to end life by requesting cessation of life support while, simultaneously, denying patients similar control when life support is not involved, the court ruled in favor of Dr. Quill. This difference, the court held, violates the Equal Protection Clause of the U.S. Constitution. Attorney General Vacco, appealing the court's decision, argued before the U.S. Supreme Court in 1997 to uphold New York State's ban on physician-assisted suicide.

While the appeals court decisions in both *Quill* and *Glucksberg* supported physician-assisted suicide, Judge Reinhardt's definition of "terminal" in the latter case as any "medical condition that is incurable and irreversible" seemed threatening to many people with disabilities and chronic illnesses.[14] As early as 1958, law professor Yale Kamisar warned of courts and physicians, even clerics, allowing family members to remove feeding tubes and respirators from people who were supposedly terminal.[15] Anticipating a movement towards active euthanasia for the socially vulnerable, Kamisar cautioned that some of those patients' lives could have been extended considerably. In his essay "Against Assisted Suicide—Even in a Very Limited Form," Kamisar quoted his former colleague, Robert Burt: "It would be ironic if [at a time when millions of Americans lack adequate health care] the judiciary selected physician-assisted suicide as the one health care right that deserves constitutional status."[16]

Strongly influenced by Kamisar's analysis, Ninth Circuit Judge Robert Beezer, in his dissenting opinion in *Glucksberg*, quoted from a 1994 report by the New York State Task Force on Life and the Law: "It must be recognized that assisted suicide and euthanasia will be practiced through the prism of social inequality and prejudice that characterizes the delivery of services in all segments of society, including health care." He noted that even if they are not dying, "persons requiring dialysis, respirators, insulin or long-term nursing care would all be candidates for euthanasia."[17]

Yet allegiances on this issue are unpredictable, as illustrated by the court challenges by the National Right-to-Life Committee to the Oregon aid-in-dying measure, an initiative approved by the voters in 1994, preventing physician-assisted suicide from taking effect until a later Oregon vote in 1997. On the other hand, three New York law firms—Arnold & Porter; Cravath, Swaine & Moore; Debevoise & Plimpton—each with a history of pro bono legal contributions to disability causes and organizations, *supported* physician-assisted suicide.[18] Also, liberal Harvard law professor Laurence H. Tribe argued before the U.S. Supreme Court in 1997 for physician-assisted suicide.

In his majority opinion in *Vacco v. Quill* validating the state prohibition on physician-assisted suicide, Chief Justice William H. Rehnquist noted that this issue is properly within the jurisdiction of the states:

14. LaSpina, "We Want To Live," 7.
15. Nat Hentoff, "Death's Enemy: Yale Kamisar," *Village Voice,* May 28, 1996, 10. Hentoff paraphrased from Kamisar's *Minnesota Law Review* article, "Some Non-Religious Views Against Proposed 'Mercy Killing' Legislation."
16. Hentoff, "Death's Enemy." Hentoff quoted from Kamisar's essay that appeared in the *University of Detroit Mercy Law Review.*
17. Hentoff, "Death's Enemy." Hentoff quoted Robert Beezer.
18. Information from annotated list of participating law firms distributed at June 19, 1997, luncheon of New York Lawyers for the Public Interest.

> The state has an interest in protecting vulnerable groups including the poor, the elderly, and disabled persons from abuse, neglect and mistakes. The court of appeals dismissed the state's concern that disadvantaged persons might be pressured into physician-assisted suicide as "ludicrous on its face." We have recognized, however, the real risk of subtle coercion and undue influence in end-of-life situations.[19]

AIDS Activists

Most AIDS activists take a position sanctioning physician-assisted suicide, contrary to the majority of other disability rights activists. Three terminally-ill patients, one with cancer and two with AIDS, as well as Dr. Timothy Quill and two other doctors, initiated the case in support of physician-assisted suicide. An amicus curiae brief supporting the patients and doctors included not only the well-known gay rights organization, Lambda Legal Defense and Education Fund, and some religious groups, but also the National Association of People with AIDS.

Larry Kramer, a vocal activist in the AIDS movement, indicates that "since the start of the epidemic, there have always been doctors one could talk to.... All of us who have been on the front line have experiences—plural—with people who didn't want to suffer anymore."[20] Although he knew many desperately ill people who had procured lethal medication, he was profoundly affected by the death of Brad Davis, the star of Kramer's AIDS play, *The Normal Heart:* "The medicine was very painful, and it wasn't working, and he just saw no sunshine ahead or anything. He was just going to get sicker and sicker, and he didn't want to put his family through that. And he did not want to suffer the pain himself." Stirred by this incident, Kramer allied with a Seattle group, Compassion In Dying, that was pursuing "a constitutional right to 'self-deliverance.'" Revealing that he felt like "the casting director," Kramer recruited two other physicians—his own psychiatrist, Dr. Samuel Klagsbrun, and an old friend, Dr. Howard Grossman—to affiliate with Quill in the lawsuit.

On October 30, 1996, for the first time a small group of medical practitioners, four physicians and a psychologist, publicly endorsed the campaign of Jack Kevorkian, initiated in 1990, for physician-assisted suicide.[21] In 1991, Quill, a mainstream physician, wrote his unprecedented public confession regarding his prescribing a fatal overdose of sleeping pills for a patient with end-stage leukemia, a woman who was seeking his assistance in dying.[22] Quill defended his action with a question: "Are we going to, as a culture, override a person's deathbed request, a person who is dying who says, 'I need some help here?'"

Supporting Quill's position, Dr. Lonnie Shavelson argued for the establishment of protocols for

19. "Excerpts from Court's Decision Upholding Bans on Assisted Suicide," *New York Times,* June 27, 1997, A18.
20. David France, quoting Larry Kramer, in "A Life-and-Death Decision," *New York Times,* January 13, 1997, 26–27. Discussion of *The Normal Heart* as a spur to Larry Kramer's support of Jack Kevorkian's assisted suicides from this source.
21. "Small Group of Doctors Supports Concept of Assisting in Suicide," *New York Times,* October 31, 1996, A20.
22. "60 Minutes," CBS Television, January 5, 1997. References to publications by Timothy Quill and Lonnie Shavelson in the *New England Journal of Medicine* from this source. See Timothy Quill, "Death and Dignity: A Case of Individualized Decision Making," *NEJM,* 324(10) (March 7, 1991): 691–94.

physician-assisted suicide: "It [physician-assisted suicide] is happening anyway, whether it's legal or not.... I see a tremendous amount of hidden, underground practice [of such suicides] in which nobody knows if there are abuses. I see potential disasters." Confirming Shavelson's assertion, a survey published in 1997 of 118 members of the Bay Area Community Consortium, an association of local AIDS doctors, revealed that 53 percent of the respondents reported helping at least one of their patients to commit suicide.[23]

Pain Management

Other medical practitioners argue that the technology to manage pain is available. Pediatric AIDS nurse Sheila Diamond states that "there is really no such thing as intractable pain, but only pain which is underrecognized, under-treated."[24] Reinforcing Diamond's assertion, hospice doctor Ira Byock explains:

> Not only do we know that people's pain of their terminal illness often goes inadequately treated, it's often not even addressed. Beyond that, as if that weren't bad enough, our current non-system of health care routinely pauperizes people simply for being chronically ill and not dying quickly enough.... When you look at the curriculum of medical training, there is very, very little attention to caring for people at the end of life. Even pain control occupies no more than a handful of hours in a four-year course of study.

Dr. Kathleen Foley, palliative care specialist at New York's Memorial Sloan-Kettering Cancer Center and a pioneer since the mid-1970s in the field of palliative care and pain management, points out that "even oncology residents and fellows are poorly trained. It's a well-documented fact that those asking for assisted suicide almost always change their mind once we have their pain under control."[25]

Both proponents and opponents of physician-assisted suicide agree that pain management is a preferable option to state-sanctioned suicide. Dr. Daniel Carr (internist and anesthesiologist at the New England Medical Center in Boston, who has helped craft two sets of pain management guidelines issued by the federal government) and Dr. Nelson Hendler (clinical director of the Mensana Clinic near Baltimore, who has written extensively on pain management) support the medical profession's movement of the 1990s from a disease-centered to a patient-centered approach.[26] For example, formerly doctors were so concerned with the cancer patient's tumor or the AIDS patient's white blood cell count that they often neglected attending to the patient's experience of the illness. Carr refers to the federal guidelines for pain control, a graded step-wise progress from less to more invasive as the medical situation requires.

23. "A Poll of AIDS Doctors Finds That Many Help in Suicides," *New York Times,* February 6, 1997, A18. *New York Times* reference to this survey of San Francisco Bay Area physicians from February 5, 1997, article published in the *New England Journal of Medicine.*
24. References to Sheila Diamond and Dr. Ira Byock from "Nightline," ABC-TV, January 9, 1997.
25. References to Kathleen Foley from Paul Wilkes, "The Next Pro-Lifers," *New York Times Magazine,* Sunday, July 21, 1996, 45.
26. Daniel Carr and Nelson Hendler stated their views on pain management on the WNYC-AM program "On the Line," March 24, 1997. References to Carr and Hendler from this source.

Hendler criticizes the multiple disincentives to pain management: insurance companies that refuse to pay for pain medication prescribed by physicians, medical societies and medical schools that remain insufficiently involved in pain management, and the Drug Enforcement Agency that aggressively pursues doctors dispensing pharmaceuticals for pain control.

Both Carr and Hendler agree that pain is frequently undiagnosed or misdiagnosed and, as a result, undertreated or even mistreated. Carr points out that for too long doctors accepted myths such as that third-degree burns do not hurt, or that children—because of their undeveloped nervous systems—do not feel pain, or that cancer pain can never be alleviated. In fact, Carr indicates that although 90 percent of instances of cancer pain can be managed successfully, at least 30 to 40 percent of these cases are undertreated. Furthermore, 30 to 40 percent of cancer patients experience clinical depression, which Carr insists can be treated and reversed. Carr and Hendler maintain that with the treatment of depression—a major cause of suicide among patients with acute physical illnesses—in combination with proper palliative care, physician-assisted suicide could well be rendered unnecessary.

Carr is concerned that managed care "threatens to take away all the hard-fought-for advances [achieved] over the last couple of decades" in pain control. While the physiology of pain requires aggressive and early treatment, managed care organizations tend, in Carr's words, to "delay, defer, and deny." Thus, he adds, appropriate pain management and managed care are "at loggerheads with what we [pain management experts] know should be done." Although in 1996 Congress required health plans to cover at least forty-eight hours of hospital care for mothers and newborns, and in 1997 President Clinton recommended similar safeguards for mastectomy patients,[27] many critics of the current health care system are skeptical about the outlook for pain management procedures. Because "a drive-by mastectomy"—breast surgery for which managed care organizations formerly covered only one day in the hospital—is a dramatic denial of an essential service, such practices received much public condemnation. Since pain management is such a complex issue, however, the mishandling of this vital service by these organizations may continue to be neglected for a long time.[28]

Focus on Cure: A Pernicious Message

Campaigning for research into a cure for spinal cord injuries, *Superman* star Christopher Reeve, who uses a ventilator and a motorized wheelchair, provokes disability advocates who believe that he is inadvertently sending a pernicious message: disabled people are not whole unless cured. Reeve notes that "until five years ago, it was believed that spinal cord could not regenerate. Now it's proved that it can. Research deserves our support, though there's a long way to go."[29] Many in the disability community, however, argue

27. Robert Pear, "Clinton Names Panel to Draft Health Consumer Bill of Rights," *New York Times,* March 27, 1997, B11.

28. Brian Lehrer, well-informed radio host of "On the Line" (WNYC-AM), offered this observation during his interview with Carr and Hendler.

29. "Reeve Feels Others Show As Much Courage," *Brainerd Daily Dispatch,* October 28, 1996, 6A.

that this costly research, whose practical application may not be apparent for many years, "could drain resources from the more realistic [and in some cases even desperate] needs of the present."[30]

Speaking in neither of her official roles—as chair of the National Council on Disability nor as president and CEO of Access Living, the Chicago independent living center—Marca Bristo does not object to Reeve's desire to encourage research or even to seek a cure for spinal cord injuries.[31] The increased survival rate of spinal cord injured people has resulted from research, she observes. Yet, uncomfortable with Reeve soliciting from the private rather than the public sector, she considers "the hype" that he uses to generate donations detrimental to the disability rights movement. Frustrated by the mass media's general inability to perceive disability in a civil rights context, many disability advocates view Reeve's March 1, 1998, two-hour television special, *Christopher Reeve: A Celebration of Hope,* as a sophisticated version of a Jerry Lewis telethon, employing pity to elicit contributions.[32]

Other disability advocates point out that although Reeve is articulate, well-informed, and socially conscious, he is new to disability culture and issues. They commend his efforts to improve funding and legislation for people with disabilities, as well as to encourage equipment suppliers to decrease costs.[33] More to the point has been Reeve's ability to resume working in his field. He directed a well-received HBO special, *In the Gloaming,* in late 1996, and in 1998 he directed and starred in a remake of Alfred Hitchcock's 1954 classic film *Rear Window,* with the protagonist in the new version using the modern technology available in the late 1990s. Yet the fact that Reeve has been able to continue his involvement in so many activities—his autobiography, *Still Me,* was published in 1998[34]—does not preclude the possibility that he may still be in the "mourning phase" for his paralysis resulting from his 1995 horseback-riding accident. Regardless of Reeve's focus on cure in his discourse, in his life he demonstrates his determination as a person with a disability to participate in the world utilizing his unique intelligence, talents, and visibility.

In his book *Moving Violations,* journalist John Hockenberry, who also has a spinal cord injury, writes: "There is much more effort put into curing spinal cord injuries or discussing the legal issues involved in suicide for the severely disabled than there is integrating disabled folks into society at large. Pray to be normal no matter how impossible it seems is the sentimental message. The alternative is too horrible to contemplate."[35] Disability activist and quadriplegic motorized wheelchair user Daniel Robert describes the quandary in which people with disabilities find themselves: "And there we are, between a rock and a hard place, between waiting for a 'Cure' (read Miracle) and waiting to be 'offed.' The sum total of all the media

30. David Peterson, "Reeve's Honesty Charms His Audience," *Minneapolis Star Tribune,* October 28, 1996, A12. When a television commercial using computer animation showed Reeve walking, "many advocates for the handicapped were aghast, maintaining that no such cure is in the offing, and that the spot cruelly offered false hope to people who should be concentrating on adapting to life with their disabilities" (Bernard Stamler, "Christopher Reeve Is Sanguine about His Madison Avenue Connections, but Some Are Skeptical," *New York Times,* June 15, 2000, C10).
31. Information about and comments of Marca Bristo from authors' April 30, 1998, interview with Bristo.
32. "Superman's Telethon," *Ragged Edge,* May/June 1998, 27.
33. "Reeve Feels Others Show As Much Courage," 6A.
34. Christopher Reeve, *Still Me* (New York: Random House, 1998).
35. John Hockenberry, *Moving Violations: War Zones, Wheelchairs, and Declarations of Independence* (New York: Hyperion, 1995), 204.

attention given to Christopher Reeve and Jack Kevorkian ... boils down to this simple formula. If they can't fix us *we're better off dead*. It's our civic duty."[36]

The Eugenics Movement and Euthanasia

Medical historian Martin S. Pernick documents the sensational story of Dr. Harry Haiselden, a prominent Chicago surgeon, who in 1916 was as well known to Americans as Jack Kevorkian is in the 1990s.[37] As Pernick explains, when Haiselden decided in November 1915 to allow a newborn baby with an impairment to die, he told a reporter for Hearst's *Chicago-American* that although he had permitted other newborns to die quietly, he wanted to make this case a public issue:

> Haiselden and his supporters were torn between passionate expressions of sympathy and love, versus, in the next breath, expressing contempt, hatred, fear and loathing for those born with disabilities.... The disabled were a menace, an evil stalking beast, that was going to devour society. Haiselden was investigated three times by different legal authorities, for allowing impaired newborns to die, and each time he was upheld, but he was expelled from the Chicago Medical Society for writing newspaper articles and making a movie, *[The Black Stork]*.[38]

Working with "muckraking" Hearst journalist Jack Lait, Haiselden was both writer and star of *The Black Stork*, a film whose storyline resembled a widely publicized incident involving a newborn girl with spina bifida:

> The main plot of this remarkable film begins with Claude, who has an unnamed inherited disease. Despite repeated graphic warnings from Dr. Dickey (played by Haiselden himself), Claude marries his sweetheart, Anne. Their baby is born so severely disabled that it needs immediate surgery to save its life, but Dr. Dickey refuses to perform the operation. Anne is torn by uncertainty until God reveals a lengthy vision of the child's future, filled with pain, madness, and crime. Her doubts resolved, she accepts Dr. Dickey's judgment, and the baby's soul leaps into the arms of a waiting Jesus.[39]

Pernick reveals why Haiselden was not only supported by so many prominent early twentieth-century Americans, but also won editorial endorsements from some of the country's most prestigious publications,

36. Daniel Robert, "A Rock and A Hard Place—Superman, Dr. Death and You and Me," *New York Able*, February 1997, 11.
37. Martin S. Pernick, *The Black Stork: Eugenics and the Death of "Defective" Babies in American Medicine and Motion Pictures* (New York: Oxford University Press, 1996).
38. Stated by Martin S. Pernick in "Tomorrow's Children: Beyond Affliction: The Disability History Project," National Public Radio, May 1998.
39. Pernick, *The Black Stork*, 5–6.

including the *New York Times* and the *New Republic*:[40] "The common progressive belief that science provided objective means for distinguishing good lives from bad ones hid the subjectivity of the values people actually used to make such judgments. And because they believed their values to be objectively proven, they could dismiss ethical or political criticisms as biased, unscientific, and therefore irrelevant."[41]

One of the most egregious examples of the perversion of medicine was the mass killing of people viewed as mentally or physically inadequate by the Nazi doctors. Robert J. Lifton links this so-called "biomedical vision" practiced by leading physicians in Nazi Germany with the eugenics movement that continued to be deemed respectable in the United States and England in the 1920s and even beyond.[42] In 1923, Fritz Lenz, a German physician-geneticist, complained that "Germany had nothing to match the eugenics research institutions in England and the United States."[43]

Lenz rebuked the German people because of "their backwardness in the domain of sterilization as compared to the United States [for] Germany had no equivalent to the American laws prohibiting marriage ... for people suffering from such conditions as epilepsy or mental retardation." Virginia Kallianes and Phyllis Rubenfeld discuss the impact, especially on women with disabilities, of the reoccurrence of the eugenics movement in the late twentieth century:

> Given the repression of sexuality and social proscription of mothering among disabled women, it is not surprising that they look suspiciously upon selective abortion or genetic technologies that are used to prevent reproduction by disabled women or the birth of disabled babies. Some of this concern arises from the legacy of sterilization abuse among disabled women, particularly in the early 20th century United States eugenics movement.... Many see in advancing reproductive technologies, such as genetic screening combined with abortion, the return of eugenics practices and claim society is reverting to attitudes such as those embodied in the 1927 United States Supreme Court case upholding compulsory sterilization in the state of Virginia which came from Oliver Wendell Holmes's often quoted statement: "Society can prevent those who are manifestly unfit from continuing their kind."[44]

J. P. Landman, in his 1932 study of the sterilization movement in the United States, refers to "overzealous and overardent eugenicists" who "regard ... the feebleminded, the epileptics, the mentally diseased, the blind, the deformed, and the criminals as inimical to the human race ... [because] these

40. Ibid., 7. Although the *New York Times* supported Haiselden on eugenics, the newspaper eventually took issue with his publicity-seeking.
41. Pernick, *The Black Stork,* 16.
42. Robert J. Lifton, *The Nazi Doctors: Medical Killing and the Psychology of Genocide* (New York: Basic Books, 1986), 23.
43. Ibid., 23. Unless otherwise indicated, references to Fritz Lenz from this source. Lenz was referring to the research, such as that at Cold Spring Harbor, New York, guided by Charles B. Davenport and financed by the Carnegie Institution in Washington and by Mary Harriman.
44. Virginia Kallianes and Phyllis Rubenfeld, "Disabled Women and Reproductive Rights," *Disability and Society,* 1997, 12(2): 212.

people perpetuate their deficiencies and thus threaten the quality of the ensuing generations."[45] Because they contended "a nation must defend itself against national degeneration as much as against the external foreign enemy," these eugenicists believed, according to Lenz, that the nation should endeavor "to exterminate these undesirables."

In their 1996 testimony delivered before Congress, Diane Coleman and Carol Gill succinctly articulated the strong objections to physician-assisted suicide by many members of the disability community.[46] Having experienced discrimination and persecution, people with disabilities and incurable chronic diseases fear a reemergence of the 1930s euthanasia movements in England and the United States. These movements inspired execution by Nazi doctors of two hundred thousand people judged deficient because of their physical and mental impairments.[47] Although Hitler rescinded this euthanasia policy on August 24, 1941, the only official order reversed in his twelve years of power,[48] the killing of people with disabilities continued by means that were not always obvious, such as withholding of treatment, medication, or food.[49] Yet the Nuremberg court did not require that reparations be paid to the families of those with disabilities who were killed, nor that their murderers be punished.

In this context, Coleman and Gill's reference to Kevorkian's admission that his suicide device was designed as an answer for quadriplegics is a chilling harbinger to many people with disabilities of "the right to die" becoming "the duty to die."[50] Echoes of Nazi rhetoric are evident in Kevorkian's defense of "medicide": "The voluntary self-elimination of individual and mortally diseased or crippled lives taken collectively can only enhance the preservation of public health and welfare."[51] Women's roles as nurtures and caretakers make them especially vulnerable when they become dependent:

> If anyone doubts that women will be exploited and endangered by assisted suicide, the doubters should study Kevorkian's "clients." The first eight were all middle-aged or elderly women with chronic illnesses and disabilities. Many said they feared being a

45. Quoted in footnote in Lifton, *The Nazi Doctors,* 23. Reference to "national degeneration" from this source.
46. Diane Coleman, J.D., and Carol Gill, Ph.D., testified before the Constitution Subcommittee of the U.S. House Judiciary Committee on April 29, 1996. References to Coleman and Gill from this source.
47. The 1996 Israeli documentary *Healing by Killing,* produced and directed by Nitzan Aviram, pointed out that without "the technical know-how from euthanasia" and "euthanasia teams" already in place, the Holocaust may not have been possible.
48. In *By Trust Betrayed* (Arlington, Va.: Vandamere Press, 1995, 202–3), Hugh Gregory Gallagher credited this reversal to many people who risked their lives: disabled people themselves, as well as others, including some clergy, some doctors and nurses, and even some Nazi party members. While the execution of Jews, gypsies, homosexuals, and others was not condemned by most German people, many were troubled by the killing of what they considered to be "German" people with disabilities.
49. Marta Russell, *Beyond Ramps: Disability at the End of the Social Contract* (Monroe, Maine: Common Courage Press, 1998), 27–28. References to the Nuremberg Court from this source.
50. In *Freedom To Die* (New York: St. Martin's Press, 1998), authors Derek Humphry and Mary Clement imply that there indeed is a duty to die: "Is there, in fact, a duty to die—a responsibility within the family unit—that should remain voluntary but expected nevertheless?" (p. 313).
51. Michael Betzold in a letter published in the June 30, 1997, *New Republic*—commenting on his May 26, 1997, *New Republic* article, "The Selling of Dr. Death"—described Kevorkian as "a man who advocates medical experiments as part of euthanasia for people who are disabled and depressed."

burden on others. An autopsy on one of them revealed no evidence of any physical illness. Women with disabilities are going to be the first to feel a "duty to die."[52]

Despite the current prosperity, opponents of disability rights always claim that resources are scarce; therefore, people with disabilities are apprehensive about being perceived as costly, unproductive expendables.[53] Campaigners for a right-to-die movement in the 1990s Derek Humphry and Mary Clement state that "in the final analysis, economics, not the quest for broadened individual liberties or increased autonomy, will drive assisted suicide to the plateau of accepted practice."[54] More radically, John Hard wig asserts, "In fact, there may be a fairly common responsibility to end one's life in the absence of any terminal illness at all. Finally, there can be a *duty to die* when one would prefer to live."[55] In reaction to this mindset, Coleman and Gill warn that assisted-suicide proponents have been feeding public misconceptions regarding the social expense of disability in their characterization of services, devices, and technology for people with disabilities as resulting in an inherently undignified lifestyle.

The Politics of Physician-Assisted Suicide

As former director of the New York City Mayor's Office for People with Disabilities, Anne Emerman and law professor Yale Kamisar predicted, the decision regarding the "Pandora's box" of physician-assisted suicide is being determined in state legislatures rather than in the Supreme Court.[56] Ezekiel and Linda Emanuel chronicle the national experience with efforts to legalize assisted suicide: "Since 1995, nearly fifty bills have been introduced in more than twenty states concerning assisted suicide, but none of the bills [until the Oregon 1994 referendum] calling for legalization have passed.... Today [July 24, 1997] thirty-five states have laws that explicitly criminalize euthanasia and doctor-assisted suicide."[57]

Although Oregon voters had approved legalizing physician-assisted suicide in 1994 by a 51 percent to a 49 percent margin, the referendum was held up by legal challenges for three years.[58] The Emanuels

52. Coleman and Gill, testimony before the Constitution Subcommittee of the House Judiciary Committee on April 29, 1996. In her July 14, 1998, testimony before the Constitution Subcommittee of the House Judiciary Committee, Coleman indicated that although Kevorkian's acts violate Michigan law according to the state Supreme Court, he is "still killing people with non-terminal disabilities, and now even harvesting their organs."
53. John Hess, formerly of the *New York Times,* argued on WNYC-AM on "New York and Company," June 6, 1996, that in the United States, the economy is currently booming, and therefore scarcity is a manufactured product of a conservative social agenda.
54. Humphry and Clement, *Freedom to Die,* 313.
55. John Hardwig, "Is There a Duty to Die?" *Hastings Center Report,* March–April 1997, 27(2): 80. Emphasis added.
56. Unless otherwise indicated, references to Anne Emerman's views on physician-assisted suicide from her January 10, 1997, conversation with authors. Wilkes, "The Next Pro-Lifers," 42. Wilkes quoted Yale Kamisar.
57. Ezekiel J. Emanuel, associate professor of ethics and medicine at Harvard Medical School, and Linda L. Emanuel, vice president for ethical standards at the American Medical Association, "Assisted Suicide? Not In My State," *New York Times.,* July 24, 1997, A21. This article appeared before the referendum victory for physician-assisted suicide in Oregon on November 4, 1997. See Timothy Egan, "Right To Die: In Oregon, Opening a New Front in the World of Medicine," *New York Times,* November 6, 1997, A26.
58. Neil A. Lewis, "Reno Lifts Barrier to Oregon's Law on Aided Suicide," *New York Times,* June 6, 1998, A1.

note the "historical precedent for blocking efforts to sanction euthanasia": Despite much public debate in the United States from 1890 to 1906 regarding legalization of physician-assisted suicide, in 1907 the Ohio legislature failed to support the measure and, as a result, "euthanasia all but disappeared from the public agenda until the last few years."[59]

While the Emanuels believe that "legislators understand that deep down the public is ambivalent about euthanasia," Emerman is profoundly concerned about this controversy. Given the common public misunderstandings about disability and assisted suicide, as well as the complexity of this contentious issue, those in the disability community who are fervently opposed have their work cut out for them, she maintains. They must embark on "a crusade to educate the public." She was referring to the Gallup survey revealing that 75 percent of Americans believe doctors should be legally permitted to "end a patient's life by painless means," as well as the poll of the American Society of Internal Medicine indicating that 40 percent of all doctors had provided assistance to their patients who sought a means to end their lives.[60]

A 60 to 40 percent vote by Oregon citizens on November 4, 1997, on a new referendum not to repeal the 1994 referendum permitting physician-assisted suicide,[61] as well as Attorney General Janet Reno's June 5, 1998, ruling removing "the last legal obstacle to the full operation of Oregon's landmark assisted-suicide law," added to Emerman's apprehension.[62] "It is ironic," Emerman says, "that at a time when technology permits people who are very disabled to be independent and productive members of society, they have to contend with this movement for assisted suicide."[63] Confirming Emerman's fears, Reno's decision signified that other states may pass comparable legislation sanctioning physician-assisted suicide without federal restriction. Though the front-page *New York Times* article describing Reno's Oregon judgment noted the strong opposition of the Roman Catholic Church to authorized assisted suicide, no reference was made to the intense and vocal objection of most of the disability community.[64]

59. Emanuel and Emanuel, "Assisted Suicide?", A21. References to the Emanuels from this source.
60. France, "A Life-and-Death Decision," 26. Sheryl Gay Stolberg, in "Assisted Suicides Are Rare, Survey of Doctors Finds," *New York Times*, April 23, 1998, A1. Stolberg, offering statistics that conflicted with those presented in France's article, indicated that although only 5 percent of physicians admitted that they have given lethal injections, more say they would do so if such action were legally sanctioned.
61. Timothy Egan, "Right to Die," A26.
62. Lewis, "Reno Lifts Barrier," A1. References to Reno's ruling on Oregon's assisted suicide law from this source. Although according to the Associated Press, November 11, 1997, "Administrator Thomas Constantine [of the Drug Enforcement Administration] warned that doctors who take part in assisted suicides would be violating federal narcotics law and risk losing their licenses to prescribe drugs," Reno reversed that position on June 5, 1998.
63. Interview with Anne Emerman, November 8, 1997.
64. Because on October 27, 1999, the U.S. House of Representatives passed a bill that would make prescribing lethal drugs for terminally-ill patients a federal crime, elected Oregon officials considered a legal challenge that could bring the issue to the U.S. Supreme Court. See Robert Pear, "House Backs Ban on Using Medicine To Aid in Suicide," *New York Times*, A1, A29; and Sam Howe Verhovek, "Oregon Considers Challenge," *New York Times*, October 28, 1999, A29.

Netherlands "Slippery Slope" vs. U.S. "Political Strategy"

Characterizing the policy of the Netherlands as a "slippery slope," psychiatrist and psychoanalyst Herbert Hendin issued a warning to the United States: "The Netherlands has moved from assisted suicide to euthanasia, from euthanasia for people who are terminally ill to euthanasia for people who are chronically ill, from euthanasia for physical illness to euthanasia for psychological distress, and from voluntary euthanasia to involuntary euthanasia (called 'termination of the patient without explicit request')."[65] In their 1996 congressional testimony, Coleman and Gill offered several illustrations of the relaxation of laws and policies protecting the lives of people with disabilities in the United States: Oregon's endeavor to ration health care based on "quality of life" judgments made by nondisabled people reveals the vulnerability of people with costly conditions; lifesaving organ transplants regularly are denied to people with rather mild disabilities; assisted breathing frequently is not presented as an option to people with disabilities who need ventilators; and many using ventilators indicate that they are increasingly requested to contemplate "do-not-resuscitate (DNR)" orders and withdrawal of life support.

Coleman pointed out that bioethicists have asked if American society is willing to allocate scarce resources to people with disabilities: "Whether it's a 'voluntary' DNR order, a surrogate decision by a family member, an involuntary 'futility guideline,' or health insurance denials, we [people with disabilities] are being eliminated through the withholding of medical treatment."[66] Futility guidelines, developed by the AMA and many individual hospitals, allow doctors to withhold medical treatment against the expressed wishes of a patient or the patient's family.[67] Referring to a statement in the December 1997 fund-raising letter of the pro-euthanasia organization Compassion In Dying, Coleman revealed that "proeuthanasia advocates are now raising funds for expansion of their advocacy efforts to openly include people with nonterminal conditions."

Unlike in the Netherlands where the assisted suicide movement was accurately described as a slippery slope, the United States right-to-die campaign is a "political strategy," asserted Coleman,[68] "as people with disabilities are regularly bombarded with messages that [they] cost too much to be allowed to live."[69] She referred to the vision embodied in a statement by the founder of the right-to-die organization, the Hemlock Society, Derek Humphry: "Like it or not, the connection between the right-to-die and the cost, value, and allocation of health care resources are part of the political debate, albeit frequently unspoken."[70] Citing well-documented physician biases about quality of life for people with impairments

65. Summary of the warning posed by Herbert Hendin—author of *Seduced by Death: Doctors, Patients and the Dutch Cure* (New York: W. W. Norton, 1996)—from Charles E. Rosenberg's "Slippery Slope," *New York Times,* Sunday, November 24, 1996, sec. 7, p. 33. In "Kevorkian on Trial," *Psychiatric Times,* February 1999, 16(2), Hendin related the "slippery slope" danger to Kevorkian's euthanasia of Thomas Youk.
66. Coleman, letter to Not Dead Yet Members and Supporters, January 25, 1999. References to Compassion In Dying from this source.
67. Diane Coleman, testimony before the Constitution Subcommittee of the House Judiciary Committee, July 14, 1998.
68. Interview with Diane Coleman, March 11, 1999.
69. Coleman's 1998 Congressional testimony.
70. Humphry and Clement, *Freedom to Die,* 313.

and chronic illnesses, Coleman fears further justifications for refusing to provide appropriate health care for the disability population: "People with disabilities have no confidence that either the civil or criminal justice system will value [their] lives enough to protect [them] equally in a society which is more and more open in its certainty that everyone would be better off without [them]."[71]

First-Year Report on Physician-Assisted Suicide in Oregon

In 1999, the *New York Times* compared two reports on assisted suicide, one in the *Journal of Medical Ethics* on the fifteen-year practice in the Netherlands, the other by the State Health Division on the one-year experience in Oregon.[72] The *New York Times* reported that the *Journal of Medical Ethics* found a "fatal confusion" in the Netherlands because assisted suicide is technically illegal but widely practiced: "In one in five cases surveyed there, euthanasia was performed on patients who had not requested it, and on patients for whom other untried treatments for their illnesses were still available." In contrast, the *New York Times* indicated that the Oregon report found no confusion or abuses resulting from the law: "Only 15 people, 8 men and 7 women, were helped to die in 1998. Thirteen were cancer patients, and many, their doctors said, were decisive personalities, or people acting on long-held principles."

Dr. Kathleen Foley and other specialists in terminal care are skeptical about Oregon's positive judgment regarding the effect of the legislation.[73] Not only was the state's report based on twenty-minute telephone interviews with the doctors who prescribed the lethal drugs, but the 40 percent of the doctors in the Oregon cases who refused to give the drugs because of their misgivings in assisting in a suicide were not represented. As Foley observes, perspectives essential to comprehending people's motives in seeking assisted suicide were omitted: "We lost the voices of the patients; we lost the voices of the families."

Although the report indicated that only one person specified fear of pain as a reason for seeking assisted suicide, Joseph Shapiro refers to others with similar objectives. Since those who opted for suicide were "several times more likely" than the norm to be divorced or never married, Shapiro wonders whether a care-giving spouse would have altered the patients' decisions. Finally, while the report underplayed the significance of fear of financial consequences in the patient's choice of assisted suicide, others disagree. As Shapiro notes, "At a recent public meeting in Oregon, Ric Burger, a diabetic who uses a wheelchair, complained that the state's Medicaid program now pays for assisted suicide [supposed "death with dignity"] but not for enough hours for in-home aids necessary for many elderly and disabled to live—in dignity—in their own homes."

71. Coleman's 1998 Congressional testimony.

72. Editorial, *New York Times,* February 27, 1999. References to this comparison from this source.

73. Joseph Shapiro, "Casting a Cold Eye on 'Death with Dignity,'" *U.S. News & World Report,* March 1, 1999, 56. References to Shapiro's discussion of the 1999 Oregon report from this source. Shapiro quoted Kathleen Foley.

Legalizing Disability Discrimination

In her 1998 testimony before Congress, Diane Coleman maintained that the Oregon assisted-suicide law not only "violates the Americans with Disabilities Act, [but] under a disparate impact analysis, may also violate the Civil Rights Act of 1964."[74] She added, "People with terminal illnesses generally qualify as people with disabilities, yet policymakers have completely ignored the ADA violations inherent in assisted-suicide laws. Unfortunately, discrimination based on health status is still fundamentally acceptable in this culture, still so deeply ingrained that it's hard for people to recognize it when it stares them in the face."

In fact, Coleman pointed out that Congress included language in the ADA stating that disability discrimination may warrant more "judicial and legislative scrutiny" than it has frequently been given: "Individuals with disabilities are *a discrete and insular minority* who have been faced with restrictions and limitations, subjected to a history of purposeful unequal treatment, relegated to a position of political powerlessness in our society."[75] She cited a dramatic example of such "unequal treatment," an experiment that occurred at Children's Hospital of Oklahoma between 1977 and 1982. Twenty-four babies with spina bifida died because their parents did not know they were being used in a study testing whether parents would accept "do-not-treat" recommendations from doctors.

Explaining that the Oregon law cannot be understood outside its social context, Coleman described the first widely reported case involving an eighty-year-old woman with breast cancer whose doctors denied her request for assisted suicide because they diagnosed her as depressed. Once Compassion In Dying found a doctor who would grant her suicidal request, her case met the explicit requirements of the law. As Coleman observed, "Nothing in the law says the individual has to be informed about independent living or social service options, nothing says that an individual has to actually be provided any medical or service alternatives he or she might prefer, and nothing says people can't shop around until they find a doctor who will do it." In addition, Coleman notes that "since there's no enforcement mechanism, there are no legal consequences for failure to report assisted suicides."[76]

Coleman described this type of discriminatory law to hasten death as tantamount to "a denial of equal protection of the law under the Fourteenth Amendment." Although she noted that courts have so far not granted "'suspect class' status to people with disabilities," the landmark U.S. Supreme Court assisted suicide ruling recognized disability discrimination: "The State's interest goes beyond protecting the vulnerable from coercion; it extends to protecting disabled and terminally ill people from prejudice, negative and inaccurate stereotypes, and 'societal indifference.'... [A] seriously disabled person's suicidal impulses should be interpreted and treated the same way as anyone else's."

74. Unless otherwise indicated, discussion of legalizing disability discrimination from Diane Coleman's July 14, 1998, testimony before the Constitution Subcommittee of the House Judiciary Committee.
75. 42 USC 12101 (a)(7); emphasis added.
76. Interview with Coleman, March 11, 1999.

Dangers of an Inflexible Law

In his article "Whose Right To Die?" oncologist Dr. Ezekiel Emanuel reveals that interest in euthanasia—which dates back to 1870—was generated not by new technologies that extend life, but rather by the discovery of pain-relieving drugs such as morphine that could also result in painless death.[77] Although drugs administered aggressively—not to hasten death but to relieve pain—may ultimately induce death, this practice, both ethically and legally sanctioned, is not physician-assisted suicide. Since depression, not pain, primarily motivates patients to request physician-assisted suicide, Emanuel notes that our usual approach to people in psychological distress is "psychiatric intervention—not ... a syringe and life-ending drugs." Moreover, patients kept alive by technology who no longer wish to live do not require new legislation permitting physician-assisted suicide since they already have the constitutional right to discontinue medical interventions.

Fearing legalization of physician-assisted suicide, Emanuel predicts that the most vulnerable will be "children, the demented, the mentally ill, the old, and others." No doubt paramount among "the others" would be people with disabilities, for frequently presumptions made by healthy people about those who are suffering, or those assumed to be suffering, would not be countenanced by the objects of those presumptions. Many people with visible impairments are concerned that the same kind of presumptions often are made by nondisabled people about the quality of life of people with disabilities.

According to a 1996 *Washington Post* poll, marginalized demographic groups, other than people with disabilities, also tend to feel threatened by legalization of physician-assisted suicide: African Americans opposed legalization 70 percent to 20 percent; people over seventy opposed it 58 percent to 35 percent.[78] Lacking the universal and comprehensive health care of the Netherlands, patients and doctors in the United States could be making decisions about physician-assisted suicide while encouraged to cut costs. The significance of this factor will be amplified "in the context of demographic and budgetary pressures on Social Security and Medicare as the Baby Boom generation begins to retire, around 2010."[79]

Believing, like Emanuel, that ethical ambiguities regarding physician-assisted suicide are better addressed on a case-by-case basis than by an inflexible rule, ethics professor emeritus Lewis Smedes maintains that "sometimes it is better just to leave things murky."[80] Harvard's Michael J. Sandel explains why even laws that are disregarded from time-to-time serve a purpose: "It [physician-assisted suicide]

77. Ezekiel Emanuel, "Whose Right To Die?" *Atlantic Monthly,* March 1997, 73–79. Emanuel's references to the danger of the legalization of physician-assisted suicide for vulnerable populations from this source.
78. David E. Rosenbaum, "Americans Want a Right To Die or So They Think," *New York Times,* Sunday, June 8, 1997, sec. 4, p. 3. "The better off financially and the better educated ... the more likely [people] were to favor legal assisted suicide," Rosenbaum noted.
79. Emanuel discusses the effect of budgetary pressures on decisions regarding physician-assisted suicide. Both Dr. Kathleen Foley and Dr. Joanne Lynn (editor of *Handbook for Mortals: Guidance for People Facing Serious Illness* [New York: Oxford University Press, 1999]) stated on "The Open Mind" (PBS-TV, aired November n, 1998, and March 3, 1999) that these demographics will forge a cultural shift in attitudes toward death and dying. As Lynn indicated, two generations ago people died suddenly, but now they tend to "die by inches."
80. Rosenbaum, "Americans Want a Right to Die," 3. References to Michael J. Sandel from this source.

should be burdened morally by the sense that we are taking a life, something that isn't entirely ours to take. Preserving the laws on the books is a way of keeping this sense of burden." Similarly, Emanuel asserts that physician-assisted suicide should remain illegal and exceptional so that those who make "moral judgments" will be "accountable before the law."

Rather than providing the technology and services that would allow people with disabilities to live productive lives in the mainstream, the health care system too frequently supports—sometimes even elicits—misguided suicidal impulses in vulnerable people. Given the many people with disabilities who may be included among the "marginalized," the warning of psychiatrist Herbert Hendin threatens the disability population in the United States: "The Netherlands? With a homogenous, pretty much law abiding citizenry, almost all of whom have medical coverage? And America, with many different cultures represented, many marginalized people, tens of millions without health care insurance? As bad as it was *there*, in other words, it could be much, much worse *here*."[81]

"A Better Solution"

Describing the popular support for physician-assisted suicide as "neither strong nor deep," Emanuel observes that answers to questions on the subject are dependent on how these queries are crafted. "For the majority of people with disabilities, whose only information about living with disability comes from health care providers, today's trends do not bode well," cautions Diane Coleman: "In those critical early hours, weeks, and months after injury, people could easily be swayed to make a so-called 'choice' for death."[82] In his article "Americans Want a Right to Die. Or So They Think," David E. Rosenbaum refers to "the opinion surveys [that] have not addressed the wrenching specifics ... that for many people first have meaning when they face them personally."[83]

Nancy Rolnick, a C1-2 quadriplegic—paralyzed from the neck down as a result of an automobile accident and unable to breathe without a respirator (or the phrenic nerve pacer she now uses)—describes her fundamental difficulty with the "right to die" movement:

> Before my accident, I saw Brian Clark's play *Whose Life Is It Anyway?* about a young man paralyzed in an accident, struggling for the right to cease living. Along with my husband and friends, I sided with the protagonist, never questioning his decision. After my accident, I saw the movie made from the play, and while I still identified with the young man, I thought, "Gee, this guy is making his move much too soon. He's not giving himself the chance to find out what it's like to live outside the hospital." In other words, as a disabled person, my perspective changed. I no longer automatically accepted suicide as a good solution to disability.
>
> So what is a better solution? I can only answer for myself. First of all, I've been

81. Wilkes, "The Next Pro-Lifers," 26.
82. Coleman's 1998 congressional testimony.
83. Rosenbaum, "Americans Want a Right to Die," 3.

> surrounded by people who fully expected me to come home from the hospital and pick up my life—my husband, my children and their spouses, a few good friends, and my nurses. Their attitude has been—do it. At crucial moments I met disabled people who inspired and guided me—a paraplegic woman when I first entered the rehabilitation hospital, and as I left the hospital, a young woman quadriplegic who became my mentor, for she had created a fantastically independent life for herself. Other disabled people along the way have been important to me, and of course working with disability advocacy groups has given a new focus to my life.[84]

Recognizing the significance of her accessible living quarters, as well as her private insurance—which provides her with care and equipment to achieve maximum independence—Rolnick continues, "Given the tools and the proper support, most people with disabilities want to continue laughing, loving, and living."

The Distinction between Severe Disability and Terminal Illness

The following examples reveal how the difference between severe disability and terminal illness easily may become obscured by the courts. In making judgments, do courts value the life of a person with a disability as much as the life of a nondisabled person? American disability rights advocates have seized upon the case of Tracy Latimer, a twelve-year-old Canadian child with cerebral palsy who was killed by her father, Robert Latimer, in 1993 by means of a lethal dose of carbon monoxide.[85] Although Tracy's father was convicted of second degree murder—a verdict usually carrying a mandatory life sentence without a chance of parole for ten years—the jury recommended parole after one year.

Not only did the jury consider Robert Latimer's deed a mercy killing, but there also was an outpouring of public support for Tracy's father. Disability advocates asked, however, why does the killing of a nondisabled child evoke outrage while the killing of a child with a disability is accepted? Another question they posed concerned the necessity for the medical procedures that Tracy was forced to undergo to improve her condition. "News accounts ... suggest the girl was relatively stable and happy before doctors started operating on her to 'correct things.'" Was it these surgeries rather than the cerebral palsy that caused Tracy's reported suffering? Disability advocates fear that the notion that killing a person with a disability is different from killing anyone else encourages courts to condone physician-assisted suicide.

Utilizing the joystick on a motorized wheelchair, twenty-six-year-old Elizabeth Bouvia, a college graduate studying for a master's degree in social work, lived independently in her own apartment with her husband until, over a short period of time, everything she sought to accomplish seemed to unravel:

84. Nancy Rolnick, "The Right to Live/The Right To Die," *New York Able,* December 1995, 12, 19. References to Rolnick from this source.

85. References to the Latimer case from "Murder of Disabled Daughter Draws 1-year Sentence," *Ragged Edge,* January/February, 1998, 5. Bioethicist Adrienne Asch at a December 5, 1997, Disabilities Studies Colloquium at New York City's Hunter College School of Social Work stated, "A father killing his twelve-year-old daughter is neither personal assistance services nor physician-assisted suicide; we have other words for that."

> The dean of the program where she had planned to get her master's degree in social work told her that no matter how well she might do, there was not going to be a job at the end of her efforts. In despair, she dropped out of school, and the state then took away the van it had made available for her transportation to and from school.
>
> Her little family fell apart as her husband left her, and she suffered a miscarriage. She retreated back to her father's house, but together they decided this arrangement would not be convenient for him. With her world out of control, she decided to take her own life. She checked into Riverside Hospital in California and made the demand that she be kept comfortable as she starved herself to death. Within a very short time, the psychiatric staff of that medical facility had officially designated her as mentally competent, and the American Civil Liberties Union was in court pleading her right to this bizarre form of suicide.[86]

Although her disability, cerebral palsy, was not progressive, the California Supreme Court judged her 1983 bout with depression as an acceptable reason for allowing the hospital to assist in her suicide. Bouvia's subsequent change of heart—her decision to go on with her life—underscored the fact that the court would be highly unlikely to accept depression of a nondisabled person as suitable grounds for physician-assisted suicide.[87]

In 1984, Mary Jane Owen, blind disability activist, editor, writer, and former faculty member of the graduate program in social work at San Francisco State College, made this observation about the Bouvia case: "What we keep telling each other about Bouvia illustrates more about how *we* feel about disability than it does about how this young woman is dealing with her depression. She is trapped by the snare of our terror and prejudices. She has come to personify our horror of vulnerability, frailty and all the 'imperfections' of disability."[88]

The highly publicized requests for physician-assisted suicide by two other quadriplegics also were sanctioned by the courts. Without having ever met Kenneth Bergstedt, a highly intelligent quadriplegic, Las Vegas District Court Judge Donald Mosley ruled in June 1990 that a physician could sedate Bergstedt and then remove the respirator upon which he depended for breathing.[89] Using peculiar logic, Mosley determined that Bergstedt's death in this manner would not be suicide; rather, Bergstedt would be regulating his medical care. Neither a newspaper reporter who covered the case, nor Mary Johnson in her capacity as editor of the *Disability Rag,* nor any disability activist was able to speak to Bergstedt directly. After Bergstedt, assisted by a physician, had committed suicide with court approval, Johnson—in

86. Mary Jane Owen, "The Elizabeth Bouvia Suicide Case: Is Psychiatry Only for Able-Bodied?" *The Detroit News,* February 6, 1984, sec. A, p. 11.
87. While Joseph P. Shapiro in *No Pity: People with Disabilities Forging a New Civil Rights Movement* (New York: Times Books, 1993), 274, indicated that in 1988 Bouvia was wishing for death, Richard B. Treanor in *We Overcame: The Story of Civil Rights for Disabled People* (Falls Church, Va.: Regal Direct Publishing, 1993), 264, stated that she was a happy person in 1988.
88. Mary Jane Owen, "We're Cowards to Think This Suicide Is Right," *The Washington Post,* February 12, 1984, B05 (in "Sunday Outlook").
89. Mary Johnson, "Life and Death: Unanswered Questions," *The Ragged Edge* (Louisville: The Advocado Press, 1994), 187–93. References to comments on this case by Kenneth Bergstedt and Edward Roberts from this source.

the September/October 1990 issue of the *Disability Rag*—revealed her impression that Bergstedt, himself, was never consulted regarding his life or death decision.

Founder of the Independent Living Movement and winner of a MacArthur "genius" fellowship, Edward Roberts, who like Bergstedt relied on a respirator, expressed his feelings about the case:

> The whole thing is outrageous. I am getting angrier and angrier about these cases. They feed on each other. The attorneys, the courts, the judges, they don't know anything. They see somebody like Bergstedt, and they say, "Of course he wants to die." What's happening is we're killing disabled people in this country and then act like we're doing them a favor. It's outrageous. I've been on a respirator for twenty-six years, and I watch these people's cases. They're just as dependent on a respirator as I am. The major difference is that they know they're going to be forced to live in a nursing home—or they're already there—and I'm leading a quality life. That's the only difference. It's not the respirator. It's the money.

Lacking the technology that would make it possible for him to live and work independently, thirty-four-year-old Larry McAfee, a quadriplegic, clearly planned to commit suicide in 1989, a decision supported by the court, the clergy, and his family. "McAfee, who became disabled in 1985, won court approval to hook up a switch to his motorized chair to allow him to turn off his own respirator and kill himself. Disability activists got involved, fought for other options for him, and showed McAfee the possibility of community living arrangements [that] no one else (including those that [were] helping him win his death) had told him about."[90] Once he acquired the opportunity to function in the community (using a puff-and-sip motorized wheelchair) and to work in the professional world (employing a voice-activated computer), McAfee changed his mind, for he found new meaning in his increasingly self-directed life. The 1992 made-for-television film dramatizing McAfee's plight made no reference to the role of disability advocates, who showed McAfee how to live rather than how to die.

Like McAfee, who could utilize his professional training and skills as an engineer when he was provided with the proper tools, many people with severe disabilities are living fulfilling and productive lives employing appropriate technologies. In 1992, a coalition of six independent living centers of New York City gave its annual award for outstanding achievement by a student with a disability to an African-American teenager with cerebral palsy. Although he was originally labeled as "retarded," once he was given the chance to use computers to operate a power wheelchair, a voice synthesizer, and a word processor, he was upgraded to very intelligent. While still profoundly disabled, the youngster was no longer handicapped in revealing his talents.[91] Disability rights advocate Professor Frank Bowe, who is deaf, draws a distinction between the words "disability" and "handicapped":

> Our disabilities are not going to disappear, but what we can work on are the handicaps. In this room today I am not handicapped. I can talk to anyone here and you can talk to

90. "Around the Nation," *Incitement*, July 1992, 8(2): 15. In chapter 9 of *No Pity*, Joseph Shapiro offers a thorough discussion of this case.
91. Republic Bank funded these yearly awards ceremonies honoring two or three students for their accomplishments, as well as several adults, who have served the disability community in New York City.

> me because I have an interpreter. I am still disabled; I am as deaf as I ever was—as I was this morning, as I will be when I go to bed tonight. But I am not handicapped in this room. And because this room is accessible, people, whatever their disability, can get into it. So the people in this room are not handicapped. They are still disabled, but they are not handicapped. This means that the people in this room can do whatever their intellect, their knowledge, their training, their ability enable them to do.[92]

Technology has allowed Stephen Hawking, the world renowned British physicist with a severe disability, to continue to pierce "the mysteries of the universe with the mind of a latter-day Einstein."[93] In 1963, Hawking, just twenty-one years old, working in Cambridge on his Ph.D. in physics, was told that he had two and a half years to live as a result of ALS, a degenerative motor neuron disease that causes atrophy of muscles throughout the body. Inexplicably, however, Hawking continues to thrive beyond any reasonable expectation. With a voice synthesizer, provided after his 1985 tracheotomy resulting from his bout with pneumonia, and a small personal computer mounted on his wheelchair, his ability to lecture and to collaborate with other physicists, as well as to publish books and articles, has not been compromised.

For Hawking, the knowledge that he had a severe disability seemed to act as a spur, focusing his intellect and his energy on his study of cosmology: "Before my condition had been diagnosed, I had been very bored with life. There had not seemed to be anything worth doing. But shortly after I came out of hospital, I dreamt that I was going to be executed. I suddenly realized that there were a lot of worthwhile things I could do if I were reprieved."[94] In fact, a colleague suggested that Hawking's illness may have made new creative possibilities available to him:

> As he gradually lost the use of his hands, he had to start carefully choosing research projects that could be tackled and solved through geometrical arguments that he could do pictorially in his head, and he developed a powerful set of tools that nobody else really had. So in some sense, when you lose one set of tools, you may develop other tools, but the new tools are amenable to different kinds of problems than the old tools. That means certain kinds of problems you can solve, and nobody else can.

As Intel vice president Stephen Nachtheim observes, "Wherever Hawking rolls along the Gothic splendor of Cambridge or anywhere throughout the world, he has constant access to the Internet, a faster voice synthesizer and infrared remote control of doors, lights and his personal entertainment center."[95] Nachtheim characterizes Hawking as "a man who does what he wants and tries to be minimally inconvenienced by his disability, so he uses all the technology he can to overcome a problem." Making only

92. Frank Bowe, "Handicapping America: Barriers to Disabled People," *Disability: Our Challenge,* John P. Hourihan, ed. (New York: Teachers College, Columbia University, 1979), 90.
93. Michael White and John Gribbin, *Stephen Hawking: A Life in Science* (New York: Penguin Books, 1993), 15. White and Gribbin quoted from Dennis Overbye's *Lonely Hearts of the Cosmos* (New York: Little Brown, 1999).
94. *A Brief History of Time,* 84 min., 1992, Paramount Pictures Corporation. Comments of Hawking's colleague from this source.
95. Howard B. Hain, quoting Stephen Nachtheim, in "Light Years Ahead: One-on-One with Stephen Hawking," *We,* October 1997, 14.

passing reference to Hawking's very apparent and well-known disability, a 1997 *New York Times* front-page article described the visit of "the brilliant theorist" to the California Institute of Technology.[96] Hawking explains:

> I regard my disability like color blindness—something that is an inconvenience but which one can live with and get 'round. Obviously, my disability is more severe than color blindness, but to me it is incidental and does not shape my world view. The way for disabled people to be appreciated is to be successful. For the physically disabled, this means being smarter than the next guy. No one is going to be impressed if you are a Paralympic champion. You have to be outstanding in absolute terms.[97]

Can the value of a life be judged by the degree of a disability? Can these lives of people with serious disabilities be described as unworthy to be lived? Too commonly, policy decisions reflect a confusion between terminal illness and disability, as well as an arrogance and complacency in judging the value of a life, even for those who have not made world-shaking contributions. As Not Dead Yet attorney Diane Coleman stated in the conclusion of her 1998 congressional testimony, "Our society is wrestling with what is perhaps the most pivotal issue of our time: whether a cost-benefit analysis will determine the value of a human life, whether people with disabilities, including terminal illnesses, belong in our society as a part of humanity's diversity, or whether we [people with disabilities] will be pushed, subtly and not-so-subtly, toward the Final Exit solution."[98]

Questions

1. Given the authors' centering of disabled experiences/perspectives on the morality/legality of physician-assisted suicide, what are you inclined to think about this bioethical issue? Is your view of it changed by the authors' discussion?
2. How could an intersectional lens be used to understand the issue of physician-assisted suicide? What are some ways in which the morality/legality of physician-assisted suicide is further complicated when we consider economically disadvantaged disabled persons and/or disabled persons of color, especially given the fact that many of them cannot afford health insurance (due to underemployment, unemployment, economic disparities,

96. Malcolm W. Browne, "A Bet on a Cosmic Scale and a Concession, Sort Of," *New York Times,* February 12, 1997, A1, A22.
97. Hain, "Light Years Ahead," 14, quoting Hawking.
98. Diane Coleman's mention of "Final Exit" is a reference to Derek Humphry's bestseller, the right-to-die movement's call to arms, *Final Exit* (Eugene, Ore.: Hemlock Society, 1991).

and other factors)?

Reading 4.2

Why Suicide Is Like Contraception

A Woman-Centered View

Dena S. Davis

Editor's Introduction

In this reading, Dena S. Davis articulates a feminist perspective on the rationality of suicide and physician-assisted suicide, using women's experiences to illuminate the complex debate over rational suicide. Davis argues that using contraception is analogous to engaging in rational suicide in cases of terminal illness or impending dementia, thus explaining how a feminist view of contraception suggests an argument for a feminist view of rational suicide. In both cases, one views an aspect of one's body (be it one's fertility or one's continued ability to live or experience full consciousness and bodily autonomy) as contingent and as a threat to one's values and interests. Davis's discussion admits that medical assistance in giving access to birth control is not analogous to medical assistance in physician-assisted suicide, and she discusses the legal ramifications of this.

Dena S. Davis is a professor at Lehigh University's Department of Religious Studies. Her research interests include bioethics and the relationships between church and state, and religion and law. She has served on the boards of the American Academy of Religion and the American Society of Bioethics and Humanities.

A feminist view of contraception suggests an argument for a feminist view of rational suicide. To use contraception or sterilization is to view one's fertility as contingent rather than given, and to limit one's fertility as a way of maximizing one's interests and goals. To resort to rational suicide when faced with terminal illness or impending dementia is to view one's body's continued ability to pump blood and oxygen as contingent, and no longer a good for one's life but rather a threat to one's values and interests in how the final chapter of that life is written.

* * *

Despite the flood of writing on assisted suicide in the last few years, relatively little has been written about suicide itself.[1] There are certainly important reasons to distinguish these two subjects. One could, for example, argue that suicide can be a good decision in some situations, but still acknowledge powerful reasons why *medical* people should not blur their mission by taking on this task. However, it is important, before tackling the issue of physician-assisted suicide, to think about suicide *simpliciter.* If one believes that suicide is sometimes a rational, even an admirable, decision, one is at least more sympathetic to the notion of assistance. Whereas someone who believes that virtually all suicides are really "cries for help," responses to social situations that could be ameliorated, or the product of clinical depression is likely to be much more suspicious of any steps society might take to make it easier. In the following pages, let me offer one feminist view of rational suicide.

Women live in a critique relationship with our bodies. Sometimes that is a negative thing, as when we judge ourselves by the "norm" of the tall, skinny model on the cover of *Vogue* and find ourselves wanting, or when we buy into male myths about how women ought to make love and experience orgasm. But it is also a positive thing. Women (at least in the West) learn in adolescence that we must take control of our fertility. We need to view that fertility as *contingent* rather than *given*; we need to evaluate our capacity for procreation with a critical eye, asking how and when that capacity fits into our plans for our lives. To use contraception is to say, "*Despite the fact that my body retains its capacity to be fertile from, say, age eleven to fifty-one, that capacity is not (now) a good for my life but rather a threat to my goals and plans; therefore, I will choose to limit my fertility.*" To choose sterilization is to say, "*My fertility has permanently outrun its usefulness for my life and is now a danger, and, therefore, I will exert control by bringing my body's physical capacities into line with my plans for the rest of my life.*"

Thus, an important piece of the feminist project has been to argue that biology is not destiny. To decide how to deal with one's fertility—whether by celibacy, pregnancy, contraception, or sterilization—is to exercise choice and will over against the passive acceptance of what would otherwise happen to one's

1. One exception is M. Pabst Battin, *Ethical Issues in Suicide* (Englewood Cliffs, NJ: Prentice-Hall, 1982).

life because of one's bodily proclivities.[2] Sometimes, of course, these are very tragic choices, as when a woman longs for another child but knows that pregnancy will risk her health or the well-being of children already born.[3]

To choose suicide, when one is facing a diagnosis of dementia or the last stages of a terminal illness, is to say, *"My body's continued capacity to pump blood and oxygen is no longer a good for my life but rather a threat to my values and interests in how the final chapter of my life is written; therefore, I will exert control by committing suicide."* These interests might include preserving my assets to use in ways consonant with my values (for example, to endow a scholarship or pay for my children's education); sparing family members the experience of coping with protracted dementia and death; preserving friends' and family's memories of me as a vital and competent person; ending my life with a final chapter that is a fitting capstone to the narrative as a whole.

Some religious ethicists, and those with natural law fidelities, will argue that it is arrogant and delusional, "autonomy run amok" as the current phrase has it, to imagine that one can control the course of one's life. In an article tellingly entitled, "Embracing Mystery, Losing Control," William F. May speaks of "a purposeful willing and waiting in the course of letting be and letting go."[4] David Novak mocks autonomy arguments for suicide when he says this:

> We want to die just as we have lived—autonomously. Since we have believed in life that our dignity is to be self-sufficient, we now believe that we must die with that same dignity. Death is no longer the ultimate horizon that teaches us that our essence in this world is not to be in control but to make our peace with an order greater than anything of our own making.[5]

Certainly, there is much that one simply has to accept—such as having terminal cancer or Alzheimer's Disease in the first place. Thus, the decision whether or not to commit suicide is often made in the context of tragedy; one would hugely prefer not to have gotten cancer, or not to live in a society where a nursing home stay will destroy one's assets, or not to be at the mercy of a medical system in which half of dying patients report severe or moderate pain at the end-of-life.[6]

Embracing the idea of suicide as one possible choice among others aligns us on the feminist side of

2. Of course, it would be highly preferable for men to take an equal interest in controlling *their* fertility, but women have far more to lose from unplanned pregnancy than do men and, therefore, a much greater interest in contraception.
3. *Infertility* can also challenge women to make very difficult choices. Feminists are divided about whether innovative reproductive technologies give women more choice or less. See, for example, Janice G. Raymond, *Women as Wombs: Reproductive Technologies and the Battle Over Women's Freedom* (San Francisco: Harper, 1993).
4. William F. May, "Embracing Mystery. Losing Control," *The Park Ridge Center Bulletin* 1: 15 (1997).
5. David Novak, "Suicide Is Not a Private Choice," *First Things* 75: 31–34 (1997).
6. The SUPPORT Principal Investigators, "A Controlled Trial to Improve Care for Seriously Ill Hospitalized Patients: The Study to Understand Prognoses and Preferences for Outcomes and Risks of Treatments (SUPPORT)," *Journal of the American Medical Association* 274: 1591–98 (1996); Joan Stephenson, "Experts Say AIDS Pain 'Dramatically Undertreated,'" *Journal of the American Medical Association* 276: 1369–1370 (1996).

two important divides that are present in the debate over contraception as well: *passive versus active,* and *natural (or "given") versus chosen.*[7]

Passive Versus Active

Not to use contraception, or rather not to include contraception as an active possibility in one's life, is to be passive, to be at the mercy of one's body. Indeed, one of the reasons "moralists" pushed for laws against contraceptives was that they "encouraged" immorality by allowing people to "escape" the consequences of their acts. To be fertile and sexually active without employing contraceptives (or abortion) is to be governed by the vicissitudes of fertility and fate. Given the impact of childbearing and motherhood on women's lives, the consequences for one's health, economic status, and career are enormous.

Conservatives opposed to contraception, especially Christian conservatives, would speak of "openness" rather than passivity, as in this illuminating quote from a woman pro-life activist interviewed by sociologist Kristin Luker:

> Because most pro-life people have a deep faith in God, they also believe in the rightness of His plan for the world. They are therefore skeptical about the ability of individual humans to understand, much less control, events that unfold according to a divine, rather than human, blueprint. From their point of view, human attempts at control are simply arrogance, an unwillingness to admit that larger forces than human will determine human fate. One woman made the point clearly: "God is the Creator of life, and I think all sexual activity should be open to that [creation]. That does not mean that you have to have a certain number of children or anything, but it should be open to Him and His will. The contraceptive mentality denies his will. "It's my will, not your will." And here again, the selfishness comes in.[8]

The idea of life as a "gift" also is common to those who argue for openness and against control. Sydney Callahan, for example, a pro-life feminist who also argues against assisted suicide, says that, "Having received the gift of life and social identity, one has a moral obligation to preserve and respect each

7. I am keenly aware that there is tremendous diversity and controversy in feminist philosophy, and to speak of "the" feminist side is a kind of arrogance. Many feminist philosophers, e.g., Rosemarie Tong, have done a superb job of delineating the many different types of feminist thought and their implications for issues in bioethics. For me, being a feminist means always asking "the woman question," always being alert, as it were, for the impact upon women of a particular policy or perspective. As a liberal feminist, I take equality, justice, and respect for individual autonomy as crucial principles which I seek to extend to women (and to other historically oppressed groups) equally with men. While I agree that equal attention to women's experience will change our notions of how those principles are applied (the abortion issue is an obvious example of this point), I reject the "relational" or "difference" feminism of Carol Gilligan, Robin West, and others.
8. Kristin Luker, *Abortion and the Politics of Motherhood* (Berkeley: University of California Press, 1984), p. 186.

human life and refrain from suppressing, killing, or destroying self or others."[9] This notion of the self as the receiver of a gift that one is then stuck with, and yet does not own, casts the self as receptive and passive.

By the same token, to allow oneself to be taken over by Alzheimer's Disease or cancer, past the point of possible cure or treatment, is to be passive. With regard to dementia, it is to be the object of others' concern, to be led by the hand, to be unable to drive a car or control one's finances—in short, to return to the infantilized notion of women that prevailed in the West in earlier times (and that still reigns in cultures such as Saudi Arabia). On the other hand, to seize control of one's destiny, perhaps especially under circumstances of great tragedy and limits, is to be active and dominant.

U.S. District Court Judge Barbara J. Rothstein and the Ninth Circuit Court of Appeals expressed the same point when they relied heavily on the U.S. Supreme Court's abortion decisions to ground the right of terminally ill persons to receive physician assistance in determining the time and manner of their deaths (an argument the Supreme Court ultimately rejected).[10] In *Compassion in Dying,* the Ninth Circuit quoted *Planned Parenthood* v. *Casey,* a 1992 decision upholding women's rights to abortion, as saying that:

> At the heart of liberty is the right to define one's own concept of existence, of meaning, of the universe, and of the mystery of human life.[11]

Commenting on the string of contraception and abortion cases that began with *Griswold* v. *Connecticut* in 1965, the Ninth Circuit noted that:

> A common thread running through these cases is that they involve decisions that are highly personal and intimate, as well as of great importance to the individual. Certainly, few decisions are more personal, intimate, or important than the decision to end one's life, especially when the reason for doing so is to avoid excessive and protracted pain.[12]

Most (not all) feminists have long argued that, in the context of abortion, their right to control over their bodies and over the shape of their future lives is supreme. Although the decision whether or not to have an abortion is fraught with moral issues, most feminists have consistently resisted mandatory counseling, waiting periods, spousal notification, and other state interference. If we insist that we can and must be trusted with the power to decide whether or not to destroy a potential human life, how can we not insist on the right to be trusted with the decision whether or not to end our own?

9. Sydney Callahan, "A Feminist Case Against Euthanasia," Health Progress, November-December 1996, pp. 21–29, at p. 23.
10. For an argument against the assertion that the constitutionally protected interest in abortion and treatment refusal embraces a parallel interest in assisted suicide, see Susan M. Wolf, "Physician-Assisted Suicide, Abortion, and Treatment Refusal: Using Gender to Analyze the Difference," in Robert F. Weir, ed., Physician-Assisted Suicide (Bloomington: Indiana University Press, 1997), pp. 167–201.
11. *Compassion in Dying* v. *State of Washington*, 79 F. 3d (9th Cir. 1996), p. 813.
12. Ibid.

Natural Versus Chosen

One of the principal ways in which women have been oppressed in our society is the identification of women with that which is "natural," and the demand that women simply accept rather than control their fertility. "Biology is destiny." Women are "made" for childbearing and childrearing. Birth control is "unnatural" (and will lead to immorality to boot!) Thus, Pope Pius XI, in the 1930 encyclical *Casti Connubii*, wrote:

> It is a divinely appointed law that whatsoever things are constituted by God, the author of nature, these we find the most useful and salutary, the more they remain in their natural state, unimpaired and unchanged, inasmuch as God, the Creator of all things, intimately knows what is suited to the constitution and the preservation of each, and by his will and mind has so ordained all things that each may duly achieve its purpose....
>
> The conjugal act is of its very nature designed for the procreation of offspring; and therefore those who in performing it deliberately deprive it of its natural power and efficacy, act against nature and do something which is shameful and intrinsically immoral.

Other arguments that rely on a divinely constructed world order are equally pernicious to women, as in the notion of male-female "complementarity" which is so often used to support a "separate but equal" argument against women's full participation in public life.[13] Natural order arguments are also frequently associated with what Charles Curran terms a "negative dualism," in which women are identified with the bodily, the emotional, and the material, while men are identified with spirit and rationality. In this tradition, men are the "head" of the family and women are the "heart."[14]

Until the advent of reasonably dependable birth control in the middle of this century, most women faced the unenviable choice of uncontrolled fertility (often associated with poverty and ill health) or some form of celibacy. For too many poor and Third World women, that description still applies. Today, most feminists believe that access to contraception and sterilization is the *sine qua non* of women's self-determination. And, while long-acting contraceptives (such as Norplant) and the shameful history of forced sterilization of poor and minority women remind us of the problems associated with contraception when it is *forced* upon women, the potential for abuse does not tempt us to give up our support for the principle of contraception itself and women's control over their own fertility.[15] This feminist commitment to a "non-

13. Margaret A. Farley, "Feminist Theology and Bioethics," in Lois K. Daly, ed., *Feminist Theological Ethics: A Reader* (Louisville, KY: Westminster John Knox Press, 1994), p. 198.
14. Charles Curran, "Sexual Ethics in the Roman Catholic Tradition," in Ronald M. Green, ed., *Religion and Sexual Health: Ethical, Theological and Clinical Perspectives* (Dordrecht, Kluwer Academic Publishers, 1992), pp. 17–36. See also Margaret Farley, "Feminist Theology and Bioethics," in Lois K. Daly, ed., *Feminist Theological Ethics: A Reader* (Louisville, KY: Westminster John Knox Press, 1994), pp. 192–212.
15. Ellen Moscowitz and Bruce Jennings, eds., *Coerced Contraception? Moral and Policy Challenges of Long-Acting Birth Control* (Washington, DC: Georgetown University Press, 1996).

natural," *controlled* approach to our fertility suggests what ought to be our approach to end-of-life decisions as well. To quote Mary Rose Barrington, past chair of EXIT, the London-based Society for the Right to Die with Dignity:

> Very little is "natural" about our present-day existence, and least natural of all is the prolonged period of dying that is suffered by so many incurable patients solicitously kept alive to be killed by their disease.... If I seem to be suggesting that in a civilized society suicide ought to be considered a quite proper way for a well-brought-up person to end his life (unless he has the good luck to die suddenly and without warning), that is indeed the tenor of my argument; if it is received with astonishment and incredulity, the reader is referred to the reception of recommendations made earlier in the century that birth control should be practiced and encouraged. The idea is no more extraordinary and would be equally calculated to diminish the sum total of suffering among humankind.[16]

Physician-Assisted Suicide

It is tempting to carry my analogy to the next step and to argue that, just as medical assistance is the *sine qua non* of access to birth control and the "right" to contraception would be empty without it, the "right" to suicide is empty without the specialized assistance of a healthcare professional to prescribe the drugs and, preferably, to be present to smooth the way and ensure success.[17] Although I am a proponent of rational suicide, I am less convinced that the legalization of physician assistance is a good policy. The many concerns expressed about the effect on the medical profession, and the move to HMOs, with their tendency to look to the cheapest solution to any problem, give me pause. I am also influenced by Joanne Lynn's point about the "routinization" of medical procedures (for example, the routine use of ultrasound and amniocentesis during pregnancy, and the difficulty many pregnant women experience in resisting that expectation).[18] One can imagine that, rather than being an option people have to ask for, even fight for a little, physician-assisted suicide becomes one more track onto which certain patients are shunted.

Thus, we may have to settle for a compromise in which certain compassionate physicians continue to break the law A better approach would be to look for creative solutions that do not involve the medical profession, for example, lay support groups, end-of-life "midwives," and so on. But this approach assumes a robust and public debate that can shake off the taboo of suicide in the same fashion that we are shaking off the taboo of contraception. Now that the Supreme Court has declined to find a constitutionally protected liberty interest in assisted suicide and left this question up to the political process in the several states, the

16. Mary Rose Barrington, "Apologia for Suicide," in M. Pabst Battin and David J. Mayo, eds., *Suicide, The Philosophical Issues* (New York: St. Martin's Press, 1980), pp. 90–103.
17. It is interesting to note that the Supreme Court cases dealing with contraception are not directly about the right of persons to use contraception, but about the criminalization of physicians' and pharmacists' prescription and distribution of contraceptives.
18. Joanne Lynn, "What You Can Do for Your Dying Patient," Presentation at the Cleveland Clinic Foundation, October 10, 1996.

time for such debate has certainly begun.[19] However, it is worth noting that, although there is widespread debate at the level of public policy and legislative action, the taboo against discussing suicide still holds in many other areas, including much of medical discourse. For example, when suicide as a response to a probable diagnosis of Huntington or Alzheimer's Disease is mentioned in the medical literature, it is characterized as an "adverse reaction,"[20] or as a "catastrophe."[21] Suicide is always described negatively as a "risk," rather than as a "response" or an "option."[22] Thus, discussions of the usefulness of certain kinds of genetic tests are truncated by the refusal to speak openly about the possibility that some people might use genetic testing to make a rational choice to commit suicide.

To date, the distinctly feminist voices in the debate have been opposed to assisted suicide. Sydney Callahan is one example; Susan M. Wolf is another. Wolf, in common with Callahan, is concerned that women will be particularly threatened by the legitimation of physician-assisted suicide.[23] Together, they note that women are more likely to live long lives, to outlive their spouses, to be poor and underinsured, and to be undermedicated for pain. The historic power inequality between (male) doctors and (female) patients makes it doubly difficult for women to assert themselves to get the medical care they need. Wolf notes that men are statistically more likely to complete acts of suicide, but women are more likely to attempt them. She hypothesizes that women may be more likely to use suicide attempts to effect changes in their environment; but, if a request for assistance in suicide becomes something to which a doctor can easily answer, "Yes," many women might commit suicide who really did not want to.[24] Both Callahan and Wolf find it significant that the majority of Kevorkians clients have been women (including many who faced diseases, such as Alzheimer's or multiple sclerosis, that made them increasingly dependent, but not close to death).

Wolf's essay has a number of objectives and arguments. The argument I want to take issue with here is her concern that women's decisions to commit suicide, and society's acceptance of those decisions

19. *Washington* v. *Glucksberg,* 117 S. Ct. 2258, 2274 (1997).
20. Medical and Scientific Advisory Committee, Alzheimer's Disease International, "Consensus Statement on Predictive Testing for Alzheimer's Disease," *Alzheimer's Disease and Associated Disorders* 9 (4) (1995): 182–87.
21. Sandi Wiggins, et al., "The Psychological Consequences of Predictive Testing for Huntington's Disease," *New England Journal of Medicine* 327 (20): 1401–1405 (Nov. 12, 1992).
22. Miriam Schoenfeld, et al., "Increased rate of suicide among patients with Huntington's disease," *Journal of Neurology, Neurosurgery, and Psychiatry* 47: 1283–87 (1984).
23. Susan M. Wolf, "Gender, Feminism, and Death: Physician-Assisted Suicide and Euthanasia," in Susan M. Wolf, ed., *Feminism and Bioethics: Beyond Reproduction* (New York: Oxford University Press, 1996).
24. On the other hand, if assisted suicide became open and legal, perhaps women who otherwise would use a suicide attempt as a "cry for help," will be forced to confront and articulate their real needs. To continue to play a societal game in which women "attempt" suicides they don't really intend, perpetuates a situation in which women are rewarded for communicating one thing and meaning another. This makes it more difficult for women to command respect for their real beliefs and wishes, as documented by Steven H. Miles and Allison August in "Courts, Gender and the "'Right to Die,'" *Law, Medicine and Health Care* 18: 85–95 (1990). I make a similar argument with respect to Jehovah's Witnesses and refusal of life-saving treatment in "Does 'No' Mean 'Yes'? The Continuing Problem of Jehovah's Witnesses and Refusal of Blood Products," *Second Opinion* 19: 35–43 (1994). (I am indebted for this point to Paul Finkelman.)

as appropriate, may be skewed by "a long history of cultural images revering women's sacrifice and self-sacrifice."[25] She worries, in other words, that women are asking (and receiving) suicide assistance for the "wrong" reasons, based on historical and cultural roles that feminists now reject.

Of course, Wolf is correct that self-sacrifice and womanhood have all too easily been considered a natural configuration. But I want to suggest a different way of looking at the content of self-sacrifice. My point is not to denigrate Wolf's picture of the historical and cultural assumptions about women that may play into suicide, but to show that these are actually multifaceted and cut in more than one direction.

Self-sacrifice can be seen, culturally speaking, along a number of different axes. The axis Wolf contemplates is that of resource use. On one end of this axis is the stereotypical mother who doesn't want resources used on her. On the other end is the person who is comfortable having time, money, and resources spent on her, even out of a limited family pool. Wolf argues that women have historically been consigned to the self-sacrificial end. Because women were traditionally expected to fulfill themselves through their families while their husbands pursued success in more public ways, women could all too easily be expected—and expect themselves—to put everyone else's needs first. But there is another sense in which, perhaps unwittingly, the opponents of rational suicide fall into another understanding of self-sacrifice. Here, the self-sacrifice expected is to undergo long periods of pain and disability, perhaps even dementia, rather than to do something as dramatic and unconventional as to put an end to one's life. The ill or dying person is being asked to forgo acting on her own interests in order to (1) avoid making her relatives look like selfish, uncaring brutes in the eyes of the more conventional world; (2) refrain from challenging the comfortable belief that life is always worth living; and (3) avoid giving society at large a push down the slippery slope in the direction of callousness toward those sick and disabled persons who do *not* wish to end their lives. Thus, one could argue that those who oppose rational suicide are asking women to shoulder yet another traditional female burden: the preservation of society's moral and religious values. The stereotypical virtues assigned to Victorian women of "piety, purity, submissiveness, and domesticity," which rightly disturb Wolf, can as easily be harnessed by traditionalists to argue against suicide as for it.[26]

Here again, we see a parallel with enforced motherhood. As Beverly Harrison points out, "We live in a world in which many, perhaps most, of the voluntary sacrifices on behalf of human well-being are made by women, but the assumption of a special obligation to self-giving or sacrifice is male-generated ideology."[27] It is, of course, often a valid argument that the interests of the individual must give way to the good of society as a whole. Although I am not yet persuaded by these arguments, we should certainly consider the concerns of, for example, the New York State Task Force on Life and the Law, which concluded that the probability of "mistake and abuse" was too high to countenance the legalization of physician-assisted

25. Ibid., p. 283.
26. Ibid., p. 298.
27. Beverly Wildung Harrison, *Our Right to Choose: Toward a New Ethic of Abortion*, quoted in Janice Raymond, "Reproductive Gifts and Gift-Giving: The Altruistic Woman," in Lois K. Daly, ed., *Feminist Theological Ethics, A Reader* (Louisville, KY: Westminster John Knox Press, 1994), p. 236.

suicide,[28] an argument the Supreme Court took very seriously when deciding that assistance in suicide was not a constitutionally protected liberty interest.[29] (We should also consider the accounts of observers in Oregon that the possibility of physician-assisted suicide has actually been *better* for patients, as doctors interpreted Measure 16 as a "wake-up call for medicine" and have been motivated to step up efforts in pain control and hospice care.)[30] But, if we are to make this sort of argument, then let us be honest about it: People are being required to forgo their own interests (and individual values) for the good of society as a whole. Women, who historically have suffered the brunt of that sort of reasoning, and who have special reasons for avoiding the indignity and dependence of being demented, pain-wracked, and bedridden, may decide that it is not worth the price.

Conclusion

There are many different ways in which women's experience can illuminate the complex debate over rational suicide. Some facets of this experience rightly suggest great caution, as women reflect on their greater vulnerability due to age, poverty, and historic oppression. My goal in this [reading], by drawing an analogy between contraception and rational suicide, is to highlight one area in which women's experience can argue in favor of support for rational suicide.

Note

I am grateful to colleagues Patricia Falk and David Forte for the opportunity to discuss these ideas (but neither of them can be held responsible for the contents of this [reading], as they disagree with me completely). The writing of this [reading] was supported by a grant from the Cleveland-Marshall Fund.

Questions

1. Davis's argument relies on an analogy between contraception and rational suicide. How strong do you think this analogy ultimately is? What are the main ethical/political lessons that you think should be drawn from this analogy?

28. The New York State Task Force on Life and the Law, *When Death Is Sought: Assisted Suicide and Euthanasia in the Medical Context* (New York: The New York State Task Force on Life and the Law, 1994).
29. *Washington* v. *Glucksberg,* 117 Sup. Ct. 2258, 2272–73 (1997).
30. Susan W. Tolle, "How Oregon's Physician-Assisted Suicide Law Spurs Improvements in End-of-Life Care," *Issues and Resources on Dying* (New York: Grantmakers Concerned with Care at the End of Life, 1977) pp. 3–4.

2. Davis discusses Wolff's concern that women might be motivated to engage in physician-assisted suicide for the "wrong" reasons given the social pressures they face. How do you think this worry becomes more pressing for women facing multiple marginalizations (e.g., queer and economically disadvantaged women or disabled women of color)?

End-of-Unit Questions

1. Given a critical intersectional lens and the centering of persons facing multiple forms of marginalization, what are some ways you think the legalization of physician-assisted suicide can lead to its abuse against multiply marginalized persons/communities?
2. What are some ways you think we might be able to prevent this abuse in circumstances where physician-assisted suicide is legal?

Conclusion

Throughout this book, we have not merely included the perspectives of those who are marginalized because of their race, Indigeneity, and/or ethnicity, their disability, and/or their sex, gender, and/or sexuality as one voice (or one chapter) among many in the bioethical conversation. Rather, we have reoriented our discussion of bioethical problems around these perspectives, thereby giving pride of place to the lived experiences of those who are most affected by these and other social justice problems and to the solutions that emerge from this centering.

When these perspectives are centered, bioethical problems become complicated in ways that require nuanced approaches to developing solutions that take seriously the experiences of marginalized persons. These include

- the causes of health and healthcare inequities among underrepresented/marginalized groups, given the layered, interacting systems of oppression in society and the long history of injustice we have inherited;
- the ethics and legality of informed consent, given racial and cultural differences in the value of patient autonomy;
- the ethics and legality of physician–patient relationship given multicultural differences in values, inherent information asymmetries, and lived experience of disabled persons;
- the ethics and legality of physician-assisted suicide, given perspectives from both feminist studies and disability studies;
- the ethics of human research, given the ongoing history of race/ism, sexism, ableism, androcentrism, and trans/homophobia in the institution of medicine (and others); and
- the ethical and moral political significance of access to birth control (and of restricting it) and of reproductive justice (not just reproductive rights), given Black women's historical circumstances.

The resources in this book thus provide the readers with valuable information and tools that can guide a genuinely more inclusive, empathetic, and humane approach to healthcare and medicine, an approach that is informed by the lived experiences of those who have long been marginalized, underrepresented, and underserved by the medical and philosophical establishment.

Our margin-centering reorientation takes part in painting a vivid picture of just how pervasive and pernicious different systems of oppression are: the shifting shadow of racism, the invisible ocean of white supremacy culture, the ever-present specter of ableism, and the toxic miasma of cisheteropatriarchy permeate every aspect of our social world, from the way we talk, think, and interact to the way that policies and laws are justified, passed, and implemented. These systems work together to systematically and unjustly privilege (in different, interacting ways) wealthy people, white people, abled people, men, straight people, cisgender people, and people in the Global North. Regardless of our identity, all of us are hurt by these systems—but in importantly unequal ways. People who lie at the intersection of multiple systems of oppression (e.g., queer disabled economically disadvantaged people of color) experience complex, interacting layers of injustice that we have seen put them in danger of experiencing "spirit murder" by the very institutions that are supposed to care for them.

Using This Knowledge to Take Action

Armed with this knowledge of the social world we live in, and the deeply unfair and uneven playing field it constitutes, readers can apply the lessons and insights from scholars represented in this book to become a greater force for good in the institutions of healthcare and medicine and in other sectors of society. With the resources in this book, readers are now armed not only with a vivid picture of the complexly unjust society we live in but also with a more nuanced and empowering intersectional conception of identity that recognizes how systems of privilege/oppression interlock around different aspects of our identity in complex, context-sensitive ways. Thus, readers are in a position to better understand other people's positions, the problems that others face, and discussions of social difference and inequality. Additionally, readers who enjoy social privilege of different kinds are now in a better position not just to acknowledge it but to use it for good by amplifying underrepresented voices and raising the visibility of problems that marginalized groups face.

Readers who work as (or aim to be) healthcare providers are now armed with tools for better understanding the ways that people who are marginalized because of their race, Indigeneity, and/or ethnicity; their disability; and/or their sex, gender, and/or sexuality experience our shared social world. Among other things, readers are more aware of the complexities of seeking healthcare from institutions that have a blemished track record of genuinely helping out. This can empower such readers to take a more informed and genuinely empathetic approach in their relationship with patients and their delivery of healthcare.

Similarly, readers who work as (or aim to be) policymakers now possess a better understanding of how different systems of oppression can often interact to make the lives of people at the intersection of them (e.g., queer, disabled, economically disadvantaged, people of color) unbearable. These readers are now in a better position to develop more inclusive, humane, and equitable top-down policies informed by transdisciplinary frameworks and an intersectional understanding of the perspectives and lived experiences of different marginalized persons. Such readers now know of a kind of strategy that can be implemented to address health and healthcare disparities/inequities. This strategy takes the form of intersectoral interventions that are guided by transdisciplinary frameworks and that jointly address different aspects of systems of injustice so as to shift the systemic dynamics of our social institutions toward a more just flow. Thus, they can help bring about transformative change. These readers are therefore now in a position to experiment with more informed, nuanced, and effective solutions to well-known and persistent problems in healthcare.

Moreover, all readers are now in a position to adopt and deliberately cultivate more inclusive language—for example, by resisting such ableist expressions as "being blind to" and by employing gender-neutral pronouns as the default. By applying the knowledge in this book, provided by scholars from marginalized groups, readers of all kinds can help build liberatory communities that can help us heal and empower each other to bring about transformative social change.

Enriching Our Moral Reasoning and Theorizing

Going forward with their own moral reasoning, all readers can put the knowledge from this book to use in articulating their preferred moral theory and implementing their preferred approach to moral problem-solving in a humane and inclusive way that is informed by the lived experiences of and problems faced by marginalized persons. Consider these examples:

- Readers attracted to utilitarianism or other forms of consequentialism now know to adopt a systemically informed view that is aware of how structural dynamics affect the way benefits and burdens are (re)distributed in society (and the importance of changing these dynamics for meaningful long-term improvement, given their inequality and injustice).
- Readers attracted to a Kantian approach to morality now realize that a key part of respecting people's dignity, freedom, and self-determination consists of respecting (and protecting) the freedom of all persons to self-determine and to ensure their gender, sexuality, and bodily autonomy.
- Readers attracted to principlism now recognize that in interpreting and weighing different major bioethical principles, they need to consider the context of deep systemic injustice in which we find ourselves, and the way people with different social identities might give different priority to those principles.
- Readers attracted to virtue ethics now know that they must aim to cultivate virtues that allow us to navigate multicultural contexts empathetically and respond to people whose lives are differentially shaped by social systems of privilege/

- oppression with a long, ongoing history of injustice.
- Readers attracted to the ethics of care and feminist ethics now know that they need to take an intersectional approach to social identity and the ways that different social systems of privilege/oppression shape our interactions and personal relations in complex ways in different contexts.

My hope is that readers of all moral inclinations are inspired to further engage with the work of scholars from underrepresented groups and build transdisciplinary frameworks that can guide our way to transformative social and moral change.

Forward Into the Future and Our Moving Moral Horizon

As we move forward and bring about such change, we must not lose sight of the fact that these systems of oppression are insidious, shifting their shape as we make moral progress. As William James notes, as we move, our "moral horizon moves with us," and "more brutal forms of evil . . . are replaced by others more subtle and poisonous" (James, 1896/2010, p. 192f). And as we have seen, this worry is confirmed by the history of the shifting shadow of race/ism. Thus, as we successfully dismantle systems of oppression, we must remain vigilant and attend to more subtle and poisonous forms of evil that may arise to try to replace them.

It may seem, especially given the recent Supreme Court decisions that dismantle federal protections of abortion rights and affirmative action, that the world is moving in an unjust direction and that meaningful change is beyond our control. Although the future may be uncertain, in times of hopelessness like these it is important to remember that every major societal change was once thought to be impossible. Monarchs were once thought to be gods. But they are not (and never were). And neither are the systems that oppress us. Dismantling and improving them may not be easy, but doing so is not beyond our control. Together, we can change our thinking, our attitudes, our choices, our relations, our interactions, and our institutions and build a more socially just world. Together, we can awaken to the injustice all around us, and awaken to our power to make a difference as we empower each other to bring about transformative social change that shapes the lives of all people—especially those who continue to be marginalized—for the better.

There is much work to be done to build a more socially just, inclusive, and equitable social world. But there is no better time to start than now. And together, we can make it happen.

References

James, W. (2010). The dilemma of determinism. In W. James (Ed.), *The will to believe, and other essays in popular philosophy* (pp. 168–207). The Floating Press. (Original work published 1896)

www.ingramcontent.com/pod-product-compliance
Ingram Content Group UK Ltd.
Pitfield, Milton Keynes, MK11 3LW, UK
UKHW051453290926
15471UKWH00008B/1178

9 781793 575807